CHRISTIAN FAITH,
HEALTH,
and
MEDICAL PRACTICE

CHRISTIAN FAITH, HEALTH, *and* MEDICAL PRACTICE

By the Fellows of the Calvin Center for Christian Scholarship
Calvin College

>   Hessel Bouma III
>   Douglas Diekema
>   Edward Langerak
>   Theodore Rottman
>   Allen Verhey

With Editorial Assistance by

>   Jan Walhout

WILLIAM B. EERDMANS PUBLISHING COMPANY
GRAND RAPIDS, MICHIGAN

Library of Congress Cataloging-in-Publication Data

Christian faith, health, and medical practice / by the fellows of the
  Calvin Center for Christian Scholarship, Calvin College,
  Hessel Bouma III . . . [et al.]; with editorial assistance by Jan Walhout.
      p.   cm.
   Bibliography: p. 376.
   ISBN 0–8028–0369–5
   1. Health—Religious aspects—Reformed Church.   2. Medicine—
Religious aspects—Reformed Church.   3. Medical ethics.   4. Christian
ethics—Reformed authors.   5. Reformed Church—Doctrines
I. Bouma, Hessel.   II. Calvin Center for Christian Scholarship.
BX9423.H43C48   1989
261.5'6 — dc19   89–1071
                                                                              CIP

Contents

PERSONALIA   x

PREFACE   xii

1. Faith in God and Faithfulness in Medicine   1

Faith in God the Creator   3
The Critique of Idolatry
The Critique of Dualism
The Reality of Evil

Faith in God the Provider   8
The Problem of Suffering
Faithfulness and Care
Faithfulness and Freedom

Faith in God the Redeemer   16
Watchfulness and Healing
Watchfulness and the Poor
The "Not-Yet" Character of Our Life and Medicine

2. Imaging God in Sickness and in Health   27

Imaging God   27
Imaging God: Beginnings
Imaging God: Endings
Imaging God in Health

Health and Life Span   53

Health and Persons with Disabilities   56

Treating Imagers of God: Autonomy,
   Informed Consent, and Paternalism   57

3. **Covenantal Fidelity in a Pluralist Society**   **67**

The Examined Moral Life   67

Main Alternatives in Western Ethics   70

Covenantal Ethics   83

Respect, Tolerance, and Cooperation   95

4. **The Character of Medicine**   **102**

Medicine as a Practice   102

Medicine as a Profession   109

Medicine as a Calling   113

The Character of Relationships in Medicine   116

5. **Technology, Tragedy, and Christianity**   **123**

Tragedy   124
   Technology and "The Sad Story"
   Technology and "The Flawed Hero"
   Technology and "The Gathering of Evils"

Tragedy and the Christian Tradition   136
   The Sad Story and the Christian Tradition
   The Flawed Hero and the Christian Tradition
   The Gathering of Evils and the Christian Tradition

6. **Scarcity and Health Care: Personal, Public,
and Professional Responsibilities**   **144**

The Financial Crisis: Scarcity and Sanctity   145

Personal Responsibility for Health   150

Stewardship and Cost Containment   156

Justice and Access to Health Care   162

The Future of Medicine   170

7. **On Having Children and Caring for Them:
Becoming and Being Parents** **176**

Human Control over Procreation 177

Public Discussion of Human Procreation 178

Toward a Christian Perspective 182
Freedom
Utility
The Future
Technology and the Mastery of Nature
Children and Parents
Society and Children
Conclusions and Cautions

8. **Abortion: A Covenantal View** **205**

The Nature and Status of the Fetus 206

Conflicts of Interest and the Nature of Childbearing 208
Appeals to the Parable of the Good Samaritan
Pregnancy and Sacrifice
Responsibility and Sexuality
Failing to Help versus Harming
Summary

Policy Implications 224

9. **Genetic Control and Counseling** **234**

Some Background in Genetics 235
Cytogenetic Conditions
Single-Gene Conditions
Multifactorial Conditions
Genetic Knowledge and Human Response

New Powers, Possibilities, and Problems
in Human Genetics 243
Diagnosis of Newborns, Children, and Adults
Prenatal Diagnosis

Diagnosis of Carriers and Genetic Counseling
The Power to Treat (or Not)
The Power to Intervene: Power to Cure and to Design

10. Death and Covenantal Caring   268

Dying Contrasted with *Being Sick*   269

General Principles   274

Questions of Competence   279

The Living Will   281
   A Critique and a Model
   Advantages and Possible Disadvantages of a
      Christian's Living Will

Allowing to Die and Killing   290
   Allowing to Die by Withholding Medical Means
   Allowing to Die by Withdrawing Medical Means
   Is Withdrawing Nourishment a Special Case?
   Suicide and Mercy Killing

The Covenantal Base of Caring   303

11. AIDS and Care   308

The Disease: AIDS   309
   The Human Immunodeficiency Virus (HIV)
   HIV Transmission
   Stages of HIV Infection
   HIV Testing
   Medical Treatments for HIV Infection
   Prevention of HIV Infection

The Response: Care   319
   Faith in God and Faithfulness in Response to AIDS
   Imaging God: Persons with AIDS and the Response to AIDS
   Covenantal Fidelity: Responding to AIDS in a
      Pluralistic Society
   The Character of Medicine and the Duty to Treat
   Technology, Tragedy, and AIDS
   Scarcity and AIDS: Personal, Public, and Professional
      Responsibilities

Children, Abortion, and AIDS
Dying of AIDS and Covenantal Caring

**Appendix A: Balancing Christian Compassion
and Clinical Detachment**   **343**

**Appendix B: Health-Care Delivery in Great Britain,
the United States, and Canada**   **346**

Introduction   346

History   347
   Great Britain
   The United States
   Canada

Health-Care Delivery Systems—A Critique   355

Conclusion   361

**Appendix C: The State of Health throughout
the World**   **363**

Appendix D: Codes of Ethics   **373**

The Hippocratic Oath   373

American Medical Association Principles of
  Medical Ethics (adopted in 1980)   374

American Nurses' Association Code for Nurses
  (adopted in 1976)   375

REFERENCES   376

Personalia

Hessel Bouma III is professor of biology at Calvin College. He received his Ph.D. degree in human genetics from the University of Texas Medical Branch in 1975 and was a National Institutes of Health postdoctoral fellow in biochemistry at the University of California, San Diego. Since 1978 he has taught in the Biology Department at Calvin College. He served as team coordinator for the Calvin Center for Christian Scholarship in the study for and production of this book.

Douglas Diekema is a pediatric resident at the University of Wisconsin Medical School in Madison, Wisconsin, where he also teaches a course in medical ethics at Edgewood College. In 1985 he received his M.D. degree from the University of North Carolina Medical School, where he was the recipient of a prestigious Morehead Fellowship.

Edward Langerak is professor of philosophy at St. Olaf College in Northfield, Minnesota. He received an M.A. degree from the University of Michigan and an M.A. and a Ph.D. from Princeton University in 1972. Since 1973 he has taught philosophy at St. Olaf College and has taught courses in medical ethics in conjunction with the Mayo Clinic staff and students. In 1978 he received a fellowship from the National Endowment for the Humanities to study technology, values, and medicine at the University of Chicago. His article on abortion that appeared in the *Hastings Center Report* has been reprinted in five anthologies.

Theodore Rottman is professor of sociology at Calvin College. He received his Ph.D. in sociology and anthropology from Michigan State University in 1965. Since 1965 he has taught sociology—including several courses on death, dying, and geriatric issues—at Calvin College. During this time he also served for ten years as director of the Calvin College Social Research Center.

Allen Verhey is professor of religion at Hope College, Holland, Michigan. He received his B.D. degree from Calvin Theological Seminary in 1969 and his Ph.D. in Religion from Yale University in 1975. He has taught as an instructor at Calvin Theological Seminary and since 1975 has taught in the Religion Department at Hope College. In 1981-82 he received a fellowship from the National Endowment for the Humanities to study medical ethics at Indiana University. He is an ordained minister in the Christian Reformed Church. Among his numerous published works are *The Great Reversal: Ethics and the New Testament* (Eerdmans, 1984) and the work he co-edited with Stephen Lammers entitled *On Moral Medicine: Theological Perspectives in Medical Ethics* (Eerdmans, 1987).

Preface

The Calvin Center for Christian Scholarship was founded in 1976 "to promote rigorous, creative, and articulate Christian scholarship." Under its auspices, a team of scholars has come together every academic year since 1977-1978 to jointly explore a topic selected by the faculty of Calvin College in Grand Rapids, Michigan. For 1985-1986 the topic was "Christian faith, health, and medical practice," and we, the authors of this book, constituted the team. It was a good year for us, and we want our first words to be "thank you" to the governing board of the Calvin Center and to Calvin College for the opportunity we have had as a team to think, talk, read, and write about this topic. We will leave it to readers of this book to judge whether the team achieved "rigorous, creative, and articulate Christian scholarship," but we want it made clear that the Calvin Center "promoted" it.

The topic was proposed to the governing board of the Calvin Center by Thomas D. Kennedy, a young scholar who had been a visiting professor of philosophy at Calvin College. His proposal was where we began; we hope that where we ended up in this book honors his vision and intention in making the proposal.

When the team came together in the fall of 1985, we began to read and to talk about what we had read, to write and to argue together about what we had written. Our conversations were not always easy. All of us had to struggle sometimes to understand or to make ourselves understood; sometimes when we did understand each other our conversations became harder still, because we didn't always agree. Even so, our conversations were always good. We engaged in a common quest: together we wanted to discern the shape of Christian obedience and integrity in the midst of the dilemmas and problems of medical care. We learned to rely upon and to trust not only the contribution of the different disciplines represented by members of the team but also the Christian wisdom and moral sensitivity of each party to our conversations, even when we disagreed.

During the year we did more than talk among ourselves. Our conversations were enriched and enlivened by others who were willing to participate in them. Two capable student fellows assisted and enhanced our work and our conversations: Ken Faber, a senior premedical student from Strathroy, Ontario, and now a medical student at the University of Toronto Medical School; and Kurt Kooyer, a graduate premedical student from Grand Rapids, Michigan, now a medical student at the Michigan State University College of Human Medicine. Three adjunct fellows also spent time with us: Peter Boelens, a pediatrician from Vicksburg, Mississippi, who also serves as executive secretary of the Luke Society and has helped establish a number of medical clinics in Korea; David Van Reken, a pediatrician who was serving as missionary-in-residence at Wheaton College and came to the team as a veteran of nine years in medical missions in Monrovia, Liberia; and Scott Vander Linde, a doctoral candidate in medical economics and an instructor in business and economics at Calvin College.

At the end of our year together, we had not discovered—much less disclosed—the last word on the Christian faith or health or medical care (much less the last word on how they are related). The quest we undertook together must be continued among the people of God; it will take more gifts than ours. To discern the shape of Christian obedience and integrity will require the very best gifts and skills of the people of God gathered together as communities of moral discourse. It is our hope that this book will stimulate and illumine that discourse, that it will nurture reason-giving and reason-hearing among the people of God so that the diverse gifts God gives—the skills, the wisdom, the creativity, the technical knowledge—may all be used to discern the medical and moral words and deeds that are worthy of the gospel.

Discourse among Christians need not result in unanimity, and it probably won't. But mutual admonition and mutual accountability can encourage and help all Christians to make every medical decision, every public-policy proposal, and every morally significant idea captive to the Lord Jesus Christ. That, at least, has been our experience as a team; that's why our conversations were always good. If this book is any good, it will be so not because it delivers the last word on medical ethics but because its words evoke and nurture discussion about medical ethics among the people of God. That conversation won't always be easy—but it is necessary, and it will be worthwhile.

Our book is not an anthology, not simply a collection of chapters written by different authors. Although each chapter was initially written by one or several of five different authors, our method of writing, review, and discussion has produced a consensus and sometimes an amalgam of our writing styles. Still evident is the fact that the book has five different authors with different writing styles and different emphases (we like to think of them as "creative differences" rather than "tensions"). We leave it to the good judgment of our readers whether to lament or celebrate these personal differences.

On two matters of style we did reach consensus. First, for biblical citation we agreed to use the Revised Standard Version of the Bible throughout the book, unless otherwise noted. Second, we agreed to jointly own the thoughts expressed in each chapter, something we attempt to reflect in our use of the first-person plural — *we (us)* — throughout the book.

During the 1985-1986 study year, we sought input from a number of academicians and health-care professionals—hospital administrators and chaplains, nurses, physicians, therapists, and social workers. We benefited considerably from these interactions, which helped to shape the course of our thought and work and to keep our academic feet on the ground. Even as we acknowledge these individuals, we remind our readers that just as the viewpoints expressed in this book ought not to be taken as positions of Calvin College or the Christian Reformed Church, so too these viewpoints ought not to be taken as positions approved by any one or all of the individuals we are about to mention. In some instances and on some issues we simply agreed to disagree. Our tribute to these individuals, therefore, is simply public acknowledgment of our indebtedness to them; it does not represent their endorsement of the perspectives expressed in this book.

The team is very grateful for the assistance we received from the individuals who made presentations to us and thoughtfully engaged in dialogue with us during the year: Martin Benjamin, Harry Boer, Harry Demissianos, Anthony Hoekema, Thomas Hoeksema, Case Hoogendoorn, Richard Houskamp, Abbyann Lynch, William F. May, Edmund Pellegrino, Neal Plantinga, Carol Rottman, James Rusthoven, Deborah and Robert Sterken, Henry Stob, Ian Taylor, John H. Timmerman, Harold Thornhill, James Vander Laan, Leonard Vander Zee, Ken Vaux, and Thomas Zeyl.

The team is also very grateful for the assistance received from those who participated in our medical-panel workshops: Judy Bergman, Karen Bottema, Harvey Bratt, Lois Breuker, Anita Brink, Robert Brummel, Ina Bulten, Nicolaas Buma, Elizabeth Carlson, Cloe Ann Danford, Mark Davies, Bruce Deckinga, Alice De Haan, Janice De Haan, Ray De Haan, William De Rose, Daniel De Vries, Dan Diekema, Jeane Diekema, Kathy Dykstra, Martina Dykstra, Gerrit Egedy, Jeanne Engelhard, John Engelhard, A. Dirk Evans, Gwenyth Evenhouse, Lynn Fagerman, Larry Feenstra, Carol Flietstra, Larry Gerbens, Laird Hamstra, Ellen Hoebeke, Janice Hoeksema, Elizabeth Klassens, Cheryle Knibbe, Joyce Kunnen, Robert LaFleur, John Leegwater, Bonnie Medema, Judith Meyer, Catherine Molenaar, Linda Northouse, Henry Ottens, Marlene Post, Mary Ratliff, Evan Reinders, Joanne Rozema, Darlene Rubingh, Laura Ruster, Robert Schindler, Lewis Schoon, Laura Schuring, Joan Sikkenga, Ruth Sipma, Vicki Slot, John Stahl, Susan Strikwerda, Kathy Teerman, Dorothy Ten Brink, Ruth Thomas, Jane Tiesenga, Barb Timmermans, Robert Uken, Tunis Vanden Berg, Eric Vander Haagen, Sandra Vander Jagt, Marie Vander Linde, Bruce Van Dop, Jane Van Drie, David Van Dyke, Kornelius Van Goor, Eleanor Van Harn, Ronald Van Valkenburg, Nick Vogelzang, Mary Voorman, Ron Vredeveld, Jane Warners, James Waun, Barb Weeber, Dottie Wiersma, Janyce Wiersema, Jane Zwiers, and Dorothy Zylstra.

The team is also very grateful for the dialogue we enjoyed in numerous adult-education presentations that we made in area churches, in the symposium that we conducted with the Attending Clergy Association at Holland Community Hospital on the topic of the prolongation of life, in the symposium that we conducted with the Institute for Christian Studies in Toronto, Ontario, on the topic of this book, and in the symposium that we jointly sponsored with the Luke Society, also on the topic of this book.

Finally, a special debt of gratitude goes to Jan Walhout, who has faithfully sought to edit and amalgamate our writing for this book; to Katie Miller, who diligently labored to type our manuscript and check our references; to all the members of the governing board of the Calvin Center for Christian Scholarship but particularly to Rodger Rice, dean of the faculty, who oversaw this work for a period of three years, from concept to finished product; and to the courteous and helpful staffs of both the Computer Center and the Calvin library.

1. Faith in God and Faithfulness in Medicine

Medical ethics is a growth industry in the academic world. It has provided new jobs, funded research and conferences, produced books and journals and study centers, and even furnished personnel for a presidential commission for the study of ethical problems in medicine.

There are good reasons for all this intellectual activity, of course. Advances in medical research and technology have furnished medicine with powers that human beings only dreamed of fifty years ago. Injections of what once were called "miracle drugs," respirators, artificial kidneys, transplant surgery, and sundry other developments have given us remarkable control over the prolongation and the endings of life. The pill and other birth-control devices, in vitro fertilization and other techniques to conquer infertility, abortion, neonatal intensive care, and various other developments have provided remarkable control over the beginnings of life. We are even assuming control over the quality of life, including the quality of the life that is just beginning. The powers to identify carriers of certain genetic diseases, to diagnose certain genetic defects in the fetus, and—soon—to intervene directly in the genetic endowment of a newborn provide an astonishing control over our genetic legacy. These new powers are fascinating to some, terrifying to others; they appear promising to some, threatening to others (Kass, "New Biology," 779). It is little wonder they have called forth considerable careful reflection and even more literature.

For all their novelty, moreover, the extraordinary new powers are being applied to the ordinary but central human events of giving birth, suffering, and dying. These events have always commanded the attention of reflective people. The account one gives of these events is intimately related to the account one gives of being human. Because the new medical technologies provide new powers to intervene in these events, they provide a new challenge to think about what it means to be human.

1

Christians have been thinking about medical ethics for a very long time. Indeed, long before medical ethics became a distinguishable discipline, let alone a growth industry, Christians were engaged in the field, because Christian doctors and nurses were conscientiously trying to bring their practice into line with their Christian profession, Christian patients were trying to make decisions about medical care with Christian integrity, and ministers and other leaders were struggling to find a Christian word of admonition or encouragement for both professional and patient. Christians continue to think and ask about these things and sometimes to write about them. However, in the last decade, during which time medical ethics has become a growth industry, Christians who have written on medical ethics and contributed to the public discussion of these issues have often been more easily identified as followers of some moral philosopher—of Kant, say, or Mill, or Rawls—than as followers of Jesus.[1]

And there are some good reasons for that development. The professional groups medical ethicists want to convince are composed of both Christians and non-Christians. The public-policy makers whom medical ethicists hope to influence are sworn to protect the freedom of religion and not to establish legislatively a particularly or peculiarly Christian policy. The society within which medical ethicists attempt to form and inform a consensus is overwhelmingly secular. In this setting, arguments based candidly on Christian convictions may be regarded as at best insufficient, and perhaps as irrelevant. Convincing arguments in these contexts will presumably be based on universal and rational principles of morality, on legal precedents, and on an impartial point of view. Christians may—indeed, they must—participate in such public discussions, and part of the agenda of this book is to articulate and defend arguments we think are convincing in those contexts.

But in response to the new powers of medical science Christians must also witness to their deepest convictions about the human condition, about the ordinary but central events of giving birth, suffering, and dying. There are good reasons for not appealing to one's Christian convictions in certain contexts, but it is lamentable if Christians never speak candidly *as Christians* about medical morality. It is lamentable both for the pluralistic society in which we live and espe-

---

1. For this complaint, see especially J. M. Gustafson's "Theology Confronts Technology and the Life Sciences," and S. Hauerwas's "Can Ethics Be Theological?" and "Salvation and Health." For an account of the contributions Christian theologians have made to establishing interest in medical ethics, see L. Walters's "Religion and the Renaissance of Medical Ethics in the United States."

cially for the Christian communities with which we identify. A genuinely pluralistic society nurtures and profits from the candid articulation and vigorous defense of particular points of view. Faithful members of the Christian community want most of all to live (and die and suffer and give birth) with Christian integrity, not just with impartial rationality.

Lately there has been a revival of interest in a candidly Christian investigation of the issues in medical ethics.[2] People are asking how Christian convictions can guide and limit their new medical powers. People are wondering what Christian identity requires in the context of new ways of having children and caring for them and new decisions about the technological apparatus that surrounds our dying. The central agenda for this book is to express our faith in God in the context of the new powers of medicine and to suggest what faithfulness to God requires of those who deliver and receive medical care.

Faith in God the Creator

God is the creator, the maker of all things. All things are from God. This affirmation has been part of the Christian faith from the very beginning. The church expressed it in the doctrine *creatio ex nihilo*. That classic expression means simply that God created all things out of nothing. It is a simple statement in a way, but its consequences have been profound. From the very beginning it forced the church to distance itself from two other explanations about the source of all things.

There were those who thought that some things, at least, were not so much from God as identical with God, not so much made by God as of one piece with God—or the gods. Therefore, these things were in some sense divine and worthy of our worship. We could earn the favor of these gods or rely on their goodwill to deal with our needs and wants and to sustain us in our giving birth and in our suffering and dying. But to these and to any others who would lift up any part of God's creation as an idolatrous object of trust and hope, the people of God have said and continue to say, "No! God is the creator. God made all things from

2. Among the signals of the revival of interest in candidly Christian investigation is "Project X," an ecumenical research and publishing venture that has already produced an introductory volume (Marty and Vaux) and volumes on the Lutheran tradition (Marty), the Catholic tradition (McCormick), and the Reformed tradition (Vaux). Seven other volumes are planned, and a journal, *Second Opinion,* has been initiated. See also S. Lammers and A. Verhey's *On Moral Medicine.*

nothing. Therefore, all that God made is not God. Therefore, nothing God made is god."

There were others who thought that there were finally *two* sources of whatever is, a good source and an evil source. Gnostic dualism, for example, said that the soul, or spirit, is good because it has a good source and that the body is evil because it has an evil source. Death, then, comes as a friend to release our spirits from a mortal prison, and we may take pride in indifference to the body's suffering. But to these and to any others who would empty any part of God's creation of goodness and make it an object of enmity and spite, the people of God have said and continue to say, "No! God is the creator of all things out of nothing. All things have their source in the goodness of God. Therefore, all that God made is good."

God is the creator. Therefore, nothing that God made is god, and all that God made is good. Not many of us know any people who belong to a Gnostic congregation or kneel before a shrine of Ba'al, but our faithfulness to God the creator continues to be challenged by new temptations to idolatry and dualism.

The Critique of Idolatry

In our sex-saturated and health-oriented society, perhaps we are not in much danger of thinking of the body as evil, but one may wonder sometimes whether we're not in some danger of making the body—and its health and vigor—some kind of idol, something worshiped, an object of ultimate concern. The health and life of the body are goods that we may and must seek, but they are not the greatest good, and they may need to be risked or sacrificed in the pursuit of other goods.

Perhaps the high god in the contemporary pantheon of idols is technology. Properly impressed with the goods technology has provided, we are tempted sometimes to expect too much from it, to look to technology to be our faithful savior. Because of the new powers medical technology provides, it can be an idol, and doctors, its priests. Patients kneel at this shrine when they visit the doctor's office to petition him or her for a piece of medical wizardry to be provided with technological grace. And physicians have sometimes for a little while basked in the glory of their techniques, profiting from and enjoying the expectation that technology delivers us from our finitude or to our flourishing. Faithfulness to God the creator can deliver both patient and physician from extravagant and idolatrous expectations of technology; it can free them both to delight in the good that technology provides without expecting technology to rescue us from mortality or finitude or from the consequences of irresponsibility; it can free them both to be human in their clinical encounter.

We should be careful, however, about accusing physicians and scientists of "playing God." It is possible to have idolatrous expectations of technology, but to presume that human technological intervention violates God's rule is to worship Mother Nature, not the creator. Natural processes are not sacrosanct, and faithfulness to God the creator can require us to exercise dominion over natural processes for the sake of God's cause in God's creation.

The temptations to idolatry are everywhere. Anywhere a good exists, it can evoke an extravagant and ultimate loyalty and prompt extravagant and final expectations. And medicine is a very real good. It touches us near the center of our fears and hopes, where we live and die, give birth and shudder with pain.

Life itself is a good gift from God, but it can become an idol. Health is a good gift, but it can become a very demanding god. The relief of pain is a good gift, but in the midst of pain it is nearly impossible to resist the temptation to make it an ultimate concern, to curse God or to damn our neighbors, to do or undo anything for the sake only of relieving our pain. Children are a precious gift, but even children can be the object of idolatrous loyalty and expectation. It is a commonplace that our children are our hope for the future, but it is nevertheless blasphemous, and a commonplace blasphemy may be the most dangerous of all. God is our hope for the future, and Christians bear and rear children out of confidence in and hope for that future. When we make our children idols, we don't love them more; we are only more embittered when they confound our expectations. When we make our children the hope for the future, we don't love them more; we only become more demanding of them and of ourselves—for then we have the impossible task of making perfect children (through our reproducing) and making children perfect (through our parenting).

The critique of idolatry will surface in this book from time to time, reminding people that nothing God made is god and calling them to depend upon God and show him gratitude for every good gift.

The Critique of Dualism

The Gnostics thought the soul, or spirit, good because it has a good source and the body evil because it has an evil source. Contemporary dualists are more likely simply to say that the body doesn't count for very much, that the soul, the mind, the rational part of us, the capacity for self-awareness and reflection is what really counts. Our reply is the same: God made all things out of nothing, and therefore, while nothing God made is god, all that God made is good. We are not to make the body—or its health and vigor—an idol, but we may and we must receive and delight in our bodies as gifts of God and temples of his Spirit. They are not gods, but God's, and they deserve our respect and care.

God created us to be embodied persons, not souls now captive to bodies, and it is as embodied persons that we may and must receive and delight in each other. Dualism divides mind or soul from body, considers them mutually exclusive entities that do not require each other to be or to be known. Descartes, for example, distinguished mind *(res cogitans)* from matter *(res extensa)*, but however convinced he was that these "substances" were ontologically distinct, he could not escape (or explain) the fact that in our everyday experience there is an intimate union of mind and body. The mind or soul or self is not "in" the body the way a taxi driver is in a cab; the union is much more intimate than that (Zaner, 187). In our embodiment the knot of our being human is tied, a knot dualism cuts rather than unravels.

The union of body and soul in an embodied self is so intimate that it makes sense to say "I *am* my body." If my arm is broken, it is "I" who am injured. There is a duality, to be sure, because it also makes sense to say "I am *not* my body." It is still *my* body that is injured, but I can experience it as something other—indeed, as a "stranger" to me, whether in delighted surprise at its eager obedience or in angry disappointment at its spiteful refusal to do what I want (Zaner, 189). The experience of illness is an experience of the otherness of our bodies. When we are sick, we tend to objectify our bodies in ways that otherwise are unusual to us. We feel uncomfortably distanced from our bodies, which suddenly seem to have aches and processes of their own. Even so, sickness points to the unity of body and self, because the experience of sickness, of the otherness of the body, is an experience of being alienated from ourselves. (For further discussion, see Gadow; Pellegrino, "Being Ill.")

If this knot is cut, two contrasting errors become tempting. On the one hand, it is tempting to reduce the embodied person to soul, to mind, to some rational part, and to count that alone as valuable. On the other hand, it is tempting to reduce the embodied person to body, to biological organism, and to count that alone as valuable. Faithfulness to God the creator will be content with neither of these reductionisms, and faithful medicine and faithful reflection about medicine will have to be vigilantly watchful against these temptations. When dealing with both the beginning and the ending of life, for example, we will want to be careful to resist the temptations to reduce the embodied human being who deserves our respect to either body or mind, to either biological organism or rational soul. It may be necessary for care-givers to objectify the body, to think of it and treat it as a manipulatable organism in order to cure it, but care-givers must also always recognize and respect the body as an embodiment of a person and treat the whole person. With respect to technological reproduction, too, it will be important to resist the temptations of dualism: because human beings are children of nature as well as children of spirit, the course of wisdom will be neither to reduce "being a parent" to a biological relationship nor to treat it as a technical accomplishment.

The critique of dualism will surface in this book from time to time, reminding people that all that God made is good and calling them to be faithful to God, who loves the embodied people God created.[3]

The Reality of Evil

Before we continue, it is important to face one very important question: Is it true that all God made really is good? The counter-evidence is all around us: disease, pain, injustice, death, and even such prosaic things as petty, quarrelsome people and hard, dreary work.

The Bible never says there is no evil in the world. What it says and says plainly, however, is that God made all things and that God made all things good: "God saw everything that he had made, and behold, it was very good" (Gen. 1:31). The creation was a free act of love that God intended to be fulfilled in free, embodied people acting in love, receiving their being and their meaning from God. The one who stands behind this world and our lives as the creator is worthy of our trust and praise. But Adam made evil of something good. The Fall was a free act of disobedience by which people stood against and withstood God's intention in creation, a free act by which people subjected themselves and their world to what is not God and to what is not God's cause. By that free act, evil entered the world—but it could enter only as a corruption of the good. There is evil because people sinned, because people refused to believe that—and to live as though—all God made was good and that nothing God made was or could be god. Evil

3. We here stress, as we do in Chapter Two, the psychosomatic unity of human persons, following H. Stob (226), G. W. Bromiley (134), and A. Hoekema (217-18). It is possible to stress the duality of *psyche* and *soma* without denying the unity, and even (but not without risks, in our view) to use the term *dualism* (e.g., Cooper; Evans, "Healing Old Wounds"). Our critique of dualism is directed against the temptation to disvalue or to ignore one or the other aspect of the psychosomatic unity of embodied persons.

is in no sense the first word about our world. God's love is. Evil is and must be a parasite feeding on the good in a world created by God out of nothing. Parasites are, however, both real and dangerous; they threaten to destroy the good.

So we have little sympathy with the position of Mary Baker Eddy. Christian Science is not science, and it is not Christian, either (Barth, 364-65). Sin and sickness, pain and death—they are real, and they are real evils. The embodied life God created is real life, and it suffers real evils.

The evil is always a corruption of the good, and no less so with respect to death. God does not create immortal souls and test them in a body; God creates embodied selves who have to depend always on God for the power to be and to live as they are created to be and to live. The embodied selves God creates never have the power to be human in the same way God has the power to be God. Human life is always a gift, and people receive it moment by moment, according to God's good will as creator. It may not be too much to say that humans were created mortal, but that since evil entered the world, when death comes, it comes as the judgment of God, as human subjection to the power of nothingness, as the eruption of chaos, as itself a power that menacingly claims people for its very own, threatening jealously to sunder relationships with friends, family, and—yes—even God. Death is real, and it has become a real evil; the death to which the Fall subjects all creation is not the creative or covenant intention of God.

There will be occasions in this book to remind ourselves of the reality of evil in practicing medicine and in reflecting on it, to remind ourselves that in a world God created good there are still real evils, death and sickness among them.

Faith in God the Provider

Evil is not the first word about our world; neither is it the last word. God did not just create the world and then leave it to be destroyed by that parasite evil. Human sin could have smashed the cosmos back to chaos, but God sustained it and restrained the effects of sin upon it. God provided—in spite of sin and evil.

God is the provider. God preserves and governs and cares for the world. This, too, has been part of the Christian faith from the very beginning. Doctrines of providence can be incredibly complex, but what the believing communities say by them is fairly simple: God's care is the world's constant companion. And, as we noted earlier, faith in God forced the church to reject some other ways of explaining the governance of things.

There were some who thought all things happen by chance. If so, there is no meaning, no purpose, no justice to be discerned in the world or in history; there is just chance. Then it makes sense to live by the simple motto "Eat, drink, and be merry, for tomorrow we die." But to those who believe in mere chance and to all of our contemporaries who think life is meaningless and history pointless, faith in God the provider says, "No. God is the provider. Things do not happen by chance. In spite of evil, God sustains and rules the world with the same loving intentions with which he created the world. God's care is the world's constant companion."

There were others who thought all things happen by fate. If so, persons are simply puppets in the hands of necessity, no human action can affect history, and any human resolve is powerless against the strength of fate. Then it makes sense not to become angry with evil or to delight too much in the good. Human freedom and virtue will be found, curiously, in willing whatever happens. But to those who believe in fate and to all of our contemporaries who urge apathy and indifference and a death to passion and to freedom, faith in God the provider says, "No. God is the provider. Things do not happen by fate. In spite of evil, God upholds and governs the world with the same intention of human freedom and fruition with which he created the world. God's care is the world's constant companion."

This world is not ruled by chance or fate, not sustained and upheld by chance or fate; it is ruled in spite of evil by God, sustained and upheld in spite of evil by God's care. And faithfulness to God the provider disposes us, too, to care, to struggle against the claims of evil to speak the last word, to celebrate freedom in life because fate does not rule and meaning in life because chance does not govern.

The Problem of Suffering

Again we must pause to ask if it is true. Is it true that God provides, that God's care is the world's constant companion? The truth about our world is dripping with blood. The truth about our world is the myriads of sad stories people tell with and about their bodies: the infant who dies of sudden infant death syndrome, the youngster who suffers her way toward death of Tay-Sachs disease, the father who, unemployed and therefore uninsured, loses his life because his injury is left untreated. It's a sad world, not transparent to meaning, and care does not seem to be written over it, at least not legibly.

The problem of suffering has always challenged our assurance that God rules, that there is justice in history or meaning in the world. Even the biblical authors struggled with this issue (Verhey, "Evil," 209-10). There were some who insisted that God is kind to the good and pays back evil for evil, that suffering is always in some sense deserved. But the wicked sometimes experience God's kindness, too, as Jonah learned to his chagrin, and more distressingly, the good sometimes suffer, as Job witnessed to his doubtful friends. Suffering is sometimes deserved, to be sure, but not always—and seldom so clearly that we can read God's justice or judgment in it. So some insisted instead that suffering is educational, that it teaches us to rely on God, that it forms character, that it is necessary if we are to learn to celebrate the good and to be properly grateful for it—that suffering is always in some sense meaningful. But people are as often broken by suffering as educated by it. Suffering is sometimes meaningful, to be sure, but not always—and seldom so clearly meaningful that we can be content with the meaning and "pedagogical value" of another's suffering (D. Smith, "Suffering," 257-59). Neither account of suffering is finally very satisfying intellectually—or very honest—and the faith does not make liars of us. Much suffering is undeserved; much suffering is pointless. It is a sad world, marked and marred by suffering. So the question with which we began this section returns irresistibly, again and again: Can it be true that God's care is this world's constant companion?

In reply, Christians do not deny the horrible reality of suffering or their own powerlessness to "justify" God and the ways of God in a theoretical theodicy; instead, Christians point to a Roman cross and to an innocent Jewish teacher who suffered there, to the truth about our world who hung there. The cross is no lie; the cross is the truth about our world, both in its revelation of the reality and power of evil and in its revelation of God's love and care. When Christians point to the cross, they point to real evil and real suffering *and* to the real presence of God and the constant care of God. In the cross we may see—and believe—that God's care is the constant companion of a world where evil is real and powerful, of a world that stands against God, of a world that can only nail God's son to a cross. In a world where evil is real and powerful, *to care* will mean "compassion," to "suffer with" another, for in the cross we see not only the reality and power of evil but also—even if we can hardly believe it—God, suffering.

So to those who suffer, our first word is not to justify God for sending evil as punishment or training; it is to say that God suffers too, in and with their suffering, so that they may cry out, "God, why?" and still be assured that they do not suffer alone. And to those who would be faithful to God in ministering to the suffering, the word is to care, to be present with those who suffer, perhaps to save their lives or to relieve their pain, perhaps simply to wipe their tears with tenderness, but certainly to assure them that they do not suffer alone. In those who suffer, the eyes of faith can see the image of the Lord.

Faithfulness and Care

If chance ruled, perhaps people could do no better than a sophisticated hedonism. But it does not rule; God's care is the world's constant companion, and so people may cherish and delight in the meaning of life. And the meaning of life, the truth about the world, hangs on a cross. The cross — where Christians see the care with which God accompanies suffering people and because of which God refuses to abandon the world to evil—is the meaning of life. Faithfulness to this God will dispose us to care as well.

The disposition to care is the motive and rule for good medicine (Ramsey, "The Nature," 20). The responsibility of physician or nurse to a patient is precisely to care for the patient. This point will be made again and again in this book, and it will bear repeating. But to emphasize the responsibility of medical professionals to care is not without its dangers or free from temptations (Hauerwas, "Care").

We will need to remember in the first place that *medical* care is not the only important form of care. There are other forms, and not all suffering can be relieved or remedied by medical care. Not every problem is a medical problem, nor is care the responsibility and province of doctors and nurses exclusively. Faithfulness to God will dispose people to care, but it will not relieve them of hard choices about whether to allocate finite resources of time, money, and energy to medical care or to some other form of care. Even the sick and dying who suffer in ways that are responsive to medical care need other forms of care as well—in fact, sometimes they need these kinds of care even more than medical care, for they suffer also in ways that no medicine can touch. It makes sense in these contexts to insist on medical care, but it also makes sense to insist that the community of the faithful not abandon the sick and dying to medicine, not even to good medical care. Those faithful to God will be disposed to care for the sick; therefore, they will nurture a medicine capable of helping the sick, but they will also respond to suffering in non-medical ways, in ways that may be like a bone crossways in the throat of those who provide *medical* care. The first temptation, then, is to reduce *care* to *medical care*. That temptation can be resisted by acknowledging that the responsibility to care is not only a responsibility of doctors and nurses, even if it is surely theirs, and not only a responsibility to provide medical care, even if it is ordinarily that.

The second temptation is to reduce *medical care* to *care*. To resist that temptation we will have to acknowledge that the responsibilities of those who provide medical care are not just to care, even if they surely include that. Perhaps it is better to say that the responsibility of medical professionals to care requires of them not just compassion but competence, that precisely because it is *medical* care, responsible medicine and nursing will involve certain knowledge and skills that must be practiced carefully and competently. The rhetorical question "If your life is endangered by disease or injury, would you prefer a competent medical professional or a compassionate one?" may not be altogether fair, since one may hope for and expect a physician or a nurse who is both. But it does have a point, because medical professionals may have to strike a balance between listening to a patient's chest and listening to a patient's sighs, between taking time to research new studies of a patient's condition and taking time to be with the patient. The medical technology that enables medical professionals to care, though not more profoundly, at least more effectually than before, may also so distance practitioners from their patients that it makes it more difficult for them both to express and to nurture the attitude of care.

This second temptation is not necessarily remedied even when competence is joined to care, for such care can still abuse. "Taking care of someone" can, in ordinary language and in sophisticated medicine, be synonymous with doing violence to that person. The responsibility to care can be used as a license for paternalistic manipulation of a patient. Faithfulness to God the provider will dispose people to care, but not to resort to the kind of care that does not respect and preserve the freedom of the person who is a patient. The next section will say more about freedom. For now, the sum of the matter is as follows. Because all things do not happen by chance, those faithful to God may delight in the meaning in life—and so they may and must care. Because all things do not happen by fate, those faithful to God may celebrate the freedom in life—and so they may and must join respect for a patient's freedom to the care they give.

We shall have cause to return to these issues later in this book, to remind ourselves that faithfulness to God the provider means to care, that a faithful medicine and a faithful policy concerning it must be governed by care, and that physician and nurse are called to care even when they cannot cure or when they, limited by the respect due the patient's freedom or by the demands of equitable access to scarce resources, may not cure.

Faithfulness and Freedom

If fate ruled, perhaps we could do no better than passivity, indifference, and apathy. But it does not rule; God's care is the world's constant companion, and so we may cherish and preserve the freedom in life.

Faithfulness to God the provider will reject fatalism, but in its defense of freedom against fate it will not acknowledge chance as lord, either. Freedom is not the arbitrary freedom of a neutral agent whimsically to will what he will. The Pelagian[4] defense of freedom takes that path, defining freedom as the absence of any restraints upon a neutral self as it makes choices. In this view the indeterminacy and chance of choices and the inconsistency and unpredictability of an agent are evidence of freedom. To Augustinians like Calvin and his heirs, however, there is no neutral self, no self in equipoise between good and evil, but there is freedom. In the Augustinian view, freedom is the capacity an agent has precisely to establish a self, to determine an identity, to secure a self upon some loyalty by choice. Augustinians believe that from the first choice on, it is an established self who faces any particular subsequent choice, and consistency and predictability provide evidence of freedom.

These different notions of freedom are associated with different visions of God and of God's rule. A Pelagian sees the sovereignty of God and of God's grace as a threat to human freedom, because a Pelagian believes that a free person must approach his choices—even his choice about God—neutrally and without external or internal constraints, even (or especially) the constraint of the sovereignty of God's grace. A Pelagian sees the relationship of human freedom and divine sovereignty as at best a paradox. An Augustinian, on the other hand, views the sovereignty of God and of God's grace not as a threat to human freedom but as its very condition and fulfillment. God's gracious invitation to human beings to establish themselves in faithfulness to God creates human freedom and determines its proper fulfillment. The paradox for an Augustinian is not the relationship of freedom and divine grace—there is no apparent con-

---

4. Pelagius, a monk from Britain, was a popular preacher in Rome. His view of human freedom was that the will is always as free to choose evil as it is to choose good, and vice versa. The will is always equipoised between the two, unaffected by the fall of Adam or even by the formation of character. Augustine of Hippo vigorously opposed Pelagius, and the Councils of Carthage in 416 and 418 judged Pelagius's teaching to be heretical.

tradiction there. The paradox is rather that, being free, a person can withstand God's grace, the very ground of freedom. This is the terrifying mystery of freedom: it is freedom even with respect to its own condition and fulfillment. When human beings sinned, when they determined in that free act (itself an *affirmation* of freedom) an identity apart from loyalty to God and to God's cause, they nevertheless *denied* their freedom. That is the contradiction captured in the very Augustinian oxymoron "voluntary bondage." And that contradictory choice might have smashed the cosmos back to chaos—and evil might have had the last word—but God freely and consistently continued and continues his project of human freedom. God, by a gracious invitation and sovereign command, continues to call people to establish their selves upon loyalty to God and love for the neighbor, to reject the identity they have established upon some "good" and to reestablish themselves upon God, on whom all goods depend and in whom all goods cohere. This inviting and commanding word from God still provides the condition and fulfillment of freedom, liberating established selves for a new identity. God's call and human freedom are, of course, ordinarily mediated in terms of this world and with respect to concrete choices in this world, but a relationship to God and one's very self are always mysteriously at stake in a choice. We meet God everywhere in the world of our choices and, above all, in our choices with regard to our neighbors. Everywhere we are called to faithfulness to God. And in this same way we establish a self, making of our choices in living and in dying one integrated whole, an identity.

God's providence, then, does not deny, disregard, or destroy human freedom. It respects and preserves it even when that freedom is culpably and paradoxically used against God and its own fulfillment. And faithfulness to God the provider will dispose us to respect and preserve the freedom God gives even when, in terrifying mystery, it denies God's claims and cause.

The issue of freedom will arise again and again in this book, because it arises again and again in medical practice and in reflection upon medical practice. Sickness, for example, can be considered and experienced as a threat to an established self, as a threat to the capacity of an agent (now a patient) to adhere to those goods on which his self is established. To restore the freedom (or autonomy) of the patient may thus be considered one of the goods of medicine, part of medical care (Cassell, *Healer's Art*). However, medical care may and must be joined to respect and also be restrained by the freedom of the patient, even in the attempt to restore that freedom. "Informed consent" procedures are an attempt to honor the freedom of patients, and they are important for that reason. We will need to be careful, however, lest we define the freedom (or autonomy) of the patient as the freedom of a neutral agent to "will what he will." The freedom we must honor is not the arbitrary freedom to will one thing one moment and another the next, but the freedom to establish an identity and to maintain integrity.

A pluralistic society cannot exist without the moral standard of equal freedom. The freedom of each may be limited only by the equal freedom of all. Faithfulness to God the provider will respect and preserve freedom and the political standard that protects it. Even so, we will need to give careful attention to whether tolerance of and compromise and cooperation with the free choices of an established self are permissible and/or required—and when. And we will want to remind ourselves and our society that the standard of equal freedom is a minimal standard, providing only a minimal account of what is morally at stake in our choices. A choice, after all, does not become right simply because it is freely made. God and God's cause remain the condition and fulfillment of human freedom—and mysteriously at stake in our choices. The simple and concrete moral question "What ought I do?" may always be rephrased as a question of identity and, indeed, of faith: "To whom or to what am I giving loyalty in this act? On what am I establishing myself in this choice?"

A final caution is called for here, lest we slip back to fatalism. God does not deal with persons as though they were puppets. God does not remove the freedom of persons by providence; God sustains it. God does not destroy the humanity of persons by providence; God preserves it. The freedom and full humanity of people are part of God's intention, and God provides with those intentions always in view—in spite of evil. In a world under the sign of the cross, faith in God's providence will often have an "in spite of" attached. "In spite of" death, we believe God provides. "In spite of" sickness, we believe God preserves. "In spite of" suffering and every evil, we believe God's care is the world's constant companion and ours. Christians sometimes talk as though death, sickness, and suffering are themselves what God's providence intends. It isn't so, and if we are to stand with God and for God's cause, then we may only ever stand *in spite of* death and sickness and suffering and poverty and powerlessness and any other form of evil. Fatalism calls us to be passionless, unsuffering, apathetic. Faith in God the provider calls us to stand with God and for God's cause in a world still marked and marred by evil; it calls us to share the passion of Jesus. He has fought with death and sin—and he has won.

Faith in God the Redeemer

The God who spoke with love the first word upon our world, and so created it, the God who would not permit evil the last word upon our world, and so preserved it, that very God has spoken the final word upon our world in Jesus Christ, and so redeemed it. When God raised Jesus from the dead, God spoke the last word. Jesus came preaching that the kingdom of God was near, that the future unchallenged sovereignty of God was at hand—and he made its power felt already in his deeds and words, especially in his miracles of healing and his preaching of good news to the poor. As he said to the disciples of John, "... the blind receive their sight, the lame walk, lepers are cleansed, and the deaf hear, the dead are raised up, the poor have good news preached to them" (Luke 7:22; cf. Matt. 11:5). And when the powers of death and doom had done their damnedest, God raised him up and set him at God's own right hand in triumph over the power of evil. When God acted to raise Jesus from the dead, death was swallowed up in victory, evil was exposed as a parasite, the power of sin was vanquished, and God's own future sovereignty was established. When God called Jesus from the grave, God spoke the last word upon our world; God established the world's destiny. All things are not only from God as the creator, not only through God as the provider, but also unto God as the redeemer (cf. Rom. 11:36). Jesus was raised from death in our world and in our history, and our world and our history have, happily, no escape. The last word has been spoken.

The last word, of course, has in another sense not yet been spoken. All things have not yet reached their destiny. People still suffer, and some suffer from ills too many to count and too powerful to fight. People still die, and some die premature and horrible deaths. The enemy forces of poverty and pain and tears and death have not yet laid down their arms and admitted defeat. God's unchallenged cosmic sovereignty is not yet. We wait and watch and pray for God's last word at the appearance of Jesus in glory. But Jesus has already been raised, and now he sits at God's right hand. And already those who would be faithful to God the redeemer own Jesus as Lord and orient their character and their conduct, their life and their medicine, to God's future sovereignty.

This has been the church's profession from the very beginning. The church was born with the claim that God raised Jesus of Nazareth from the dead, and it lives by the knowledge that in the resurrection God spoke the last word. From its very beginning the church has said that the world's destiny was already won but not yet reached, that God's final word had been spoken and yet remains to be spoken. So faith in God the redeemer always looks back to Jesus' resurrection and forward to his appearance, and here and now and all the time between those times, it struggles to be faithful to God's future sovereignty already made known in Jesus. Faithfulness to God the redeemer requires that we be a watchful people and nurture a watchful medicine.

Watchfulness and Healing

God raised Jesus from the dead in mighty triumph over death and Satan and sin. The same Jesus had already gestured the same triumph over death and Satan and sin in his healing ministry. The people who celebrate God's rule and watch for it will orient their lives and their medicine toward God's good future, already made known in Jesus.

The resurrection of Jesus was, first of all and most obviously, a victory over the power of death. In the healing ministry of Jesus, the future reign of God over death and its domain already made its power felt. The dead were raised, and those thought to be "like dead" or under the power of death—the lepers, the blind, the paralyzed—were healed (Luke 7:22-23; Seybold and Mueller, 123). In Jesus and his resurrection, God acted to disclose and to assure God's cause—which is life, not death; health, not sickness. So a watchful people will celebrate and toast life, not death, but be able to endure even dying with hope. A watchful people will delight in human flourishing, including the human flourishing called health; they will not welcome the dwindling of the strength to be human—including the loss of strength called sickness—yet they can endure that in the confidence that God's grace is sufficient (2 Cor. 12:9) and that God's power is present even in our weakness.

A watchful people will not condemn medicine, as if to turn to natural and scientific remedies were to turn against God and God's grace. A wise and prudent Jewish teacher instructed the people of God long ago, "Honor the physician . . . for the Lord created him. . . . The Lord created medicines from the earth, and a sensible man will not despise them" (Ecclus. 38:1-4). Medicine is a good gift of God the creator, a gracious provision of God the provider, and a reflection and servant of God the redeemer. To condemn medicine because God is the healer would be like condemning governments because God is the ruler or condemning families because God is the parent. Of course, if medicine arrogates the role of faithful savior or presumptuously thinks of itself as the ultimate healer, then its arrogance may be and must be condemned. Perhaps the doctor—at any rate, the good and honest doctor—is less tempted to have this sort of extravagant and idolatrous expectation of medicine than many patients are. A modest medicine may be granted its modest—and honorable—place under God and alongside other measures that protect and promote health and life (good nutrition, public sanitation, a clean environment, etc.).

A watchful people, then, will not condemn medicine, but neither will they turn to it as an alternative to faith and prayer. Because the victory has been won, watchful people may now pray boldly for a foretaste of God's final triumph (as the Lord taught us) even in and through such ordinary things as daily bread ("Give us this day...") and forgiveness ("Forgive us our debts...")—and medicine. And because that final triumph is not yet, watchful people may pray still no less boldly for the presence of the one who suffers with us while we watch for that last day on which the redeemer's intentions of life and health will be at last fulfilled.

Watchful people will not condemn medicine or idolize it; they will nurture a watchful medicine, a medicine disposed to serve life and not to practice hospitality to death, disposed to serve health and not to welcome the loss of the strength to be human, disposed to acknowledge the limits of medicine's powers and to hope in the greater power of God, and, yes, disposed to pray for or with patients that God be present with the redeemer's healing intention in their therapy and present with the provider's care in their suffering.

The resurrection of Jesus was not only a victory over the power of death. It was also a great victory over the power of Satan. In the healing ministry of Jesus the future reign of God over Satan and his hosts already made its power felt, for that ministry included exorcisms. Jesus himself gave his exorcisms this interpretation: "If it is by the finger of God that I cast out demons, then the kingdom of God has come upon you" (Luke 11:20).

"Possession" was widespread in the ancient Mediterranean— or, more precisely, the demonological understanding of sickness and psychosis was widespread (Seybold and Mueller, 116). What was new in Jesus was that possession was linked not to magic but to the future sovereignty of God. Jesus' exorcisms were of one piece with God's final triumph over the powers of evil, and they already diminished Satan's dominance. And watchfulness for the future reign God established will already celebrate and express the exorcisms. That does not mean that a watchful medicine will or must account for pathologies and psychoses in the strange and alien terms of the first century, as the power of demons at work. The biblical stories are not addressed to twentieth-century scientific or clinical questions and may not be used to prescribe either the way to understand such suffering today or the way to provide therapy (Seybold and Mueller, 119).[5] Nevertheless, the exorcisms do point to an important feature of the human flourishing God intends. One decisive characteristic of demon possession was precisely "possession." The sick did not have control of themselves. They were possessed, subject to the power of the demons; their speech and action had no genuine connection with who they were. The cause of God includes human flourishing, and human flourishing requires identity and integrity. A watchful medicine may use its best medical skills and

5. There is no Christian ethic which is not tied somehow to Scripture, no Christian medical ethic not formed and informed somehow by Scripture; yet the world of sickness in Scripture is strange and alien, and forging a Christian medical ethic out of it raises a number of difficult methodological questions. The bridge between the strange world of sickness in Scripture and a contemporary Christian medical ethic will be fashioned of judgments about the nature of Scripture, the questions appropriate to Scripture, the message of Scripture, and the relevance of other sources. This book can neither treat these questions adequately, piling brick upon brick to fashion a bridge, nor ignore them. Only a sketch of the bridge can be offered here in the form of summary responses to the methodological questions implied in our discussion.

First, what is the nature of Scripture? Scripture is the Word of God *and* the words of men. As the Council of Chalcedon said of the union of divine and human natures in Christ, so we say of the union of the word of God and human words: the human words—with all their historical particularity—may be neither identified and confused with the Word of God nor divided from and contrasted with the divine Word. The human words of Scripture involve a process of tradition; indeed, Scripture is part, albeit the normative part, of a continuing tradition in the churches. The development of tradition may not be ignored if we are to hear the Word of God.

Second, what questions are appropriate to be asked of Scripture? Questions about nature are appropriate, but the sorts of questions about nature that a natural scientist or a clinical practitioner would ask will receive quaint and curious replies. And questions about morality are appropriate, but not the sort of questions an Enlightenment philosopher would ask in the quest for an impartial, rational, and autonomous ethic. Within the realm of moral inquiry, furthermore, questions concerning which concrete deed I should do or leave undone in a particular context may receive only a quaint reply from Scripture. However, Scripture does speak with authority to questions about the dispositions and intentions and principles and convictions that should form our character and finally shape our conduct.

Third, what is the message of Scripture? What do you understand when you understand Scripture? The key to Scripture is the resurrection of the crucified Jesus of Nazareth. There God acted to unveil God's own good future. Any contemporary use of Scripture must be consonant with that disclosure of God's purpose.

Finally, what about the use of other sources besides Scripture? Other sources, including natural science and "natural" morality, may and must be used. No use of Scripture may violate the natural principle of justice or contradict the "assured results" of medical science. Of course, there are disagreements about how to interpret and articulate the principle of justice and the "assured results" of science as well, and Christians may and must use the affirmation of the resurrection to qualify and illumine the use of these other sources.

These judgments may allow us to search the Scriptures without being surprised at finding there a world of sickness strange and alien to us, nevertheless confident to find there the Word of God, a light to our path even through medical revolutions.

See further A. Verhey's *The Great Reversal* (153-97).

knowledge to explain what is happening in and to the sick, but a watchful medicine will use those skills and that knowledge in ways that honor God and serve God's cause, including God's cause of each individual's identity and integrity.

✱   [A watchful people will nurture the strength to be human, including the strength to have one's own identity and the power to have integrity with it. A watchful medicine, too, will serve and respect identity and integrity, serving identity when sickness threatens, respecting integrity when medical care threatens] We need not repeat what was said earlier about issues surrounding care of the whole person and respect for the freedom of established selves, but we may observe that those who share the faith in God who raised Jesus from the dead may not adopt any disposition they please toward the embodied integrity of persons. -Faithfulness to God in Jesus will sustain in us and in our medicine a readiness to protect and nurture the integrity of all people and their capacity to embody it in their living and in their dying.

The resurrection of Jesus was also a great victory over sin. Already in his ministry Jesus forgave sins, in token of God's good future. Already in his healings Jesus broke the power of sin and the assumption that sickness is a consequence of sin—not just of Adam's sin but of the sin of the one who suffers (Seybold and Mueller, 126). The stories of Jesus point in more than one direction here. On the one hand, Jesus rejects the connection between sin and sickness presupposed in the question about whether a man's blindness is caused by his own sin or the sin of his parents (John 9:1-9; cf. Luke 13:1-5). Jesus does not explain suffering in terms either of its being deserved or of its being meaningful; instead, he points to the power of God to heal, and he makes that power felt. People faithful to God the redeemer will follow Jesus in disowning the putative connection between sickness and sin whenever it is used to distance themselves from the sick, to renege on their obligation of solidarity with the suffering, to justify refusing to be present with the sick or to use their powers against disease. A watchful medicine will be disposed to cure the sick, not to condemn them, and to practice the caring presence of God even when (or especially when) their powers to cure are too limited to provide a token of the final triumph of God.

On the other hand, we have the astonishing reply of Jesus to a request for healing: "My son, your sins are forgiven" (Mark 2:5). Here the connection between sin and sickness is accepted, but it is not used to segregate, judge, and condemn the sick. On the contrary, Jesus already makes known God's total and unqualified acceptance of this sick young man, and the whole person is already renewed in earnest of God's final victory. Watchful people and watchful medicine will not use a person's responsibility for his own sickness to disown their duty to care or their desire to cure, but they will be ready to recognize and to deal with the whole person, refusing to isolate and reduce a person's suffering to its physical manifestations or its clinical symptoms.

In summary, then, the healing ministry of Jesus makes known God's cause. God's cause includes life, human flourishing (including that aspect of flourishing we call "health"), and embodied integrity. A faithful people nurturing and practicing a faithful medicine will be disposed to protect life, to sustain health, to respect the embodied integrity of people, to attempt to cure the sick, to care for the suffering. The last word has been spoken: that word is *life*, not death; *health*, not sickness; *freedom*, not bondage; *care*, not condemnation. So all of us watch and pray, and some of us use or practice medicine, watching and praying.

Watchfulness and the Poor

A watchful people will care for the sick, and so they will nurture a watchful medicine to care skillfully and effectively for the sick. A watchful people will also care for the poor, and so they will nurture in a watchful medicine the capacity and the disposition to care, skillfully and effectively, especially for the sick who are poor.

The resurrection of Jesus was also, after all, the vindication of the one who was the Christ, "anointed," as he said, "to preach good news to the poor" (Luke 4:18), the one whose words to the poor and whose compassion for them were a token and a promise of God's eschatological blessing (e.g., Luke 6:20). There is no watching for this Jesus to return and no calling this Jesus "anointed" (i.e., "Christ") that may be unaffected by Jesus' compassion to seek justice for the poor and to practice kindness toward them.

No evangelist represents this feature of Jesus' ministry more elegantly or emphasizes this requirement of watchfulness more powerfully than Luke, the physician. From the very beginning Luke emphasizes Jesus' solidarity with the poor. Jesus' own parents were poor, offering the sacrifice of the poor (Luke 2:24; cf. Lev. 12:6-8); in the Magnificat (Luke 1:46-55), Mary rejoices in God's action to exalt the humble, the hungry, and the poor, and to humble the exalted; humble shepherds (Luke 2:8-20), not rich magi (cf. Matt. 2:1-12), visit Jesus in an animal stall, not a house (cf. Matt. 2:11). In Luke's gospel the Beatitudes of Jesus announce God's eschatological blessing on the physically poor and hungry, not just the "spiritually" poor and hungry (Luke 6:20-21; cf. Matt. 5:3-6). To welcome

Jesus and to watch for the future that he promised require love and mercy (Luke 6:27-42), which includes showing carefree generosity to the poor (Luke 6:30) and lending to them without expecting a return (Luke 6:34-35). A number of parables of Jesus in Luke's gospel develop this theme: the parable of the good Samaritan explicates the love command in terms of mercy and concludes with the instruction "Go and do likewise" (Luke 10:25-37); the parable of the rich fool condemns the concern of the wealthy for their own ease and their failure to do justice or practice kindness in faithfulness to God (Luke 12:13-21); the parable of the great supper includes a reminder of God's intention to bless "the poor and maimed and blind and lame" and follows an exhortation to practice hospitality toward the same (Luke 14:15-24); the parable of the rich man and Lazarus announces an eschatological great reversal with its blessings upon the poor and its woes upon the ungenerous rich (Luke 16:19-31). Zacchaeus's choice to do justice and mercy is commended by Jesus in words which suggest that in such justice and mercy toward the poor the future reign of God has begun to take effect (Luke 19:1-10).

The physician Luke continues the same focus in Acts. All the heroes give alms—Peter and John (Acts 3:1-10), Cornelius (Acts 10:1-4), and Paul (Acts 11:27-30; 12:25; 24:17). Those in the faithful community share their goods (Acts 2:44-45; 4:32-37); the fact that "there was not a needy person among them" (Acts 4:34) is a clear allusion to Deuteronomy 15:4-5 and a clear indication that in this sharing community the promises and requirements of covenant are kept.

Luke does not represent Jesus as legislating any of this; he gives no legal rulings, and he has no social program. Nor does Luke represent Jesus as an ascetic. But the story the physician tells of Jesus, "anointed . . . to preach good news to the poor" (Luke 4:18), can shape, sometimes has shaped, and always should shape the dispositions of the faithful toward the poor. To follow this Jesus is to do justice and kindness to the poor; to watch for the future reign of God that he announced is to anticipate and already to participate in his blessing upon the poor; to keep faith with Jesus as the one in whom God's cause is made known is to practice hospitality toward the poor.

There are too many whose spirits are crippled, whose lives are ended, and whose strength to be human is destroyed by their poverty. Such poverty debilitates both the souls and cells of embodied persons. These people live—and die—not only in Third World countries but also in North America. A watchful people will be ready to defend the poor, to insist on justice for them, and to practice kindness toward them. Justice for them may not require access to high-technology medical care, and kindness toward them might not even suggest it, not when their health and flourishing depend on satisfying more fundamental human needs. A watchful people will not be disposed to defend an economy that has the resources to meet fundamental human needs but fails to meet them, especially when the same economy that accepts debilitating poverty also promotes and generates unrestrained excess. Watchfulness will urge entry into public-policy discussion and economic-policy debate in defense of the poor.

The needs of the poor are not all (or even mainly) medical; even their health-related needs are not all (or even mainly) medical; but the poor do have medical needs, and they do not all have access to medical care. In the United States, for example, while many of the poor are protected by Medicaid, many others are uninsured and have no access to medical care. Medicine, meanwhile, is adopting a corporate image. For-profit hospitals are increasing, their stock on Wall Street is advancing, and the uninsured are dumped in the emergency rooms of community hospitals. A marketplace medicine will do great things for those who can pay, but the poor and powerless who are sick will be left to their own resources—and to despair. Watchful people will commend stewardship in the use of resources, but they will also insist that public policy join a concern for the poor to a concern about cutting costs. Watchful medicine will work toward a medical-care delivery system that includes the poor, and it will nurture a medical identity that is committed to helping all the sick, be they rich or poor.

In the parable of the rich man and Lazarus in Luke's gospel, the rich man begs Abraham to send Lazarus to warn his rich brothers to repent and to do justice and love kindness. Luke, the physician and evangelist, knew Jesus had been raised from the dead. Were any of the rich brothers convinced? The one who preached good news to the poor has been raised from the dead. The public-policy recommendations, the health-care delivery systems, and the public identities of a watchful people ought all to keep faith with this risen Jesus.

This book will need to return to these issues, especially when it examines the allocation of health care. For now it is sufficient to say that a watchful community and a watchful medicine will be disposed to do justice and to love kindness toward the poor, at least as long as the gospel of the physician Luke remains a part of the church's canon.

The "Not-Yet" Character of Our Life and Medicine

The last word has been spoken—but the last word remains yet to be spoken. God's cause has been made known and its triumph assured—

but God's cause is not yet the case. The victory has been won—but the enemy powers of pain and tears and death still assert their doomed reign. The ancient foe still seeks to work us woe; "His craft and power are great, And armed with cruel hate, On earth is not his equal" (Martin Luther, "A Mighty Fortress"). It is not yet the promised age of God's unchallenged sovereignty, when "death shall be no more, neither shall there be mourning nor crying nor pain any more" (Rev. 21:4). We still wait and watch and pray for that day.

The last word is not death — but people die still. A watchful people and a watchful medicine may celebrate human powers, including the power of medicine, to intervene against death. Faithfulness to God, after all, will not practice hospitality to death. But they may not pretend or presume that the final victory over death is within human powers. The victory over death is finally God's victory, not medicine's; Jesus is the Messiah, not medicine; in living and dying and in medicine the people of God wait and watch and pray for God's final triumph. So they need not fear death. They need not stand in dread of it. They need not use all their resources or all human powers against it. In the confidence of God's final word, they may sometimes permit it its apparent triumph.

The last word is not suffering—but people suffer still. A watchful people and a watchful medicine may and must celebrate the human powers, including the power of medicine, to intervene against suffering. Faithfulness to God, after all, will not delight in the suffering of others. But a watchful people and a watchful medicine may not pretend or presume that life can be altogether freed from suffering or that medicine can altogether liberate those who suffer from afflictions too many to name or too powerful to fight. The victory over suffering is finally God's victory, not medicine's; medicine's powers are not messianic. In suffering and in care for those who suffer, the people of God wait and watch and pray for God's final triumph. So they have resources of hope to continue to struggle against the suffering of others, resources of faith to share in Jesus' suffering with those who suffer, resources of love to be present in care and in prayer even when they cannot cure.

The last word is not tears—but many still weep for the child they never had. The last word is not mourning—but many still grieve over the child of promise they lost by never having it. Childlessness hurts—but hurt is not the last word. A watchful people and a watchful medicine may celebrate human powers to intervene against infertility, at least as long as they think of children as a gift of God. But they may not pretend or presume that either a child or the medical procedures capable of helping the infertile to have a child are messianic, that such powers can deliver them to their flourishing. *The* Child has been born —and to the childless, too. So Christians may and must delight in children, not as means to their own flourishing and surely not as human accomplishments or the products of medical technology, but as "the little ones" whom Jesus loves. The burden and the duty of having children is lifted by the birth of the one Child in whom God's cause is made known and assured. In a world like this one, to have children is to express our confidence in God's last word. And the burden and bitterness of childlessness is also lifted, for since Jesus was born, to be infertile cannot be a fault. Now both having children and not having them can be an occasion for waiting, watching, and praying, for delighting in the powers of medicine without expecting too much from them, without expecting medicine to deliver the childless from their childlessness to their flourishing.

The last word is not ambiguity—but here and now, even as the people of God welcome God's cause and serve it, they face conflicting goods and confront gathering evils. Here and now, even as they seek to consent to God's future rule, part of what they know to be God's cause comes into conflict with another part of what they know to be God's cause. In allocating finite funds, for example, "good news to the poor" disposes people to meet basic needs before they allocate money for expensive medical care (to provide decent minimum health care for all before the very best is provided for any), but "healing the sick" disposes people to seek the very best medical care for those who need it. In deciding about the medical case of one patient, the disposition to preserve life can come into conflict with the disposition to relieve suffering. Here and now, between the times, the disposition to honor embodied integrity and respect freedom, to care, to heal, to do justice and show kindness, and to preserve life—all belong to faithfulness, and all can conflict. Faithfulness itself provides no neat and easy resolution to such conflicts. Watchfulness does not usher in the new heaven and the new earth, either. Here and now there is ambiguity. Here and now it is not yet the kingdom of shalom even among the goods that all belong to God's cause. So the faithful wait and watch and pray for God's triumph. And medicine waits, too.

This book is an attempt to nurture a faithful people and a watchful medicine while it deals with the choices that must be made in the midst of genuine ambiguities. It does not pretend or presume to say the last word about medicine or about the choices Christians confront when they use or practice medicine. We hope it says a helpful word, a word that will encourage Christians to think and talk and pray together about what faithfulness to God requires, about what it means to be a watchful people in our use and allocation of medical resources, in our living and in our dying, in our giving care, in our weakness and in our powers, in the ambiguities between the certainties of Jesus' resurrection and his final triumph.[6]

---

6. Parts of this chapter are revisions of parts of A. Verhey's *Living the Heidelberg* (51-55), "Calvin's Treatise 'Against the Libertines,'" and "The Strange World of Sickness in Scripture." For further reflection about many of the issues raised here, see D. W. Shriver, Jr.'s "Interrelationships of Religion and Medicine"; D. H. Smith's "Theological Context for the Relationship between Patient and Physician" and "Suffering, Medicine, and Christian Theology"; S. Hauerwas's "Salvation and Health" and *Suffering Presence;* H. Stob's *Ethical Reflections;* K. Vaux's *Health and Medicine in the Reformed Tradition;* and J. M. Gustafson's *Contributions of Theology to Medical Ethics.*

2. Imaging God in Sickness and in Health

God and God's cause were the focus of the first chapter. Now we turn to the nature of those beings who were created to be faithful to God's cause, because *how* human beings are faithful to God depends upon the nature given them in their creation. God created human beings in God's own image. Our ethical responsibility, then—what is fitting and appropriate for us to do—is to act as imagers of God and to keep ever before us that those upon whom we act and with whom we act are also God's imagers. Faithfulness to God requires that what we do be representative of what we are.

Imaging God

During the 1960s, civil-rights marchers would sometimes carry signs saying "God made me, and God doesn't make junk." This message is a good place to begin. The biblical story of creation, fall, and redemption tells us that what is happening in our world is not a struggle for survival among the fittest of animals that randomly developed from a chance coalition of atoms. Instead, we were *made*—by a God who does not make junk. Remembering both that we are creatures *and* that God declared the creation to be fundamentally good is enough to help us avoid both the self-deification and the self-debasement that are common though contradictory tendencies of secular thinking. But to understand our place in creation and to avoid lowering ourselves to mere stimulus-response mechanisms or to machines made of meat—a reductionism that is all too common in science and medicine—we must constantly recall the biblical theme of being created in God's image (Evans, "Healing Old

Wounds"). This theme establishes some "control beliefs" (Wolterstorff, 67) about how we should perceive ourselves and other persons, beliefs that can have great importance for how we relate to others and for our ideas about health and human flourishing.

What is it to be an imager of God? One way to answer this question is to notice that the Bible portrays God as making people in God's image *after* the creation of the other animals, and to infer that we image God in and only in the way we are different from the rest of creation. One can combine this inference with the observation that God does not have a body and conclude that the way we image God can have nothing to do with our bodies. This conclusion would then lead us to look for creaturely features that are nonbodily and are unique to persons. If we conduct this search within an intellectual tradition that interprets biblical talk about flesh, body, soul, and spirit in terms of the dualisms deriving from Plato and Descartes, we may too quickly infer that to be made in the image of God is to have an immaterial and immortal soul that loosely resides in a disease-prone mortal coil.[1] Fortunately, this view will conclude, a person's true essence—the real "I"—is the soul, which is immune to the diseases of the body and which can be graciously saved from the sin that infects it. The consequence is that the health of the body is perceived as distinctly secondary to the health of the soul. Medical missionaries subscribing to this view may be tempted to use the wonders of modern medicine mainly as means to an end—perhaps as miraculous signs that confirm the truth of the message, or perhaps as a means for getting sick people to listen to the preaching of the Word, or perhaps even as a witness of what Christian discipleship involves—the real goal being the salvation of souls.

We believe that this view goes well beyond and largely against much of what the Bible teaches about imaging God. First, the initial inference is invalid: the fact that God created God's imagers last does not imply that they image God solely in their uniqueness. It may just as well imply that something about them enriches or transforms, in a God-imaging way, some of the very features and capacities they share with other creatures. And the fact that God lacks a body is compatible with our imaging God in a fundamentally embodied way. God may have chosen to incarnate God's own image in bodies, in a way analogous to

---

1. This view, we hasten to add, is not that of many, perhaps most, theologians today, who believe that the Bible is best interpreted as implying that persons are unified wholes rather than conjoinings of two separate types of substances. For discussions of the Bible's language about persons, see J. R. Nelson's *Human Life*, A. Hoekema's *Created in God's Image*, and C. Van Peursen's *Body, Soul, Spirit: A Survey of the Body-Mind Problem*.

that in which an artist uses material to convey to us a nonmaterial element,[2] such as the mysterious amusement in the smile of the *Mona Lisa*.

✸ Second, the anthropology required by the previously mentioned inferences contradicts what we know about human nature. We share some of our finer features with animals, and it has turned out to be difficult to specify a human capacity that is not, in some sense, possessed by some other species. Some researchers have argued that playfulness, imagination, deceptiveness, friendliness, tool making, reasoning, language using, the expressing of emotions, the capacity to mourn the death of others, and perhaps even having a self-concept—capacities that were once thought to be uniquely human—have been discovered in other species (Midgley, 203-317). Of course, there is room for debate about these "discoveries" in animals, and, in any case, there may be uniquely human ways of exercising these capacities—ways that have to do with imaging God. But we have no biblical or scientific reason to think we image God only in those features we do not share with other animals. Moreover, it seems that we image God in a fundamentally embodied way. What we know about biology and how it relates to the choice-making involved in stewardship and covenantal love implies that human beings need brains *and bodies* to carry out these God-imaging activities. We do not merely *have* bodies; we *are embodied*, as organisms whose integrated functioning involves God-imaging capacities, perhaps as a characteristic that emerges when the organism's functioning reaches a certain level of complexity and integration.[3] Some Christians might even say that human beings *are* bodies, that what we essentially are dies with our bodies, though some of these same Christians may also have the hope of being resurrected as spiritual bodies. This view generates some interesting questions about personal identity with respect to bodies (If I completely disappear at death, is it *I* who will be resurrected or a replica of me?), and it also contradicts the belief of many Christians that we exist in some sort of intermediate state between death and resurrection. This latter belief seems to imply that, at a minimum, God can separate some aspect of persons from their original embodied state and sustain them at some level of existence while they await spiritual bodies.[4]

2. This analogy comes from Harry Boer, who is writing a book on how persons image God. The book is titled *An Ember Still Glowing: Humankind as the Image of God.*

3. Of course, one can talk about "my body" just as one can talk about "my mind." I can move my body, and I can change my mind. But in both cases it is I as an embodied mind that act. It is not just my face that frowns; I frown, though I need a face in order to do it (Sprague, 47). See W. Hasker (72-76) for a theory of how a person's God-imaging capacity could be an emergent phenomenon, one that is produced by but is distinct from (and not reducible to) the brain's neural activity.

4. W. Hasker (74-75) argues that the emergent mind could be a self-sustaining substance of some sort, just as the gravitational field of a black hole (or collapsed star) continues

✱ ⓐ For purposes of this book, we need agree only on two things: first, that the resurrection hope implies that death is not our end, and, second, that the embodied way by which we image God implies that our physical health is directly and importantly related to what God calls us to be and do. In other words, we must avoid any dualism that suggests that the real "I" is separate from the body, that ill health affects the body without affecting the person, or that the image of God in the person is a soul serenely unconcerned with and unaffected by death.

What the Bible says about the image of God reveals a number of important points. First, it gives embodied human beings a special moral status, as Genesis 9:6 makes clear, by prohibiting murder because persons are imagers of God: "Whoever sheds the blood of man, by man shall his blood be shed; for God made man in his own image." Wrongfully spilling human blood is viewed as the iconoclastic desecration of God's image. In fact, even cursing persons is forbidden because it is a contradiction to praise God and curse God's image: "With [the tongue] we bless the Lord and Father, and with it we curse men, who are made in the likeness of God. . . . this ought not to be so" (Jas. 3:9-10). And the Heidelberg Catechism (Q. and A. 105) forbids insulting our neighbors in deed or in thought as well. In other words, not just certain behaviors but certain attitudes are unfitting toward other human beings. Or, to put it positively, some of the attitudes we have toward God we should have, in a derivative way, toward God's imagers. Thus, some of the same kind of fear we have toward God is also appropriate toward those who bear God's image. Experiencing the fear of God should not be reduced to being scared, but it should be associated with feelings of reverence and awe, feelings elicited by God's goodness, holiness, majesty, power, and kingship. Creatures who represent God both by mirroring God and by being God's delegates (having the authority to rule in God's name) should be valued and loved; love of God and neighbor, after all, is Jesus' basic ethic. And seeing our neighbors as bearing God's image can help us love them, even when they are otherwise unlovable. As John Calvin advises, we should ". . . look upon the image of God in them, which cancels and effaces their transgressions, and with its beauty and dignity allures us to love and embrace them" (*Institutes* X.vi.31). It is important to

---

to exist after the star's matter apparently disappears. Christians, of course, can appeal to the sustaining activity of God to argue that some aspect of a human being is *separable* if not *separate* from the body (Evans, "Separable Souls"). J. Cooper argues that the Bible and the Reformed creeds teach at least this sort of minimal dualism. C. Plantinga, in a conversation with the authors of this book, argued that *being embodied at a certain point in time* (rather than simply being embodied) may be an essential property of human persons.

notice that Christian love is influenced by awe for the nature of its object—an imager of God. "Sanctity" is the term many religious persons use to characterize that which elicits their reverence. As Richard Stith writes, the sanctity of personal life calls for a love that has a "stand-back-ish" element and not just an urge to value, to nurture, or to control:

> Reverence, by contrast [to valuing], eschews domination. It steps back before the "sanctity" of that which is revered, and thus necessarily before every particular which has sanctity. A limit is given to us and to our schemes of domination. We can no longer destroy and rebuild as we wish, but must accept and accommodate being, even the being of individuals. If I revere human life, if I say it has sanctity, then rather than making and controlling it, I acknowledge and defer to it, I let it be (p. 6).[5]

Thus, those who image God are to be loved reverentially, even deferentially, a point that will be relevant when we discuss such topics as violating a person's right to informed consent or killing a person out of love. Of course, there may also be secular reasons for reverencing the sanctity of persons and perceiving them as having a dignity beyond price (Kant, 103), but the biblical theme of being created in God's image implies that the basis of a Christian's disposition toward people is fundamentally a religious feeling and responsibility.

The second biblical point to notice is that God's decision to create human beings in itself designated their suitability for a specific role: "Let us make man in our image, after our likeness; and let them have dominion over the fish of the sea, and over the birds of the air, and over the cattle, and over all the earth, and over every creeping thing that creeps upon the earth" (Gen. 1:26). The psalmist celebrates both the human role and the special nature of those called to it: "Yet thou hast made him little less than God, and dost crown him with glory and honor. Thou hast given him dominion over the works of thy hands; thou hast put all things under his feet" (Ps. 8:5-6). The implication of these passages is that God did not ar-

---

5. Stith himself seems to contrast reverence with love, as if the sanctity of life were a religious or moral disposition separate from that of loving one's neighbor. But reverence can also be interpreted as a quality of the type of love appropriate to persons, a point emphasized by Rev. R. Brummel at one of the workshops held by the CCCS team (5 Dec. 1985). The phrase "sanctity of life" comes out of the Hindu tradition, where it refers to all life. As L. Smedes argues, Christians should probably use the phrase "sanctity of personal life" (*Mere Morality,* 105). Sometimes, especially in the Jewish tradition, "sanctity" is interpreted as infinite value (see H. Brody, 249; Veatch, *Theory,* 30). In addition to confusing the distinction between valuing and revering, this interpretation would seem to imply that one could never risk one's life, no matter how small the risk or how great the potential benefit, and that no costs or pain should ever be spared in squeezing one more minute of life out of a person's dying process. We think it is more coherent to think of personal life as *incommensurable* with mere valuing or pricing than as valued infinitely or at an infinite price.

bitrarily select a species of creatures for special status, conferring on its members an "alien dignity."[6] Rather, we human beings are specifically constituted for the role of representing God both in the sense of mirroring God as rulers and in the sense of being God's delegates and having the authority to be stewards over creation. Since our suitability for this stewardly role requires the capacity for reflective choice-making, we infer that we image God by virtue of our being givers and hearers of reasons, beings who not only make choices but also reflect on them and make choices about our choices, who not only have desires but also have desires about our desires, who not only evaluate but also evaluate our evaluations, who not only think but also think about our thinking. These capacities, in turn, require not just consciousness but self-consciousness, the sort of "reflexivity" (Van Leeuwen, 127) which provides us with the freedom and creativity that enable our choices to be more than previously determined responses to stimuli. Other organisms may, in some sense, think and choose, but the integrated functioning of the human organism provides for a referring to itself that constitutes a capacity for choosing how to choose. With this capacity comes the responsibility to exercise it in the way that our good and wise creator intended, and consciousness of this responsibility is the foundation of our moral sense. So an important part of imaging God is recognizing and accepting the exhilarating freedom and the sobering burden of making moral judgments about proper stewardship.

The third biblical point to note about the image of God is that God's imagers were created both male and female, implying both that stewardship will be exercised in community and that community will be created through human sexuality. As with other creatures, this sexuality is natural and instinctive, but in self-reflective humans it is also controllable by the very stewardly responsibilities and moral sense by virtue of which we image God. This responsibility is part of the larger responsibility that we have toward one another as communal individuals—that is, as individuals whose identities are not just those of individual atoms but are constituted by deep, caring relationships with others. We are not simply individuals who happen to have relationships with other individuals; in an important sense we *are* those relationships. Our identi-

6. "Alien dignity" is a phrase used by some writers (Ramsey, "The Morality of Abortion," 72; Thielicke, 231; D. Callahan, "The Sanctity of Life," 186-87) to convey the idea that it is our relationship with God rather than our inherent worth or characteristics that gives us a special status. The trouble with this phrase is that it might connote that God arbitrarily chose certain creatures for this relationship rather than creating them with a special nature specifically suited for it. Celebrating our special nature is, of course, compatible with the humility appropriate to creatures.

ties can overflow into others because our relationships involve not just the capacity to sympathize, to feel *for* others, but also the capacity to empathize, to feel *with* others, to transcend ourselves and "get inside" the viewpoint of others. We are "embodied" not just as individuals in physical bodies but also as "relatives" in a moral and spiritual body of which we are members. The depth, creativity, and character of these caring relationships are in turn conditioned by our ability to symbolically interact with each other, not just to exchange signs but to communicate by infusing these signs with infinitely rich and textured meanings, meanings that can be passed on and developed into profoundly interesting and distinctive cultures. Genesis portrays Adam's naming of the creation as the beginning of his caring for it, caring that for us involves the ability to envision reality, to imagine how it might be different, and to use aesthetic and moral sensitivities to desire and create changes in it (Gaylin, "In Defense"). These characteristics enable us to converse with God, and they presumably have to do with why God wants to converse with us, although they may not entirely answer the psalmist's question "What is man that thou art mindful of him?" (Ps. 8:4).

So the Bible implies that human persons are all in a fourfold relationship: we are in relationship with God as created representatives, with the rest of his creation as stewards, with each other as community members, and with ourselves as self-reflective creatures. And these relationships interpenetrate and condition one another: it is as self-reflective, free, and responsible beings that we recognize our caring relationship with others, our stewardly relationship with creation, and our creaturely but imaging relationship with God. Losing sight of any one of these relationships or misconstruing its character will warp the rest of them, as we will suggest when discussing the covenantal ethic that flows from these relationships.

A fourth biblical point to notice is that we are imagers of God who live in a fallen condition. Our hearts—the biblical term for the center of our being, including our minds and our affections—are directed away from God and therefore away from our proper relationships with God, with ourselves, with others, and with God's creation. Idolatry and self-deification alternating with self-debasement, hatred and depersonalization alternating with deification of others, and destructive exploitation of nature alternating with pantheism (deification of creation)—these have become the dispositions of the human heart. This does not mean we have completely lost our imaging of God: neither Genesis 9:6 (which, as we saw, forbids murdering any person because that would be an iconoclastic desecration of God's image) nor Psalm 8 (which, as we saw, celebrates the ruling status of humankind) is restricted to pre-Fall persons.[7] Many

Reformed theologians distinguish here between imaging God in a broader, structural, or static sense and imaging God in a narrower, functional, or dynamic sense (Hoekema, 83-85). In the former sense even fallen persons have God-like capacities, but in the latter sense fallen persons do not exercise those capacities in true knowledge, righteousness, and holiness. We fallen persons still represent God, but we do so in a perverted way, as funhouse mirrors distort images, making them recognizable but twisted. Even our instincts retain a vestige of human nature as it was created: nurturing, caring, and stewardly dispositions are common in fallen humanity, as are a sense of moral obligation and, as Calvin says, a longing for God *(sensus divinitatus)*. Ruined nobility can often be recognized—not only as ruined but also as nobility (Plantinga, 11).

5   The fifth biblical point to note about imaging God is not only the good news that in Jesus we have a new model for imaging God—"He reflects the glory of God and bears the very stamp of his nature . . ." (Heb. 1:3)—but also that we have in that model one whose reconciling and redeeming work can save us and restore to us the ability to image God as God intended—"And we all . . . are being changed into his likeness from one degree of glory to another" (2 Cor. 3:18). So there are in human beings not only a created and a fallen imaging but also a redeemed and, eventually, a perfected imaging of God (Hoekema, 82-95). Because Christians will be informed not only by *natural* dispositions (which, because they are distorted by the Fall, can also be called *unnatural*) but also by what the biblical story reveals about the creator's intention for those dispositions, Christian ethics, including medical ethics, should ignore neither what God has written on the hearts of all people (Rom. 2:15) nor what has been revealed in the biblical story.

Imaging God: Beginnings

We have avoided speaking of the image of God as a separate entity—a soul—that human bodies passively receive at some point in their development, say at conception, quickening, or birth. Our use of such phrases as "imaging God" and "imager of God" is meant to convey the idea that

---

7. Hebrews 2:5-9 gives a Christological interpretation of Psalm 8:4-6. Apparently the recipients of this letter were interpreting the chaos of their times in a Gnostic way: evil cosmic spirits were at war with the good forces. The writer of Hebrews argues that even these spirits (angels) are under man's control, but it is man in the form of Jesus Christ, whose kingdom is established even if the forces of evil have not yet laid down their arms (Jewett, 11-12, 42-43; Hewitt, 65-68). But this passage from Hebrews does not imply that fallen human beings are no longer in God's image.

the image of God is less like something that human beings *have* and more like something they *are* and *do*. But even if we avoid asking when the soul enters and leaves the body,[8] we cannot avoid asking when human beings are or become embodied imagers of God and when they cease being embodied imagers of God. Since the human capacities we referred to as essential for imaging God (self-consciousness, moral and religious sense, symbolic interaction, and having and acting on desires about our desires) are much the same as what many philosophers think of as "person-making capacities" (Frankfurt; Dennett; Tooley, 50-157; Warren; Feinberg, "Abortion"), we can rephrase the question "When do human beings become imagers of God and when do they cease to be?" to "When does personhood begin and end?"

One straightforward answer to the question of when personhood begins and ends is the assertion that a being must *actually* have and be able to use those capacities that distinguish persons from other creatures (Warren; Tooley, 50-157; Feinberg, "Abortion"). To protect itself from the charge of arbitrariness or of having "a do-it-yourself kit for constructing a 'moral community' to [one's] own taste" (Donagan, 170), this view should specify nonarbitrary criteria of personhood such as those capacities the Bible implies are necessary to imagers of God.[9] And to protect itself from implying that some people are lesser persons than others (because they have these capacities to a lesser extent than others), this view should specify a nonarbitrary "threshold" level of having personal capacities, a minimal level at which all who attain it are equally persons and beyond which one can have more of these capacities but cannot be thought of as more of a person. This view, which we will call the "actualist" view, implies that personhood is not like a substance that characterizes an entity throughout its physical existence (analogous to being a piece of iron) but a state or capacity, a property or phase (analogous to

---

8. In this book we cannot give an extended argument against thinking of the soul as a separate entity that enters and leaves the body. We have briefly objected to one way of inferring that the image of God is a separate soul (p. 28) and have referred to discussions that provide what we believe is a more biblical and unitary understanding of human persons (see footnote 1 of this chapter). And we have claimed that what we say is consistent with believing that at death some separable part or aspect of a person can be sustained by God (see footnotes 3 and 4 of this chapter). It is possible that some ways of thinking about the soul as a substance separate from the body are consistent with most of what we say about imaging God.

9. Those holding this view would argue that slaves in the antebellum South and Jews in Hitler's Germany clearly imaged God in the biblical sense and were persons under any criteria that the slave owners and Nazis could nonarbitrarily apply to themselves. Thus, they would claim, the discrimination against slaves and Jews was the result of deeply corrupted social consciousness rather than of an effort to arrive at reasonable criteria of personhood.

being magnetized) that human beings achieve or acquire sometime after birth and lose at the point when they irreversibly lose personal capacities. With modern medical technology, the latter point can be reached well before the death of the whole human organism.

The actualist view also implies that fetuses,[10] newborn infants, and those human beings with profound mental retardation are not persons. Of course, one holding this view might argue that there are some good reasons for *conferring personhood* on some of these human beings or for *treating them as if they were persons*. One might argue, for example, that not treating them as persons would put society on a slippery slope, with the result that the rights of persons would be endangered. Or one might argue that showing respect toward "near persons" cultivates the sort of dispositions that are important in a civilized society. But such arguments imply that the respect accorded some human beings is not what they are *due*, is not elicited by virtue of what they *are*, but is conferred on the basis of debatable human reasoning about the possible effects on other persons of respecting or not respecting these "nonpersonal" human beings. This implication seems morally dangerous to many people. Moreover, the actualist view implies a duality between human beings who are persons and those who are not, which is philosophically and theologically suspicious to many who do not accept the actualist position.

Anyone who believes that God is a person (or three persons) cannot believe that being human is a necessary condition for being a person. But can one argue, without merely assuming an arbitrary species chauvinism, that being human is a sufficient condition for being a person and that all human beings are persons or imagers of God from their conception until their death? We will discuss three ways of arguing that personhood (or being an imager of God, with all that that implies morally and theologically) begins at conception. In the next section of this chapter we will evaluate views about when persons die.

One way to argue that human beings have the moral and theological status of persons is to make exegetical appeal to biblical texts that imply that God establishes a personal caring relationship with human beings from the moment they are conceived. Consider, for example, Psalm 139, which beautifully portrays the believer's sense of God's providence:

> . . . my frame was not hidden from thee, when I was being made in secret, intricately wrought in the depths of the earth. Thy eyes beheld

---

10. Rather than *baby* or *product of conception,* we generally use the comparatively less-loaded term *fetus* to refer to an unborn human being. When it is important to be more precise about early gestational development, we use the terms *zygote* (first two weeks after conception) and *embryo* (third through eighth weeks).

my unformed substance; in thy book were written, every one of them, the days that were formed for me, when as yet there was none of them. (Vv. 15-16)

Why do such texts not settle the issue for all Bible-believing Christians? Primarily because such texts are interpreted by many Christians not as teaching something about when human beings have the status of imagers of God but as celebrating God's prior gracious call extended to each of God's children. The latter interpretation seems to be the required one for Jeremiah 1:5: "*Before* I formed you in the womb I knew you" (our emphasis). One might reply that this latter text does not imply God knew Jeremiah before he was conceived, but merely implies that between his conception and his taking on human form (say, six weeks after conception), God already knew him. The latter interpretation is certainly possible, but it cannot apply to such texts as Judges 13, where God announces to Manoah's wife that she "shall conceive and bear a son" and that this son will be a Nazirite and will deliver Israel from the Philistines. This text implies that God knew and called Manoah's son Samson even before he was conceived, and no one wants to argue that this fact implies that the sperm and unfertilized egg which later united to produce the promised child already had the moral status of persons. So, although we respect interpretations which infer that human beings are persons from conception, we do not believe such interpretations are required by the texts. Those texts do not seem to speak to the moral or theological status of everything that goes into a person's formation or to state precisely when a zygote, embryo, or fetus has the status of person, or imager of God.[11]

A second way to argue that a human fetus is a person from con-

---

11. This point is relevant quite apart from our reservations (pp. 18-19) about using a proof-text approach to the Bible's message. Consider another text that has the distinction of being used by both those who assert and those who deny that the fetus is a person. The Revised Standard Version translates Exodus 21:22-23 as follows:

When men strive together, and hurt a woman with child, so that there is a miscarriage, and yet no harm follows, the one who hurt her shall be fined, according as the woman's husband shall lay upon him; and he shall pay as the judges determine. If any harm follows, then you shall give life for life.

This version seems to imply that the accidental death of a fetus, while significant, is less serious than the accidental death of a woman. If so, the fetus would seem to have a different moral and theological status than that of a woman, so aborting a fetus could not be morally the same as murder. But in the New International Version this passage suggests that the fetus has the same status as an adult:

If men who are fighting hit a pregnant woman and she gives birth prematurely but there is no serious injury, the offender must be fined whatever the woman's

ception is to appeal to scientific facts. This way does not rely on distinctive theological convictions and thereby has the advantage of persuasive appeal in legal and legislative discussions in pluralist societies. Several facts are frequently cited. It is a fact, for example, that conception is the beginning of a living, unique, individual member of the human species, an individual that, in the normal course of its development, will become an adult.[12] It may also be a fact that there will not be any later stages in an individual's development that compare with the dramatic shift in potential and character that occurs during the several hours of the fertilization process, when the gametes unite (Grobstein, "Early Development," 214).[13] But the problem with appealing to these and similar facts is that they are well known to those who hold the actualist view. The latter typically distinguish between "human being" in a genetic sense and "human being" or "person" in a moral or legal sense. Actualists grant that zygotes are human beings in the former sense but argue that they are not persons in the latter sense because it is a scientific fact that they do not have the capacities that everyone associates with personhood. Rather than recite scientific facts that are compatible with the actualists' distinction between human beings and persons, those who believe all human beings are persons should formulate an argument that calls into question any such distinction. Providing such an argument is the third way of demonstrating that human beings are persons from conception.

Perhaps the most powerful argument appeals to the implications of membership in a "natural kind," a species. According to A. Donagan, "If respect is owed to beings because they are in a certain

---

husband demands and the court allows. But if there is serious injury, you are to take life for life.

This version implies that a miscarriage would result in the death penalty and suggests that the fetus has the same status as an adult. The King James Version translates the phrase ambiguously as "and her fruit depart from her." The Hebrew words here *(yalad, yatsa)* are susceptible to any of the three translations. Those who think that enough study could arrive at the correct interpretation should notice that this passage is directly preceded by a passage which says that the mere beating of a slave is not cause for punishment (assuming the slave can get up after a few days) because a slave is property. It is doubtful that either of these passages should be the basis of moral or legal policy today. The same could be said about Numbers 5, which some interpret as calling for abortion in cases of infidelity.

12. This statement should be made with some qualifications for monozygotes, since "twinning" can occur up to two weeks after conception.

13. According to C. Grobstein ("External Human Fertilization," 59), 75 percent of all fertilized ova are spontaneously aborted, usually as the result of genetic deformities (Boue et al., 3). This claim poses an interesting consideration for those who believe personhood begins with conception.

state, it is owed to whatever, by its very nature, develops into that state. To reject this principle would be arbitrary, if indeed it would be intelligible" (Donagan, 171). Although Donagan phrases his principle in terms of respect that is due certain kinds of beings, we will see later in this section that his consideration seems consistent with what we will call the "potentiality principle"—namely, that what a being naturally becomes is relevant for what attitudes are appropriate toward it. A more direct way to argue for the "species membership" view is to assert that a being essentially *is* what it is meant (by God or nature) to be or become:

> An individual who is a member of a species of persons, such as human beings, is still a person even if the person has not actualized those capacities. In fact, one should say that an individual human being is a person even if he or she cannot actualize those capacities. We must distinguish between being a person and functioning as a person. (Evans, "Human Persons as Substantial Achievers," 15)

In this view, all human beings are essentially the kind of beings with the capacities, say, to reason or to see. When a human being actualizes the capacity to reason or when an operation restores sight to a blind person, the correct description is that the individual has actualized a capacity which, in an important sense, he or she always had by virtue of the kind of being he or she is.

We think that the preceding consideration is intuitively plausible. In particular, we appreciate the implications that profoundly retarded human beings are, in an important sense, meant by God to be reflective reasoners, and we will point out later in this chapter that this consideration should influence attitudes toward those with serious disabilities. On the other hand, we find it more plausible to say that human zygotes are not beings that already have human capacities (waiting to be actualized) but that they are the kind of beings that will acquire these capacities in the normal course of their development. We will argue that this latter fact certainly should influence our attitudes toward developing human beings, but we do not think that we should disregard what seems to us to be a distinction between what they already are and what they will become.

We already noticed that a troubling implication of the actualist view (that human beings become persons when and only when they actually acquire personal capacities) is that infants are not persons. The view that human beings are persons at conception also has some troubling implications. It implies, for example, that the spontaneous abortion rate creates tragic prenatal victims of up to 75 percent of the people that are conceived (see footnote 13). If a plague were causing that high a percentage of children to die, we would be obliged to launch a major effort to save them, an effort in which we would be obliged to use much of our medical resources. Thus, if zygotes are persons, we would seem obliged to spend much—perhaps most—of our scientific and medical resources in an effort to save the high percentage of them that die early. Moreover, the use of intrauterine devices—which probably prevent implantation rather than conception and which have been used by a higher number of women in the United States than the number of those who have obtained postimplantation abortions (Fuchs and Perreault, 76-78)—would have to be viewed as a slaughter of innocent people much greater than the Nazis caused or than is allowed by current (postimplantation) abortion policies. With each IUD user killing up to twelve people every year, it would seem that anti-abortion forces should direct more of their efforts against the makers and users of IUDs than against abortion clinics. (Or at least they should have done so before most manufacturers stopped selling IUDs to avoid lawsuits resulting from the bad health effects some users experienced.) Finally, if human zygotes are persons, it would seem to call for a radical change in our practices with respect to the products of early miscarriages or spontaneous abortions, which we do not now treat the way we treat the remains of persons who die.

None of these alleged implications are, in themselves, refutations of either the actualist view or the view that human zygotes are persons, because holders of these views may be willing to accept such implications. But they seem problematic enough that, unless these positions can be defended with premises less debatable than those discussed earlier, many Christians are motivated to consider an alternative position, one that has implications somewhere between the implications of these two views and that can be defended with highly plausible premises. Middle positions on the beginning of personhood can be classified into at least three categories: first, various "stage" or "decisive moment" positions; second, various "gradualist" or "developmental" positions; and, third, the "potentiality" position.

The stage positions assert that there is a decisive point or stage in its development before which the embryo or fetus lacks personal status and after which it has an inherent moral status equal (or almost equal) to that of all other persons. Proponents of various stage positions differ on what the decisive point is. The points most often suggested are also those commonly appealed to by the gradualist position, which argues that these points mark incrementally significant rather than decisively "all or nothing" changes. They also are appealed to by those who argue that stages are relevant to how we should be disposed to treat the fetus, even if these stages do not mark decisive inherent changes in the fetus itself. Thus much of what we say about the stage positions will be relevant to our later discussion of other positions.

The earliest suggested stage for the beginning of personhood (beyond conception) is that of implantation, which occurs approximately one week after conception, when the 150-cell zygote "roots" itself in the uterine wall. This position has what many people regard as the advantage of allowing the use of IUDs and "morning after" pills, but this implication is not in itself an argument, because convenience should be the *result* of justification, not the justification itself. One argument is that we often think of the beginning of growing things as occurring when they are rooted and sprouting rather than when they are capable of being rooted; a flower, for example, probably begins its life no earlier than when it is rooted rather than when an ovule is fertilized by pollen. But it is not clear that this is a good analogy for the beginning of a human being; a zygote seems to have an inherent natural tendency to implant itself in a way that flower seeds do not seek fertile soil. So it is not clear that asserting this stage as morally crucial—vastly more significant than conception—avoids some element of arbitrariness. A logically distinct consideration for this stage is that soon after implantation comes the last point at which a zygote can "twin," or divide into separate individuals. But, granting that the twinning phenomenon creates fascinating metaphysical puzzles about individual identity, we are not convinced that its mere possibility[14] affects the moral status of the more than 99 percent of zygotes that do not divide.

Two logically distinct considerations are used to point to sometime around the end of the first trimester as the stage at which personhood begins. First, by this time the brain structure is complete. Although the cerebral cortex activity we associate with self-consciousness may not begin until after birth, electrical activity in the brain stem can be detected as early as eight weeks after conception. Some have argued that, since the absence of any electrical activity in the whole brain is often used as a criterion for the irreversible loss or death of a person, we should use the presence of any such activity as a criterion for the beginning of the person. Both actualists and those who believe that personhood begins at conception worry about arbitrariness here. The latter point out that, unlike a human who has irreversibly lost brain waves, the early fetus has

14. It's not even clear what actual twinning implies for the status of the predivided zygote: if a full-fledged person somehow divided into two persons, it would be at once fascinating and disconcerting, but would it affect the moral status of the predivided person? The same question applies to a similarly interesting phenomenon: at least six human beings, with the genetic karyotype of XX-XY, were the result of a combining of two genetically distinct zygotes (Hellegers, 4).

the potential for having them. The former point out that a criterion for death requires the irreversible absence of only one *necessary* condition for being a person, whereas a criterion for personhood requires a *sufficient* condition (or *all* of the necessary conditions) for being a person.[15] If we were to accept electrical activity in the brain as the beginning of personhood, we would need a separate argument that brain activity is not only necessary but also sufficient for personhood.

The other consideration in favor of claiming the end of the first trimester as the point at which personhood begins is that by then the fetus has attained human shape. Of course, it is obvious how both those who believe that personhood begins at conception and the actualists will argue that human shape is neither necessary nor sufficient for personhood. But everyone must admit that human shape signifies something of importance; otherwise, pictures of second-trimester aborted fetuses would not have the emotional impact that they do. At minimum, a fetus that has attained human shape is an "icon" or "natural symbol"[16] of imagers of God, and mistreatment of it arouses at least as much revulsion and shock as that aroused in patriots seeing their country's flag abused. And a flag is just a symbol; it is not a potential country the way a fetus is a potential person. So the shuddering and horror at the abuse of fetuses is even more understandable and appropriate. Thus, although human shape cannot be plausibly urged as a necessary or sufficient condition for personhood, it may imply something about how beings in the process of becoming persons ought to be treated.

A similar point can be made about a third suggested crucial stage — namely, the traditional appeal to "quickening," the point at which the fetus begins to make spontaneous movements. It is easy to see how one can criticize the assertion that this is the point at which a fetus receives a soul[17] or becomes a person. And the ambiguity of when

15. Both sides can make the same point about the proposal that heartbeat (which can be detected a few weeks after conception) is a vital sign for both the beginning and the ending of persons, or that brain waves can be associated with sentience, or simple consciousness (the ability to have sensations like pain and not simply to exhibit unfelt reflex reactions to stimuli). Those who believe that personhood begins at conception can point out that fetuses are in the process of developing these features from conception, while actualists can claim that heartbeat or sentience is a necessary but not sufficient condition for personhood. Actualists can agree that the ability to feel pain gives fetuses *some* rights or interests (such as the right not to suffer pain unjustly) without implying that they thereby have the status of persons.

16. See J. Feinberg's "Sentiment and Sentimentality" and R. Selzer's report of his feelings when he accidentally stepped on a discarded fetus (*Mortal Lessons*, 153-60).

17. The *fetus animatus/fetus inanimatus* distinction was used by some Roman Catholics, including Thomas Aquinas, in claiming that God infuses the soul into the fetus at quickening. This view opposed the traducianism of Tertullian, who taught that the soul

"quickening" occurs is worth noting: although the fetus actually begins spontaneous movements around the tenth week, these movements cannot be felt by the mother until as much as a month later. So appealing to when the fetus has achieved the capacity to move would imply that personhood occurs earlier than the traditional notion of quickening suggests. However, there is significance in the traditional notion of quickening as that point when the movements are felt, and *feeling* the fetus as an active and reactive being is what begins to bond it as an interactor within the social community, even if it does not communicate with symbols. So, as with attaining human shape, attaining the ability to move probably is not a necessary or sufficient condition for personhood, but it may imply something about the appropriate attitude toward the fetus.

Perhaps the stage between conception and birth which is most commonly suggested as the beginning of personhood is that of "viability," the point at which the fetus can live biologically (though not socially) independent of anyone else. The United States Supreme Court, in its *Roe v. Wade* decision of 1973, designated this as the "compelling point" at which the state's interest in protecting fetal life begins. The court seemed to recognize the problem implicit in the fact that this point is relative to available technology,[18] since it did not stipulate a particular gestational time for viability (currently somewhere around the end of the second trimester). The court's reason for designating viability as the compelling point was that at the stage of viability the fetus presumably has the capability of meaningful life outside the mother's womb. It is easy to fault this logic: if the phrase "capability of meaningful life" refers to the fetus's current capabilities, then "meaningful" implausibly reduces to "biologically independent," but if the phrase refers to its potential capabilities, then the fetus had such life well before viability. And it seems implausible that biological independence by itself can so dramatically shift the fetus's moral status that killing it in the act of removing it one week and allowing it to die after removing it the next week amount to the difference between therapeutic surgery and homicide. It is difficult to see how viability so radically changes the inherent status of the fetus. On the other hand, it takes little imagination to appreciate the psychological difference between a previable and postviable abortion. If we want to nurture a sense of sanctity and avoid so callousing ourselves that we lose our ability to shud-

---

is biologically transmitted (at conception) from Adam. In 1930 Pope Pius XI denied any importance to the distinction between preanimated and postanimated fetal life.

18. This relativity can be minimized by defining "viability" as the capacity to survive and mature using only those treatments thought obligatory for full-term or nearly full-term neonates. Some might think this definition is a bit arbitrary.

der[19] when human life is taken, then this psychological difference becomes morally relevant. And a similar point can be made about the difference between postviable abortions and postnatal infanticide: even if the inherent status of those killed is not different, the different psychological and social effects may imply that the fetus should, at certain points, be treated *as if* its status were different.

Distinguishing between when a human being attains personhood and when it should be treated as if it has attained personhood brings us to another common way of thinking about beginnings. This is the "conferral" position, which argues that, rather than debating the issue of when personhood begins, society need only decide when to confer personhood on developing human beings. This need not be an arbitrary decision; one can appeal to the likelihood of bad psychological and social effects if personhood is not conferred by a particular stage and thereby argue that by conferring personhood at that stage society can protect itself, its character, the interests of those related to the developing human being, and those persons whose interests might be threatened if society and especially its medical practitioners became callous to the mistreatment of young human beings. Sometimes those holding the conferral position argue for a single stage as the crucial, all-or-nothing point at which personal status should be conferred (usually viability or birth [Lomasky; Brandt]), but more often they argue for a gradualist position (Bok, "Ethical Problems"; R. Green, "Conferred Rights"; Langerak, "Abortion"), claiming that the psychological and social effects of abortions become incrementally more serious and dangerous after each of the stages just discussed and that therefore it behooves society to confer on the fetus an incrementally more protected status. The gradualist version of the conferral position may account for the widely shared belief that the status of late-term fetuses is more significant than, say, the status of zygotes, but it does have two difficulties. Any conferral position requires the plausibility of empirical claims about dangerous psychological and social effects of abortions, claims that are debated almost as much as claims about the inherent status of the fetus. And it does not account for the widely shared belief that something about the fetus itself, and not merely the consequences of how it is treated, grants it an inherent moral or theological status.

---

19. W. May discusses a Brothers Grimm tale about a man incapable of horror. His ashamed father sends him away "to learn how to shudder" so that he can become truly human ("Attitudes toward the Newly Dead," 141). We can accept J. Feinberg's criticism ("Sentiment and Sentimentality") that sometimes these feelings must be "educated," as in those performing autopsies, while accepting May's point that sometimes they should be cultivated.

Gradualists who hold the conferral position sometimes appeal to the principle that if some beings have a special status by virtue of certain characteristics, then any beings that possess those characteristics to some extent have a proportional claim to that status. We might grant that this "proportionality principle" (Gewirth, 121) accounts for our feelings that chimpanzees, for example, should have a more protected status than fish, because their sign-using ability is so sophisticated that it perhaps begins to share in the symbol-using ability whereby persons image God, and the proportionality principle might also be relevant to the status of "beginning persons," such as young children who are beginning to be caring and not just cared-for members of the community. But it is doubtful that this principle accounts for the protected moral status of the fetus; although its *potential* for God-imaging characteristics is greater than that of, say, a chimpanzee, the degree to which it *actually* possesses those characteristics may compare unfavorably with the degree to which many animals possess the same characteristics.

Some gradualists simply assert that the moral status of the fetus grows, in much the same way as does the value of a house under construction. When the stud frame is up, the potential house has grown in value even though it fails to perform any of the valued functions of a house, such as shelter or comfort (Quinn, 37). Likewise, as the frame of the fetus is woven together in the womb, the status of the fetus grows in strength quite apart from capabilities it exhibits. But can we be sure the analogy is appropriate? Some may wonder whether the instrumental value of the house frame is analogous to the inherent status of the fetus, and others may wonder whether the internally directed and stimulated growth of a fetus is analogous to the growth of a house.

The "potentiality" position attributes moral and theological status to the fetus from conception, but it does not argue that the fetus is an actual person from conception. We believe that attending to the implications of a developing human being's potential is a less problematic way of accounting for its moral and theological status than is the effort to find some point before birth (or even after birth) when it becomes a person. We accept the following potentiality principle: if, in the normal course of its development, a being *will become* an imager of God, then by virtue of this potential it already deserves some of the reverence due imagers of God.

Perhaps, in its ordinary usage, the term *potential* is too weak to capture the implications of the potentiality principle. Some people fail to appreciate the status of what we call *potential* persons because they confuse them with what we call *possible* persons. A possible person is an entity that *could,* under certain causally possible conditions, become an actual person (or at least part of one—for example, a human sperm or egg), but a potential person is a being that *will* become an actual person in the normal course of events or in the normal course of its development.[20] Most Americans are possible presidents, but we do not salute one another because of that. However, a potential president would be a candidate who has won the election and is preparing to be inaugurated (on a somewhat arbitrarily selected date). Potential presidents do get saluted, and some of this additional respect is a recognition not just of their current abilities but of the high office and sacred trust they are in the process of attaining. To dismiss the importance of potentiality by observing that a potential president is not yet commander in chief (Benn, 143; Feinberg, "Abortion," 267) is to let a half-truth collapse the distinction between potentiality and mere possibility.

The appropriateness of granting increased respect because of what a being will become may be just a function of probabilities: although potential presidents might get assassinated or die of heart attacks, it is extremely likely that they will achieve the high office of president. This is not true of possible presidents. Likewise, although an embryo or especially a not-yet-implanted zygote might be spontaneously aborted, the chances are very good that it will achieve the high office of imager of God. This is not true of possible persons.[21] The moral relevance of potentiality may also be a function of seeing the creation and its creatures in a radically temporal way. When we perceive things, especially interesting

20. See E. Langerak's "Abortion" for a defense of the potentiality principle. H. Stob (228-36) uses the phrase "in the process of becoming" rather that "potential." We are indebted to his discussion for some of what we say about potential persons. The class of *future* persons is not identical with either that of possible persons or that of potential persons; it consists of those beings that *will* exist as actual persons. In the notion of "potential," using the phrase "in the normal course of its development" rather than "in the normal course of events" emphasizes the teleological ("nature's aim") rather than the statistical-probability aspect of "normal development," but one may assume that generally even a teleological notion of "normal" has statistical implications: if the natural end of (a) is to become (A), then it is highly probable that, without interference, (a) will become (A). Of course, one must distinguish "potential for personhood" from what we might call the "possibilities or potentialities of a person." The latter refer to accomplishments a person might achieve that elicit admiration or esteem from others. These accomplishments are analogous to the varying quality of, say, a president's performance while in office. But the respect or awe due presidents (or other persons) by virtue of their office has to do with the *type* of authority and status they have, not with how well they perform. Of course, certain capabilities or characteristics that resulted in their achieving the office may be related to the capacity for gifted performance, but once a certain "threshold" of capacity is reached, one will never be *more* of a person or a president, even if one becomes more capable of exercising the authority of one's office.

21. A woman may have up to 10,000 ova, of which perhaps 390 become mature. Of these only a small percentage can become potential persons. The odds for sperm are perhaps 31,000,000,000 times worse. So J. Noonan ("An Almost Absolute Value," 56) is cor-

things like people (or even buildings), we see something of what they were and will be as well as what they are. Humans are temporal beings and not just in the sense of having a history and a future; we are probably the only earthly creatures who internalize this temporality and make it a significant part of our subjective and intersubjective worlds. As we will argue in the next chapter, covenantal ethics incorporates this temporality; our obligations have a dynamic, historical, changing dimension to them, so that both the past and the future are directly morally relevant and, indeed, are an intrinsic part of how we perceive ourselves, others, and our privileges and responsibilities.

Can the potentiality principle be used to argue that the zygote has the *same* moral standing as adults (Wade) and thereby to collapse any moral or theological distinction between potential and actual persons? Perhaps, but such an argument would need highly debatable premises about the metaphysics of potentiality, and it would be at odds with some of the analogies and examples we use to establish the plausibility of the potentiality principle. The status of a potential president is different from that of a merely possible president, but it is not the same as that of an actual president. And we pay for garden seedlings because of what they will be, not because of what they already are, but we do not price them the same as mature plants. (In fact, we sometimes pay even more for young plants than for those that are mature, which shows we must be cautious about analogies between the status of potential persons and the value of other things in the process of their development.) So we believe that the burden of proof is on both those who deny that a being's potential is relevant to its current status and those who equate a being's current status with what it will become.

We conclude that we do not have a precise or unquestionable answer to our question of when human beings are or become persons, or imagers of God. But we believe that the potentiality principle, the conferral considerations, and the covenantal ethic we will outline in the next chapter provide us with enough well-grounded guidance that we can think through some of the practical issues we will confront in later chapters. When we confront such issues as abortion and infanticide, we will argue that the basic question is not just whether fetuses or infants image God, but whether we image God in responding to their presence and

___

rect in seeing conception as the dramatic shift in probabilities. But he should not conclude from this that abortion is like shooting into a bush when there is an 80 percent chance (or even a 20 percent chance) of there being a person in it; abortion involves not a high probability of killing an actual person but a 100 percent probability of killing a potential person (one with a high probability of becoming an actual person).

their needs. We now turn to the question of when human beings cease being embodied imagers of God.

Imaging God: Endings

It has been said that we begin dying the moment we are born. But this observation is, at best, a misleading way of saying that human beings are mortal, that they will die sooner or later. Of course, some people live through a long dying process, but even these people usually first live through a number of phases during which they are mortal but definitely not dying. These phases—as easy to recognize as they are difficult to delineate—include growing, maturing, and aging. We can even recognize a phase appropriately called "withering," in which aging makes the organism reach the stage of significant physical decline but which is still not the process of dying. The latter probably does not begin for an organism until it has a biological condition that sets it on a declining trajectory and will inevitably cause its death unless something else does so first. (One's death, of course, can be caused by something one was not dying of—for example, a person dying of cancer can be killed in an accident. And one can die suddenly without ever living through a dying process.)

When does the death of a person occur, and how can it be determined that it has occurred? Is death, like dying, a process (Morison), or is it an event (Kass, "Death as an Event") that can be more or less pinpointed? The death of an *entire organism* is usually a process that takes several days: some human cells continue to live for days after the brain and heart have died. In fact, some human cells have been kept alive and multiplying indefinitely in artificial environments. But nobody wants to argue that death occurs only when the entire organism is in a state of putrefaction. Rather, it has long been recognized that death occurs when the functioning of the *organism as a whole* is irreversibly lost. For most of human history, this loss was associated with the irreversible loss of the "vital signs"—namely, heartbeat and respiration—perhaps because their loss implied the loss of the "vital fluids"—blood and oxygen—that are the biological substratum for the functioning of the organism as a whole. Of course, today's technology can keep the vital signs going for days and even weeks after the entire brain has died, so society has been forced to consider whether, at least when mechanical respirators are used, the irreversible loss of total brain functioning is the event at which death occurs. The well-known report of the Ad Hoc Committee of the Harvard Medical School suggested in 1968 that physicians can determine that the brain is "*permanently* nonfunctioning" by observing such signs as unreceptivity, unresponsiveness, lack of movements or reflexes, and a flat (or isoelectric) electroencephalogram (EEG) (337-38). Variations of this proposal have been adopted in "brain death" statutes in most states and by the Law Reform Commission of Canada (Lamb, 31; Carrell, 20-21).

We believe that Christians should endorse the brain-death criterion of the point at which death occurs, although they may vary on their reasons for doing so. Those who believe that all human beings are persons can reason that human beings die when their brains die because the integrated functioning of the human organism as a whole is irreversibly lost at that point. This position is not the view that human beings inevitably *will* soon die after their brains die (despite the ability of respirators to keep much of the body alive for many days after the whole brain dies); a prediction of death, even with absolute certainty, is not the same as a determination that it has occurred. The acceptance of the brain-death criterion for death acknowledges that technology enables us to keep alive for a time the living remains of human beings, remains that one might call "former human beings" but not "dying human beings." It may be, as we will suggest in our tenth chapter, that sometimes the moral and medical implications of determining that death is imminent are the same as those of determining that it has occurred (removal of extraordinary treatments, for example), but one should not confuse the two different determinations and thereby seek to evade the difficult moral issue of how to treat dying people.

Christians who do not believe that all human beings are persons —such as those who accept the actualist view that one must have the capacity to image God in order to be a person—can accept the brain-death criterion by reasoning that, with the death of the brain, the person dies even if in some sense a human being continues to live. However, here an important issue arises. The logic of the actualist position seems to imply that persons die when they have irreversibly lost the higher brain (cerebral and neocortical) functions that are the necessary biological substratum for consciousness and symbolic interaction. This loss can occur much earlier than the loss of all other brain functions, including the brain-stem functions that control spontaneous respiration and heartbeat. For example, Karen Ann Quinlan's brain stem kept her lungs and heart alive for ten years beyond what seems to have been the irreversible loss of consciousness. The record for being in a (presumably irreversible) coma is over thirty-seven years (Lamb, 6). Perhaps up to 10,000 patients in the United States are in a "persistent vegetative state" (M. Rust, 8) and, with artificial feeding tubes, can be kept alive for years and even decades before "whole-brain" (including brain-stem) death.

The actualist position seems to imply that these individuals died *as persons* when they irreversibly lost the higher brain functions that allow consciousness and symbolic communication and that they live on *as former persons,* though they are still human beings. But our treating them as if they were essentially dead, perhaps allowing or causing them to "die all the way" and perhaps harvesting their usable organs (Gaylin, "Harvesting the Dead"), would seem to require a dramatic shift in our notion of death and our attitudes toward the newly dead. This shift would be much more dramatic than the shift that occurred with the acceptance of the whole-brain criterion for death, which involved recognizing that the bodies of whole-brain-dead patients can be kept alive for a few days or weeks. The bodies of such patients are certain to die shortly in spite of any heroic technological treatments, and they are definitely beyond any capacity for responsiveness. However, those in a permanent vegetative state have brain-stem activity; they can live indefinitely with artificial feeding tubes, can show a variety of reflex reactions, and can show reticular activity, including the opening and closing of their eyes. Human beings in this state can even give birth to infants (Dillon, 1090), and there is at least one case of conception in a comatose woman ("Abortion Done on Comatose Woman"). There is even debate about whether some patients in a permanent vegetative state have a capacity for feeling pain (Annas, "Nonfeeding," 20), a debate that really becomes a discussion about whether all those in a permanent vegetative state are in a coma beyond consciousness.[22] Moreover, sometimes patients regain consciousness after they were thought to have irreversibly lost it (President's Commission, *Deciding,* 179). Such "miraculous recoveries" are very rare, but they do raise the question of whether physicians have the technological capacity to determine higher-brain death (as opposed to whole-brain death) with the sort of assurance society needs on life-and-death matters.

Those supporting the higher-brain criterion for death can reply that these difficulties are not a refutation of their position but simply dem-

---

22. The categories of "permanent vegetative state," "irreversible coma," and "permanent loss of consciousness" are not well defined in the literature. Indeed, the Harvard Committee equates whole-brain death with "irreversible coma," whereas others equate the latter with "permanent loss of consciousness" and even with "permanent vegetative state." Probably "permanent loss of consciousness" is the category relevant to our discussion (Gervais, Chap. 6; President's Commission, *Deciding to Forego Life-Sustaining Treatment,* 174); it becomes an empirical question whether and to what extent the other categories overlap it. The logic of the actualist position might seem to imply that even a permanent vegetative state in which there is a low level of consciousness is compatible with the death of the person, but this position can also be interpreted as implying that, once personal identity has been achieved, it continues as long as there is consciousness, even if such capacities as choice-making and symbolic interaction are lost.

onstrate the need for education and caution (Veatch, *Death, Dying;* Gervais; M. Green and Wikler; Shrader). They can urge society to think hard about the implications of respect for former persons and to be conservative about determining which patients in a vegetative state have suffered higher-brain death. We support a different view, arguing that, although in theory there may be something to be said for the higher-brain-death criterion, using a higher-brain criterion for death in practice is susceptible to confusion and abuse and could foster callous attitudes toward senile persons and those only partly conscious. This view appeals to the inability of our technology to determine the *irreversible* loss of consciousness, to likely motivations for erring on the side of false negatives rather than false positives, and to examples of how carefully restricted and acceptable practices can lead to careless and unacceptable ones. We cannot provide the details of our argument here, but we believe that they are fairly obvious and that even those who accept the actualist position have good reasons for accepting the whole-brain criterion rather than the higher-brain criterion for the point at which persons die and cease being embodied imagers of God. In our tenth chapter we will address the moral issue of what is the appropriate medical treatment for those patients who have brain-stem functioning but who have lost higher-brain functioning and are diagnosed as having permanently lost consciousness.

Imaging God in Health

What is it to be healthy? Christians are comfortable with thinking of health in a very broad way, being concerned with psychological and spiritual health as well as with physical health. If we combine this breadth of health concerns with our unified view of human nature, we could insist on a notion of health even broader than that of the World Health Organization, which is much maligned for being too broad. WHO defines health as "a state of complete physical, mental, and social well-being and not merely the absence of disease or infirmity" (Preamble to the Constitution of WHO). Complete health, we might add, would include a right relationship with God — spiritual health. And our claim is not simply that people are made of many parts. We would try to avoid the hyphens of the phrase "physico-psycho-socio-spiritual being" in favor of an integrated view of human nature, recognizing that it is impossible to affect one aspect of a person without also affecting the others.

But there are dangers in an all-inclusive definition of health, dangers that lurk even in the WHO definition, incomplete though it is. First, this definition proposes an ideal of health that can never be completely attained in any given individual. Thus, seeking this kind of health for ourselves and others can only lead to disappointment and failure. It provides us with what Rene Dubos has called a "mirage of health," a view of health toward which we strive but at which we will never arrive. This mirage provides medicine with a goal on which to set its sights, but it may become dangerous if its unattainable character is forgotten: "It can then be compared to a will-o'-the-wisp luring its followers into the swamps of unreality" (Dubos, 346). If the good of health becomes everything that is good, health becomes a god, and the worshipful pursuit of it, like all idolatries, will collapse into bitter disappointment. The victory over suffering and death must be sought elsewhere.

Another danger in an overly inclusive definition of health is the equating of health and happiness. To make health a necessary condition for happiness already creates confusion, but to make happiness a necessary condition for health is to put the medical professions in an impossible position with patients who seek deliverance from their social and personal ills as well as from their high blood pressure. It leads to the notion that it is unhealthy and abnormal to be sad or angry or bored, a notion that fails to recognize these as important human emotions for those living in a fallen world. Becoming a drug-drenched culture is just one of the dangers of turning to medicine for deliverance from our unhappiness. A greater danger may be the "medicalization" of society (Illich, 39-124) as we seek therapeutic solutions to all our problems. By defining all of our deficiencies in terms of health, we may lose our sense of responsibility for our well-being and even for our actions, putting ourselves into the hands of health professionals whenever we have a problem.

A first step in the direction of focusing on that aspect of health which is within medicine's domain is to think of health as *well-working* (Kass, "Regarding the End"), as *well-functioning,* rather than *well-being.* Persons can be functioning in a perfectly healthy way even when they are not happy or do not have a sense of well-being—for example, when they cope with the loss of loved ones. Indeed, in certain circumstances, people would not be functioning healthily unless they were unhappy. Health is a state of *accommodation* (Pellegrino, "Being Ill," 158), and healthy functioning involves coping with problems that impinge on one's sense of well-being.

Of course, the well-functioning of an organism depends on the type of organism it is, and the integrated functioning of the human organism is a many-splendored thing, involving social and spiritual aspects as well as physical aspects. So a second step in focusing on the health that is medicine's domain is to notice that there are dimensions of health and illness that the medical profession may be able to diagnose but must recognize as outside of its expertise. Psychologists, social workers, and chaplains may have more expertise than physicians on illness as it affects the psychosomatic, social, and spiritual dimensions of persons. In Chapter Four we will distinguish between illness—the subjective experience of physical, psychological, social, or spiritual dis-ease—and disease—the anatomic, physiologic, or biochemical malfunctioning. We will assert that the distinctive expertise of medicine tends to focus on disease and that this focus is appropriate. Still, we will argue that it is ill patients that medicine should treat, not just diseases, and that the value of wholistic medicine (whatever problems there may be with some representations of it) is the recognition that health, even when defined as well-functioning rather than well-being, is a multifaceted phenomenon that often requires an interdisciplinary, team approach.

Health and Life Span

Our suggestion is that Christians view human health and flourishing as the well-working of imagers of God in their multiple relationships, well-working that often involves accommodating themselves to problems caused by the not-yet character of a fallen world. The dynamics of this well-functioning will vary throughout the life span, as will the related role of medicine. Earlier in this chapter we noted that the human life span typically involves such phases as growing, maturing, aging, withering, and dying. The relevance of these phases for medicine is that attitudes and therapies appropriate at one phase may be inappropriate at another. Shortness of breath, for example, may be related to serious illness and call for extensive therapeutic intervention at one phase of our lives, but at another stage it may simply call for a recognition of our declining physical prowess. Accordingly, sometimes physicians have to impress on patients the need for active treatment, whereas at other times they need to lower patients' expectations about medicine's capacity to "fix" inevitable decline. After all, between the ages of thirty and seventy-five, we may lose perhaps 44 percent of our brain weight (including a loss of perhaps 100,000 brain cells per day),[23] 20 percent of our blood flow to

23. A figure often stated but debatable; see A. Smith (284). Of course, since we have billions of brain cells, this figure would imply that even after forty years of losing thirty-six million of them per year, perhaps only 10 percent of one's brain cells would be lost (A. Smith, 285). (The fetus gains an average of 1,300 nerve cells per second while the nervous system is growing [A. Smith, 285].) For mental vigor, blood flow to the brain is more important than the number of brain cells (A. Smith, 285).

the brain, 30 percent of our cardiac output, 50 percent of our kidney plasma flow, 37 percent of our nerve trunk fibers, 60 percent of our maximum oxygen uptake during exercise, 57 percent of our maximum voluntary breathing capacity, 64 percent of our taste buds, and 45 percent of our handgrip strength (Shock, 101).[24] We do not know why this sort of aging and withering process is part of being human, but any medical expectations that ignore it will be as futile as they will be expensive.

We should not conclude, however, that concern for health and use of medical resources should be cost-effectively restricted to the young. Rather, we should conclude that what it means to be a healthy (i.e., well-functioning) human being will vary according to age, and so will appropriate medical goals and interventions. Recognizing the inevitability of physical decline calls for realism about our life span and, as we will argue in another chapter, it calls for a medical-care system which allocates its services in a way that recognizes different types of needs. In addition to preventive and curative services, it will provide services aimed at maintenance of the chronically ill, frail, and disabled, as well as specialized care when people are dying—when medical care is urgently needed but when pushing for some of the goals appropriate to earlier life stages is sometimes cruel, often terribly expensive, and always unrealistic. Christian realism admits that health will often primarily be a matter of accommodating one's self to problems; well-functioning can be appropriate coping when there can be no curing.

Such realism would avoid futile overuse of technology, especially in terminal illness, but would also avoid any notion that, once we are "over the hill," we should not demand resources and should accept some sort of responsibility to die or to avoid inconveniencing the young. Christians have two separate and sufficient reasons for rejecting such an attitude.

First, the essential ways in which we image God can flourish in adversity and frailty. So the issue is not what we are losing as we grow older, but which aspects of God's image we are becoming more able to reflect. This attitude is difficult in a mortality-denying society that worships youth and physical vigor. Perhaps the biggest problem with which older people must cope is not their aging but how their aging is perceived by others. We are not here advocating compassion so much as open-minded appreciation of differences and a willingness to perceive and receive the distinctive contributions that imagers of God can make at the different stages of their life spans. Can we see in aged persons less

---

24. Of course, these are averages; particular individuals can become more rather than less proficient at some of these functions during at least part of their aging. Moreover, all of this "decline" is quite compatible with living a vigorous and flourishing life while aging.

passionate elbowing in the pursuit to establish themselves and their projects? Can we see a more reflective attitude, a willingness to put things into perspective? Can we learn from what we see—if we are receptive—something about what it means to image a God who views all things from the perspective of eternity?

The second Christian reason for responding to the distinctive health needs of the elderly applies even when celebration of differences and receptive mutuality seem impossible. Sometimes interdependence, even when it is not confused with independence, seems to give way to the sheer dependence of the elderly on others. Then we must remember not just the self-interested point that we ourselves may be elderly someday, but also the Christian point that we image God by responding with compassion and respect to the most vulnerable members of the community. A Christian can imitate God by reaching out in compassion to share the suffering of another. Imitating God by refusing to abandon another person requires decision-making about the appropriate use of technological intervention and requires recognizing that sometimes heroic technological intervention is a way of caring but that at other times it is a substitute for caring, a sophisticated, subtle way of abandoning a terminally ill patient. In short, when Christian realism is combined with Christian compassion, the question is not *whether* we invest in caring for the terminally ill and those who seem utterly dependent but *how* we care for them.

Sometimes when we appropriately care for others we become able to see in them a mutuality and capacity to give that we otherwise do not notice. Relevant here is the psychological fact that how we respond to others will affect how we perceive them—even as how we perceive them affects how we respond to them—so that compassion and respect become lenses through which we see aspects of other people we would not otherwise see. We should notice a sobering implication of the fact that compassion and respect affect how we perceive others: our perceptions of and judgments about others are reflections on the categories and values we use to perceive others, so our judgments of others are also self-judgments. "Judge not, that you be not judged" (Matt. 7:1) is probably not a warning to avoid making decisions about others but a warning that our value judgments about others are, in effect, judgments about our own character. If so, a good way to find out what kind of persons we are is to look at how we perceive others. What categories do we use? What determines acceptance or rejection? What underlies our willingness to include or exclude? This point gives added meaning to the notion of mutuality in a relationship; what others are to us will depend on the categories we use to perceive them, which will depend on the values with which we respond to them, which will depend on our own virtues and character. For this reason Christian health professionals may see a close relationship between understanding themselves and understanding their patients. What we see of the needs and capacities of others depends on who or what *we* are and not just on who or what *they* are.

Health and Persons with Disabilities

Especially when relating to persons with disabilities, Christians should be sensitive to the fact that how we respond depends upon those aspects of our own character that influence how we perceive others. First, we should notice that the relationship between health (as well-functioning) and disability is far from simple. An *impairment* can be thought of as a disease since it is an anatomical or physiological condition or a mental condition resulting from a biological condition. All of us carry defective genes, which in most of us sooner or later cause impairments of sight, hearing, or movement that we simply adjust to in healthy ways. A *disability* is an impairment that one cannot simply adjust to; it significantly interferes with the ability to perform some normal human functions. If one of these functions is a major life activity, the person with the disability is often thought of as *handicapped* (Reich, 258). But, of course, many persons with disabilities and handicaps can be equipped with technologies or cared for in ways that overcome their biological limitations, making their well-functioning more complicated than usual but healthy nonetheless. Indeed, the extent to which they will be healthy—that is, well-functioning—will often depend largely on how others react to their condition. In this sense, a society that builds steps without ramps, for example, ensures that an impairment becomes a handicap which cannot be coped with in a healthy way. So whether persons with disabilities can be healthy depends on both their impairments and their social environments.

Of course, not all impairments can be technologically and socially coped with in ways that allow for an adjusted well-functioning in all of the major human activities. It goes without saying that the loving response is to help persons with these disabilities, not to shut them up in custodial environments, out of sight and mind. But Christians should notice that if their primary motive in helping is always one of pity and compassion, they may be responding with a pagan rather than a biblical notion of human flourishing. When we reflect on what it is to be an imager of God, we can see not only that most persons with disabilities are fully capable of imaging God but also that often their God-imaging activities of forgiving, accepting, working, appreciating, celebrating, trusting, and, in short, living in faith, hope, and love put to shame those without physical disabilities. Care-ful reaching out will reveal that persons with disabilities first and foremost are persons and only secondarily are disabled. And the Christian emphasis on "celebrating differences" and on "mutuality" reminds us of how much we can learn from and receive from persons with disabilities.[25] It reminds us as Christians that the body of Christ has many members and that the well-functioning of that body involves giving and receiving in many different ways.[26]

Although it is true that we can learn to appreciate the God-imaging character of persons with disabilities and can learn and receive much from them, we cannot be sentimentally or overly optimistic. The burden of meeting special needs can be crushing as well as inspiring, and sometimes the possibilities of mutuality are so limited that compassion and pity become the main motives for heroic sacrifice. So Christian care for those with disabilities will often translate into helping their families as the latter struggle to provide as much opportunity as possible for the flourishing of the family members with special needs. And in those rare cases when the disability is so great that the mental functioning simply does not allow for symbolic interaction between those caring and those cared for, perhaps the motivation for caring cannot be that these profoundly retarded humans distinctively image God. Even here, however, pity and compassion mingle not only with respect for what these victims were meant to be but also with the desire to imitate a biblical Father who shows a bias toward the most vulnerable victims among his children.

Treating Imagers of God: Autonomy, Informed Consent, and Paternalism

Knowing what it means to be an imager of God can help us think through two of the most debated issues in contemporary discussion about medical practice—that of patients' autonomy and informed consent. Medi-

25. This point is emphasized by T. Hoeksema ("Christian Responses") and the articles he shared with us by R. Uken ("My Teachers—The Retarded") and J. Vanier ("How the Weak Heal Us").

26. The claim that we image God as a corporate collectivity and that we see different aspects of God's image in different types of people is urged by, among others, R. Mouw (*When the Kings Come Marching In,* 47) and H. Boer (*An Ember Still Glowing: Humankind as the Image of God,* forthcoming).

cal people (and even some lawyers) are becoming glassy eyed at the bur-geoning literature, discussion, and litigation involving these two ideas. The implications of our discussion about imaging God reveal why au-tonomy and informed consent are important concerns for Christians and also the limitations and dangers of letting them become the defining fac-tors in therapeutic relationships.

When physicians and nurses enter into relationships with patients, they find themselves bonded with people who not only are imagers of God but who also typically are already bonded in union with other people and, if they are believers, with God. That they are imagers of God already controls which models or metaphors we should use in perceiving what we are doing and to whom we are doing it. Many of us remember childhood stories about helping or refusing to help another person who, in the story, eventually turned out to be an angel (or Jesus) in disguise. The telling of such stories would change, if only for a few days, how we treated strangers—just in case. . . . But the bib-lical message about imagers of God is that in treating persons we are in an important sense treating God. Thus Proverbs 14:31 reminds us that "he who oppresses a poor man insults his Maker, but he who is kind to the needy honors him." This point is made even more vivid by Jesus in the parable of the sheep and the goats (Matt. 25:31-46): "Truly, I say to you, as you did it to one of the least of these my brethren, you did it to me" (v. 40).

What kindness or love requires, of course, is relative to the type of being we are loving. We love God differently than we love pets be-cause of what God is and the resultant awe and reverence we feel. Inso-far as this awe is also appropriate to God's representatives, it will con-dition the way we express our kindness and nurture, as we noticed when we discussed the idea of sanctity (see p. 31). In particular, we will recog-nize that we are dealing with givers and hearers of reasons who have the privilege and responsibility before God to choose how to live and how to consume resources and therefore have the privilege and responsibility before God to be importantly involved in cost-risk-benefit judgments about the treatments they receive. Of course, these patients are in rela-tionship with medical professionals who also have the privilege and re-sponsibility before God to choose how they practice medicine, includ-ing how they respond to patients whose choice-making capacities are diminished because of illness. But even the nature of this latter response will be informed by the recognition that patients — including those whose ability to give and hear reasons is greatly diminished or even non-existent—are also typically bound in union with family, friends, pastors, and confidants, whose welfare not only interpenetrates that of the patients but who also may have special insight into what the patients would choose if they were able. Thus we have a strong and distinctly Christian rationale for obtaining the informed consent of patients, including, whenever necessary and possible, proxy consent.

The preceding considerations are congenial with secular arguments for respecting a patient's autonomy rather than simply doing what is perceived as being in the patient's best interest. In the next chapter we will discuss autonomy-based ethics, but here we should note that autonomy has not had good press among Reformed thinkers because autonomy, by definition ("self-rule"), seems to imply that we are to decide our own laws and essence without divine guidance, without any preconception of what is proper to persons, and without concern for others. Some thinkers may employ the term in this way, and we would not defend them, but we should notice that choosing one's morality can be compatible with—and may even require—commitments to others and to objective moral law or, at least, to some conception of what is proper to persons.[27] This latter view of autonomy can admit that circumstances and relationships can *saddle* us with responsibilities and that higher authority can *assign* them to us. But this view of autonomy would insist that there is also an important sense in which even these responsibilities can be and are *assumed*, not merely *imposed*. They are not inherited like the color of our eyes; we must, at some level, *choose* to accept the responsibilities that circumstances thrust on us, *affirm* those relationships that call for response, and *accept* as an authority anyone who legitimately assigns us responsibilities. Choosing not to choose is itself a choice for which we are responsible. Only a life of deep ignorance or incompetence can escape the assumption of some responsibility, but the unexamined life, while perhaps worth living, is not the life for which God created givers and hearers of reasons. Feeling gratitude toward God and perceiving that God and his laws favor us[28] amount to sufficient reasons for conforming our wills to God's. To insist that we must *choose* that conformity is not to usurp God's authority but to image him and to recognize that our distinctive creaturely role involves choosing to become what God intends us to be. That such a role is open-ended enough for things

27. See G. Dworkin ("Autonomy and Behavior Control," 25-26), R. Mouw ("Biblical Revelation," 372), and A. MacIntyre ("Theology, Ethics," 436).

28. R. Mouw and A. MacIntyre (see previous footnote) appeal to the belief that God's commands are for human welfare. This belief is challenged by James Gustafson's *Ethics from a Theocentric Perspective* (88-99) but is supported by such texts as Deuteronomy 10:13 ("Keep the commandments and statutes of the Lord, which I command you this day for your good") and Psalm 56:9 ("This I know, that God is for me").

to go terribly wrong is precisely what the freedom and the burden of being a giver and hearer of reasons are all about.

A finite and sinful choice-maker will make mistakes, but there are important limits on the ways and extent to which another finite and sinful choice-maker may override those mistakes and still respect the former's imaging of God. Herein lies the appreciation Christians will have for those who argue that, in a pluralist society, the primary moral question in medical decision-making is not "What ought to be done?" but "Whose decision is it?" However, this appreciation will be limited and critical, because Christian medical providers are in relationship not only with their patients but also with their God and with members of a profession that itself professes certain values. Moreover, their patients are not just givers of reasons; they are also hearers of reasons. And in the dialogue that is part of a medical relationship, medical profession-als may have reasons that they want their patients to hear. Depending on the situation, these reasons may follow from their Christian identity or from their professional identity or from both. The point is that Chris-tian professionals are concerned with *what* the decision is and not just *whose* it is, because their relationships with their patients are part of their identities. This fact makes their interest in the decision something much deeper than that of curious onlookers, commodity purveyors, hired technicians, or animated tools of a patient's desires. They want it to be a *good* decision—one in the patient's best interest—and not just the patient's *own* decision.

So Christian medical professionals are motivated both to seek their patients' best interests and to respect their patients' decision-making authority. This creates the potential for complicated and uncom-fortable conflict (Verhey, "Christian Community," 149). It would be sim-pler if they could merely ensure either that patients make their own choices or that patients' best interests are served. Ever since Hippocrates the medical profession has tended to reduce this conflict by emphasiz-ing the obligation to pursue patients' best interests, even at the price of ignoring, overriding, or denying patients' decision-making authority (Veatch, *A Theory*, chaps. 1 and 6). This tendency, usually called *paternal-ism*, is defended in two distinctly different ways.

One way—called *strong paternalism*—claims that the value of doing what is good for patients simply outweighs the value of respect-ing their freedom to choose. In the language of the next chapter, this is the claim that the principle of beneficence outweighs the principle of autonomy. Given what we have said about the need to respect imagers of God, we are not sympathetic with this ranking of values; we insist that manipulating patients into the "right" direction by using undue

---

Box 2.1   Commonly Cited Elements of Informed Consent

1. Comprehension of information: ability to understand the diagnosis, therapeutic alternatives, and the relevant costs, risks, and benefits of alternatives. Standards for disclosing information:
   a. Professional-practice standard: what the profession traditionally discloses
   b. Reasonable-person or "objective" standard: all information that an average reasonable person would regard as relevant to the decision
   c. Particular-patient or "subjective" standard: what a particular patient with a distinctive identity and viewpoint would regard as relevant to the decision
2. Effective reasoning: ability to reach a decision based on relevant reasons
3. Reflective deliberation: ability to affirm a decision that is consistent with one's past identity or a considered change in it
4. Voluntariness: decision is free from coercion, manipulation, and undue influence

---

influence or by disclosing relevant information in a highly selective way (see Box 2.1, "Commonly Cited Elements of Informed Consent") is to strip them of their God-given privilege and responsibility to be stewardly choice-makers. Moreover, we think that deciding what is in a given patient's best interest is often not simply a medical decision but is instead a value-laden and personal decision, one on which the patient is often as much an expert as the medical professional is. For example, if an operation has a 40 percent chance of relieving some of a patient's pain and a 5 percent chance of increasing it or eliminating it, the patient is usually in the best position to know whether it is worth the cost and risk. The patient probably knows best even when the outcome is so uncertain that percentages cannot be given. Of course, many decisions are primarily medical in nature, such as which procedures are most effective for particular results, and on these the medical professional is the expert. It is in those decisions about whether a particular result is worth the cost or risk that the patient's viewpoint becomes authoritative.

Strong paternalism asserts that patients sometimes *ought not* participate in decision-making. The second and more common way of defending paternalism—often called *weak paternalism*—is to assert that patients by and large *cannot* meaningfully participate. The reasons usually given are that medical professionals cannot provide all the relevant information or cannot do so in a neutral way or that patients cannot effectively comprehend or use the information. Of course, if something truly cannot be done, there is no responsibility to do it. But we should be careful about allowing what we think is wrong or inconvenient to determine what we think is impossible.

It is true that time constraints alone prevent presenting all the information that bears on a decision. But standards of disclosure (see Box 2.1) have evolved that help one select the information that is most relevant. Our objection to strong paternalism militates against simply using the "professional standard," which would require giving only the information that professionals have traditionally given.[29] Sincere efforts can and should be made to provide the information any reasonable person would consider relevant and, when the distinctive values of patients are known, to provide any information particular patients would consider relevant.

It is also true that information is often "packaged" in ways that bias its reception: "Almost everyone survives this procedure without serious complications; only 20 percent of patients get worse" will be received differently than "This procedure kills or maims at least one out of every five patients." But, again, sincere efforts can be made to present the information in a way that avoids manipulating patients into passive acquiescence to whatever medical professionals have already decided is best.

There certainly are difficulties in enabling patients to understand the relevant information. Sometimes this difficulty results from a medical practitioner's not sincerely trying to translate turgid prose and medical jargon into understandable English. Like many professionals, medical personnel do not always realize when their specialized terminology is opaque to others. One study found that only 15 percent of consent forms were written in language as simple as that of *Time* magazine and that in 75 percent of the forms fewer than 10 percent of the technical or medical terms were explained in lay language (President's Commission, *Making Health Care Decisions*, I: 110). Another study found that almost half of the physicians surveyed thought that, if reasonable time and effort were devoted to explanation, over 90 percent of their patients could understand the relevant information, and an additional third of the physicians

---

29. Courts in the United States have lately tended to favor the "reasonable person" standard and to reject the "professional practice" standard. See *Canterbury v. Spence* (464 F.2d 772 [D.C.C.A. 1972]) and *Cobbs v. Grant* (104 Cal. Rptr. 505. 502 P.2d1 [1972]). The appropriateness of the "particular patient" standard can be considered by asking whether a patient who is a Jehovah's Witness should be informed about a remote possibility that a blood transfusion might be needed during a proposed treatment, even if the remoteness of the possibility implies that this information would not be provided under the other standards.

thought that over 70 percent of their patients could understand.[30] These data suggest that much of the difficulty with patient comprehension is due more to what *is* or *isn't* done than to what *can* or *can't* be done. If sincere efforts are made, it is quite likely that the majority of patients can be treated not only as hearers of reasons, who can be informed about diagnosis and prognosis, but also as givers of reasons, who can participate in the decision about which treatment to choose.

This hopeful vision of respect for patients as choice-making imagers of God leaves room for legitimate exceptions. Emergencies often require swift decision at times when patients are unable to think straight or even to think at all. And often illness so incapacitates patients that they simply are not themselves. An integrated view of human nature implies that illness is not just a burden people bear while everything else about them remains the same. The whole person is ill, often writhing in pain and sick with worry. Even granting that competence is *always* a matter of degree, we can appreciate that sometimes illness so diminishes competence that the only way to respect autonomy is to recognize its diminishment or absence and seek to restore it.[31] Even here, however, patients' choices can often be indirectly respected by consideration of their formerly expressed values or consultation with family members in an effort to find out what they would likely decide if they could. And sometimes patients with diminished competence can participate in some decisions even when they cannot participate in all of them.

Another exception to insisting on informed consent exists when patients waive it, telling the medical professional not to bother them with difficult details and to do whatever the professional thinks is best. Sometimes such a waiver should be resisted as an irresponsible effort to escape from God-given freedom. But at other times it may be a responsible decision about deciding: patients may sometimes have good reason to think that a trusted authority will make decisions that not only enhance their best interests but also are in accord with their values. Moreover, they may be correct in thinking that, under the circumstances, their own participation would only make things worse. But such delegating of authority over

30. Three-fourths of these physicians preferred the "reasonable person" or "particular patient" standards of disclosure. Other things being equal, the more experienced physicians tended to think more of their patients could understand; however, those treating many poor patients tended to think fewer of their patients could understand (President's Commission, *Making Health Care Decisions*, I: 59, 73, 106).

31. This point is made by E. Cassell ("Function of Medicine"), who has often found that ill people are mentally confused enough to think that a taller, narrower tube has more water in it than a shorter, wider tube even after they observe the same amount of water being poured into both tubes (Cassell, *Healer's Art*, 38-39).

something as integral to one's identity as one's health is so problematic that, at minimum, medical professionals should be sure that the patient truly wants to do it. The mere fact that patients avoid asking for information should not be taken as an implied waiver of informed consent. There is good evidence that many patients believe physicians resent being questioned, especially if it heightens emotion, takes time, or implies lack of trust (Angell, "Respecting Autonomy," 1115). Feeling vulnerable and dependent, such patients avoid what they think would upset physicians or lose their goodwill. Surveys suggest that perhaps only 2 percent of patients ever want their physicians to withhold "bad news," while 94 percent want to be told everything, and 72 percent want to make decisions jointly with their physicians after treatment alternatives have been explained. Meanwhile, 88 percent of physicians think that patients want physicians to choose the best alternative for patients, and only 9 percent think that informed consent involves patients' stating their own preferences (as opposed to simply understanding and acquiescing to the physicians').[32] These physicians can point to studies indicating that only 12 percent of patients actually use disclosed information when consenting to treatment. But the same studies show that 93 percent of the patients thought they benefited from the information (Beauchamp and Childress, 77). Perhaps, even when patients do not use information, giving it to them prevents their feeling used. So, apart from the prudence or morality of waiving informed consent, we can wonder whether patients truly waive it as often as is sometimes thought.

One more exception to insisting on informed consent is the *therapeutic privilege* exercised by medical professionals. Sometimes they have good reasons to believe that disclosing dreaded information would so upset patients that they might be seriously harmed or they might reject treatment which they not only clearly need but would certainly accept if they were in a calm frame of mind. Although the evidence tends to be anecdotal, undoubtedly there are some legitimate exceptions of this sort. Studies suggest, however, that virtually all patients go ahead with treatment even after upsetting information is disclosed (President's Commission, *Making Health Care Decisions*, I: 99). Probably the amount of harm caused by bad news is less a matter of *whether* it is disclosed than of *how* it is disclosed. Indeed, reliable evidence suggests that disclosure of

---

32. The President's Commission (see footnote 30 of this chapter) hired independent researchers to conduct and review a number of surveys that use valid scientific methodology and to compare the results with the anecdotal evidence frequently mentioned in the literature. Our references to the Commission's report include references to some of these independent surveys (President's Commission, *Making Health Care Decisions*, I: 18, 46, 72, 75, 97, 99).

threatening information not only is not harmful but often is therapeutically beneficial (President's Commission, *Making Health Care Decisions,* I: 100). Therefore, we think medical professionals should be very careful about paternalistically overriding informed consent by appealing to the therapeutic privilege or their responsibility not to harm their patients.

A dramatic pendulum swing seems to be occurring during the 1970s and 1980s. For at least three reasons, many practitioners are regarding the traditional paternalism of the medical profession as outmoded.

First, there seems to be a resurgence of individualism in Western (especially American) values, which encourages us to "do our own thing" and to allow others to do theirs as long as nobody (unwillingly) gets hurt. It is not clear whether this attitude derives more from greedy self-absorption or from noble respect for the dignity of others, but, in either case, it does involve an awareness of the diversity of values. This recognition of pluralism seems to stimulate both a relativism about values and, somewhat paradoxically, an absolutizing of the value of autonomy. The result in medicine can be summed up in the title of a recent play which was also made into a movie—*Whose Life Is It, Anyway?* The focus of decision-making is now on proper procedure, on *whose* choice it is, sometimes at the expense of concern for proper content.

Second, this shift in values—at least the expression of it in medicine—is reinforced by economic constraints. One reaction to these constraints is the attempt to drag medicine into economic efficiency by making it a commodity. If a professional becomes a profit-maximizing purveyor of market goods or a technician for hire, the emphasis will not be on paternalistically safeguarding patients' best interests.

Third, the legal climate encourages patients to sue for malpractice as soon as something goes wrong. This litigiousness makes it prudent for medical professionals not to exclude patients from participating in decisions; it even makes it prudent to force patients to participate. Thus we see a dramatic increase in the use of consent forms, which are sometimes used so routinely that many people fear the forms have become a substitute for the very informed consent process they were supposed to substantiate (President's Commission, *Making Health Care Decisions,* I: 106). In fact, 79 percent of patients and 55 percent of physicians believe that consent forms are used primarily to protect doctors and hospitals from lawsuits rather than to protect patients from uninformed participation.[33] In spite of this perception—or because of it—few com-

---

33. However, a majority of both patients and physicians thought that the consent forms improve physician-patient communication (President's Commission, *Making Health Care Decisions,* I: 109).

petent patients now get treatments against their wishes, and patients are increasingly participating in decisions.

We worry that these powerful motivations against paternalism may overwhelm several important features of good medicine. They may diminish rather than enhance respect for the image of God both in those who are ill and in those who care for them. The attitude of "do your own thing" combined with concern for cost-effective use of time and fear of litigation may dispose medical professionals to agree too rapidly to ill-conceived patient decisions. It is good that we avoid the arrogance of assuming that, when patients disagree with professionals, patients are incompetent. But it should not be replaced with the assumption that all patients' requests are authentic decisions flowing from their identities and values. We use the term *patients* rather than *clients* because many times (though not always) illness ruptures wholeness and warps perceptions. Our notion of the "sick role" assumes the presence of incapacities. Illness can let loose deep-seated psychodynamics in which refusals of treatment can be masquerades for guilt, depression, and feelings of dependence and abandonment (Marzuk). Sometimes a patient's "No" means "Do you think I'm worth anything?" (Burt, 10-11). Of course, at other times it means precisely what it says. Accordingly, only loving and respectful dialogue about a patient's "No," rather than high-minded dismissal of it or hurried acquiescence to it, can discover whether that answer is an authentic decision or a cry for help.

Since Christian medical professionals have special motivation both for respecting patients' choice-making and for seeking patients' best interests, they often feel caught in the middle of powerful and conflicting forces. While rejecting uncritical paternalism, they will also resist economic and legal pressures that undermine their patients' best interests while pretending to respect their autonomy. The Christian community should ask itself how it can encourage and help its medical professionals in this struggle. At minimum, it should recognize that sometimes professionals may and must refuse to cooperate with decisions or policies that violate their Christian conscience or their professional integrity. Christian professionals have the awesome privilege and responsibility to image God's love and regard for God's imagers, especially when they are most vulnerable. When Christians nurture this identity in their professionals, they can hope to be treated as imagers of God in sickness as well as in health.

3. Covenantal Fidelity in a
Pluralist Society

It is tempting to stereotype Western religious ethics in the following way: Protestant ethics emphasizes painful wrestling with difficult dilemmas, Catholic ethics emphasizes careful application of detailed principles, and Jewish ethics emphasizes sagacious telling of illuminating stories. This book will suggest that biblically based ethics involves all three activities, especially when it confronts the moral problems of modern medicine.

The Examined Moral Life

But before we confront the problems of medical ethics, we should remind ourselves that most of our moral life does not involve our consciously thinking our way through difficulties. Every day we make hundreds of moral choices that simply flow from the dispositions — which include both virtues and vices—that constitute our character, dispositions that derive largely from our genetic endowment and our upbringing. Indeed, we worry about people who have to think too much before doing the right thing. We like to think that proper character-building—through careful approval and disapproval of behavior as well as through inspiring stories about moral heroes—should give us a head that knows what is right and a heart that is disposed to do it without a lot of agonizing over what to do and whether to do it. Many of us also like to think that our lives are like stories, or narratives, in which our characters and our very identities are shaped by the stories of others, including those around us whose stories interrelate with our own. And we hope that being raised in a Christian community will appropriately shape our identities—shape them through stories of the heroes of faith as well as through biblical accounts of our being created in God's image, redeemed in Jesus' life and death and resurrection, and sustained and guided by the Holy Spirit. Such character-building will, we hope, result in distinctive virtues—dispositions toward caring, gratitude, humility, faithfulness, reverence, and hope. When dispositions become habits, we typically make our everyday moral choices so naturally that others can quite accurately predict what we will do.

It is often wiser, then, to trust people who have demonstrated good character over those, say, who merely have read the latest books on ethics. Similarly, if we want to get a good idea of how a professional in any field will conduct professional activities, knowing the role models that he or she emulates will be more helpful than knowing which courses he or she took in college.

On the other hand, explicit consideration of moral theories should not be ignored. The previous chapter argued that we do not inherit our characters the way we inherit the color of our eyes or even the way we inherit our nationalities or ethnic identities. God did not create image bearers to be merely products of their genes and environments. As self-reflective choice-makers who evaluate our evaluations, we are not just the actors of our life stories; we are also, to an important degree, the authors and critics of them. The moral development of a responsible choice-maker does involve the nurturing of distinctive dispositions, but perhaps the trickiest and toughest part of moral development is that one of these distinctive dispositions is the disposition to examine one's own dispositions.

One reason to cultivate the examined life was discussed in the previous chapter: although creatures do not create the moral law, those who are image bearers have the responsibility to consciously affirm their identity and to exercise their autonomy by accepting God's will for their lives. A second reason to examine one's moral character is to become clear about what one's moral character is and what its implications for living are. The previous chapter made a modest effort at this when it discussed such ideas as sanctity and informed consent. A third reason derives from what might be called the problem of "gaps." Inevitably, it seems, we encounter new situations for which our dispositions have not prepared us. This is the case even when our dispositions have been formulated into rules, such as the Ten Commandments, which do not automatically tell us exactly what to do in specific instances—for example, when informed consent or force feeding is the issue. Especially in medicine, technological development and other changes are forcing us to confront new situations that demand decisions.

A fourth motivation for the examined life is the problem of conflicts. We sometimes disagree with other choice-makers, of course, especially in professions that require a great deal of teamwork and require it precisely when decisions are the most difficult and delicate. But we also disagree within ourselves. We find ourselves having conflicting loyalties when we cannot simultaneously meet obligations we have toward different persons or groups. And even when we consider just one other person to be the focus of our responsibilities, we sometimes find that our own dispositions are at odds with each other or that we cannot simultaneously pursue all the goods and avoid all the evils. Sometimes all three kinds of conflict occur in a single situation—when, for example, two physicians disagree over whether to send a hospital patient home, one physician being torn between loyalty to the patient and the hospital's need to economize, the other weighing the patient's desire to go home against the possibility of a medical emergency that could best be handled in the hospital.

In short, the urge to examine our morals can be sparked by the stewardly responsibility to be self-reflective or clear about our decisions, but it is also often fueled by conflict. Indeed, perhaps most people are first stimulated to think hard about their values when they experience some sort of conflict with regard to a decision of their own or between their decision and others' decisions. Although much of the moral life is a matter of simply living in integrity with one's character, and not a matter of wrestling with dilemmas, most people encounter enough conflicts or new questions that they are forced to become self-conscious about their morals. This self-consciousness can be uncomfortable, especially when other persons and groups have deeply different and contradicting beliefs about what the world is and what it ought to be. When people clarify their own beliefs in such a society (a "pluralist" society), they often discover that there are many alternative beliefs, some of which are understandable and well-reasoned and held by intelligent and decent people. Their effort to become clear about what they believe, then, leads them to ask whether their beliefs are the most appropriate and whether they can justify their position.

Difficulties in applying values or clarifying them thus lead to the basic questions of ethical theory. What are the fundamental dispositions or principles that should give structure to people's lives? How can people justify their answers to this question? And how should they respond to those with different answers to the same question? The section that follows will discuss some of the main alternatives that those in the Western tradition will encounter when answering these questions.

Main Alternatives in Western Ethics

A moral (or ethical) theory provides one or more basic guides, guides that serve as the basis from which other guides and judgments are derived. In some theories basic guides are formulated as basic *virtues*—that is, as dispositions of character that incline people to act in right ways; in other theories the basic guides are formulated as basic *principles* or *rules* about right action. A theory of the former type might claim, for example, that cultivating a benevolent disposition is one's basic moral responsibility, whereas a theory of the latter type might claim that one's basic moral obligation is the duty to avoid actions that harm others. Some inclusive theories combine both virtues and principles as the corresponding elements of the moral life. According to these theories, *virtues* are used in judgments about good character and praiseworthiness, and *principles* are used in judgments about right action and obligation. These theories see a close connection between the questions of what we ought to *be* and what we ought to *do*, although there may be disagreement over which question is primary. Discussion of moral theories can quickly lead to meta-ethical questions about the meaning, character, and justifiability of moral claims, including such questions as whether these claims are expressions of knowledge or expressions of feelings, whether they are discovered or invented, and whether they can be rationally justified.

We cannot examine all of the important moral and meta-ethical theories in Western theology and philosophy, much less consider alternatives found in Eastern civilizations. As far as meta-ethics is concerned, we will simply assume that revelation and reason can enable us to discover moral knowledge. And we will assume that although few moral principles can be either refuted or justified to everyone's satisfaction, most of them can be evaluated as more acceptable or less acceptable, both within a Christian framework and in terms of the traditional criteria of rational theory selection, criteria such as clarity, consistency, and comprehensiveness. As far as moral theory is concerned, we will consider several types of the two main moral theories encountered when people debate medical ethics, focusing on their affinities with and differences from the view we eventually endorse, a view we will call *covenantal ethics*.

In concentrating on those views that are most often defended in debates on medical ethics, we will avoid a separate discussion of egoism, the theory that every agent ought to act always and only in that agent's long-term, enlightened self-interest. Egoists are indirectly concerned about others' interests (indeed, intelligent egoists are often eager to help others) but only as a means of helping themselves. Although egoism is a stance that often motivates medical providers and patients, especially when medicine is viewed as a commodity for sale in a free market, it is less frequently used as a defense for decisions in medicine than are those views that directly take into account the interests of all those affected by a decision.

The main theoretical division we find in moral debates—especially those of ethics committees and case studies—is between teleological (from the Greek *telos*, or "goal") ethics and deontological (from the Greek *deon*, or "what is required") ethics. The oldest form of teleological ethics goes back to Aristotle. It was adapted by Saint Thomas Aquinas and has heavily influenced Roman Catholic ethics. Today it is having a revival in both theological and secular forms. What characterizes it is the effort to understand the natural or proper ends of human existence and to cultivate the virtues and character conducive to these ends. It further seeks to understand the natural ends of human activities and practices and to base relevant virtues or principles on understanding the goods naturally sought in those activities and practices. Appeal is often made to "natural law," which is understood by "natural reason" or perhaps is both revealed in Scripture and understood by natural reason. The ethics of human activities (such as sexual intercourse) and human practices (such as medicine) are a matter of cultivating virtues or following principles that are consistent with and conducive to the proper ends of these activities and practices. Intramural disagreement among those holding to this form of teleological ethics focuses on proper ends and which virtues or principles contribute to them. For example, it is difficult to agree on a common end or set of ends for medicine (or even for sexual intercourse). Still, there is enough plausibility in deriving ethics from discovering the natural ends of persons and activities to make this type of ethics attractive to many thinkers.

During this century, the most common type of teleological ethics has been utilitarianism, which teaches that people have the single fundamental moral duty of producing the greatest general good. It was elaborated in the nineteenth century by Jeremy Bentham and John Stuart Mill as a scientific way to decide social-policy issues; people need only calculate the good and evil consequences of alternative actions or policies to determine the right one. In teaching that agents must be directly concerned with (and only with) the effects of their actions on the well-being of everyone affected by them, Bentham and Mill tried to provide a scientific way for people to love their neighbors as themselves. Bentham and Mill thought that by producing the best balance of good consequences over evil consequences, people could avoid the pitfalls of both selfishness and blind adherence to old-fashioned rules, both of which (they thought) produce more harm than good.

Bentham and Mill thought of utilitarianism as a scientific way to calculate moral decisions because it is a technique for making cost-benefit analyses. One weighs the costs to everyone affected by an action against the benefits to everyone affected by it and acts in the way that maximizes net benefits. Herein lies what the critics of utilitarianism regard as a crucial moral flaw: the maximum net benefit may occur when the rights of a minority are overridden in order to produce the greatest general good. For example, when potential organ donors are dying, one might decide to hasten their deaths in order to use their organs for (otherwise healthy) patients who desperately need them. This decision might be justified on the grounds that the donors will die soon anyway, and the greatest good for the greatest number will come about if they die in time for the "desperate need" patients to benefit. Of course, utilitarians might argue that the side effects of such actions — such as increased anxiety among the terminally ill—must also be weighed in the balance, and that these effects might imply that the general good would be maximized by not hastening the donors' deaths. But critics worry that predictions about consequences are a shaky way to defend the rights of the vulnerable, that some actions are wrong *apart from* their effects on the general good, and that the *distribution* (and not just the net balance) of the costs and benefits must be directly considered. Such critics believe that in treating individuals as simply the experiencers of an intrinsic good (the production of which must be maximized), utilitarianism does not take seriously enough the distinctions among persons, who are ends-in-themselves and not just contributing parts of a larger whole.

Even if proper distinctions and careful weighing of *all* the consequences of actions can help utilitarianism avoid the charge that it allows injustice, it must answer an important question: Which consequences are good and which are evil? Bentham and Mill thought it was obvious that only pleasure (or happiness) is good in itself, but other utilitarians have thought that experiences of such things as freedom, knowledge, beauty, and friendship are good in themselves (intrinsic values) and not merely means to happiness (instrumental values). This is not a trivial disagreement. Take, for example, freedom and knowledge. Whether they are intrinsically valuable or only instrumentally valuable can make an important difference when one is calculating whether a proposed action, such as overriding another's freedom to know something, will maximize good consequences. Lack of agreement or even of hope for agreement on what is intrinsically valuable has led to what is currently the most common type of utilitarianism, the type that identifies intrinsic value as the satisfying of individual preferences, whatever they may be.

This theory is thought by many to be a powerful decision-making tool in a pluralist democracy, one that combines the principle of majority rule with a scientific way of deciding what the majority wants. If one could measure the relative intensities of the different preferences of all those affected by a proposed action or policy, one should be able to calculate whether the proposal would, in the jargon of this theory, "maximize preference satisfaction." To help policy planners use this technique, social scientists have developed highly sophisticated analytic tools for measuring public preferences on social-policy issues. Of course, preference utilitarians believe that, for everyday personal decisions, fair-minded people can usually make rough but accurate enough estimates of how to satisfy the most and strongest desires of those affected by their decisions. Thereby, they believe, an agent can do good for others without imposing on them the agent's own notion of what is good.

However, one may wonder whether people should or even can act without making value judgments about which preferences ought to be respected. Perhaps some preferences, such as those of child abusers or racists, are so irrational that no thoughtful person would allow them to count in the balance. But what about those mildly irrational or biased preferences that we encounter daily? Consider the following case, which received much publicity in 1978 in the United States.

Thirty-nine-year-old Robert McFall needed a bone-marrow transplant; without it, he would die in a few weeks. The only relative who was found to be tissue compatible was his first cousin David Shimp, who was a good tissue match. But Shimp, at first cooperative, suddenly refused to be tested for genetic compatibility or to undergo the transplant operation. The latter could be done painlessly and with little danger to Shimp, whose major risk would be the one-in-ten-thousand chance of death from anesthesia. The newspapers indicated that Shimp was influenced by his mother, who was said to have a grudge against McFall's side of the family.[1] Shimp denied this rumor, but let us suppose it was true. What would a preference utilitarian advise Shimp to do, assuming he could not change his mother's extremely strong preference that he not benefit McFall? If her preference was to count at all, it would seem to have to weigh rather heavily in the decision. This implication is troublesome. Although everyone might understand why Shimp would not want to go against his mother's wishes, few of us would think that her grudge should count heavily in deciding what would be the morally proper thing for

---

1. The information about the McFall/Shimp case, which is referred to throughout this chapter, is taken from Beauchamp and Childress (315-17) and Meisel and Roth.

him to do. But it would be difficult for preference utilitarians to eliminate the mother's preference from the moral decision without imposing some values. So even preference utilitarians have trouble avoiding the intramural utilitarian debate over what is intrinsically good.

McFall sued Shimp to compel him to undergo the operation, arguing (among other things) that laws in the Anglo-American tradition sometimes allow society to force one individual to help another. Judge John Flaherty said Shimp's refusal was "morally indefensible" but ruled against McFall anyway. Understanding that the judge's decision is consistent from a utilitarian viewpoint can help us understand another important division within utilitarianism, one that cuts across the differences over what is valuable. One side believes that the moral question is this: Which particular *action* will maximize the good in a given situation? These are called *situational*, or *act*, *utilitarians*. The other side believes that the moral question is this: Which *practices* will maximize the good in that type of situation? The latter, called *rule utilitarians*, believe that actions should follow rules — namely, those rules that would result in the greatest general good if everyone were to follow them. Judges and legislators who are utilitarians are generally rule utilitarians, because they have to worry about setting precedents and about mandating or allowing a type of action, not just a single action. A rule utilitarian could justify Judge Flaherty's decision by noting that he was deciding not whether Shimp should give bone marrow to McFall but whether there should be a certain type of practice. And the practice he was considering was not the practice of giving bone marrow but the practice of coercing one person to give bone marrow to another.

Especially on matters of legal coercion, rule utilitarians are cautious about setting a precedent that would justify or stimulate a practice. Because professionals, especially medical professionals, also worry about precedents and are very leery of situational ethics, the professional ethics espoused by utilitarian professionals tends toward the rule type. For example, utilitarian professional ethics will typically forbid breaking confidentiality even when, in a given situation, it looks as if to do so would maximize the well-being of all concerned. Rather, it will generally advocate a rule that includes exceptions to confidentiality (reporting communicable diseases, gunshot wounds, a serious threat to an identifiable person, and so on) and will forbid any breaking of this qualified rule, no matter how well-intentioned such a breaking might be.[2]

Utilitarianism is primarily future-oriented. In fact, events that

2. For an instructive example of a rule-utilitarian policy on breaking confidentiality, see the majority opinion in *Tarasoff v. Regents of the University of California*. The ruling

happened or actions that were performed before a given moral decision is made are morally relevant to that decision only if they affect the consequences that can reasonably be predicted to result from the decision. Even past promises are relevant only to the extent that their having been made affects the consequences that can reasonably be predicted to result from the keeping of them. This dependence of utilitarianism upon calculating future consequences seems to make utilitarianism a slim basis for establishing a relationship of trust. But rule utilitarians point out that the consequences that must be considered in decision-making are the (hypothetical) consequences of everyone's making the same decision in a similar situation, not the consequences of a specific instance of keeping or breaking a promise. Thus their position on promise-keeping would not be situational, nor would it insist that promises be kept regardless of consequences. Rather, their position on promise-keeping would look something like their position on confidentiality (as stated previously), which would be consistent with a relationship of trust.

Rule utilitarians can also reply to the charge that utilitarians cannot account for the belief that roles and special relationships are of moral importance. Shimp, for example, said he would likely undergo the operation if McFall were his own child. And most people think that the role of parent implies stricter responsibilities than the role of cousin. But this belief seems to contradict simple (act) utilitaritanism, because it seems independent of beliefs about the probable consequences of donating to one's child as opposed to donating to one's cousin. Rule utilitarians reply that parents' responsibilities to their own children are greater than their responsibilities to cousins because of the good consequences of the rule that people should take more care of their own children than of their cousins.

Since they apply a single-minded consequentialism to rules and practices, rule utilitarians often rely on "slippery-slope" arguments (also called "wedge" or "domino" or "camel's-nose-in-the-tent" arguments). The logic of these arguments deserves special attention because they are probably the most common arguments found in medical ethics. They can be very powerful arguments, and, since they are frequently used by proponents of all moral theories, they serve as a universal kind of argu-

---

requires a psychiatrist to break confidentiality when he or she determines that a patient presents a serious danger of violence against other specific persons. The minority opinion opposes this policy because it predicts that the duty to warn will interfere with therapy in a way that will actually increase net violence. Both opinions use what look like rule-utilitarian premises, but they disagree on the predicted consequences of the majority opinion. Excerpts from both opinions are reprinted in Mappes and Zembaty (119-27).

ment in debates on ethics. These arguments claim that a proposed decision or policy would put those who accept it on a "slippery slope" which would result in their sliding into a practice or condition that is bad. To use and evaluate such arguments, we must distinguish two very different forms of them (Beauchamp and Childress, 120-22). One form is to claim that a particular justification of a decision or policy also justifies something that is bad. For example, some people claim that if the prevention of suffering is justification enough for allowing people to die, it also is justification for killing them. This form of the argument assumes that people should be consistent and therefore be willing to accept the implications of their positions. The second form of slippery-slope argument is to claim that a particular practice or activity will likely slide into becoming something that is bad. For example, many people fear that what we know about history, psychology, and sociology shows that the practice of voluntary euthanasia (acceptable to many people) could slide into the practice of nonvoluntary euthanasia (unacceptable to many people). Whereas the first form of the slippery-slope argument is based upon logical implications of arguments, the second form is based upon empirical beliefs[3] about human nature.

These two types of arguments should not be confused, because evidence for or against one of them will be irrelevant to the other. For example, one cannot rebut the first argument—that a particular justification for allowing death also justifies killing—by appealing to the empirical belief that many physicians do the former without doing the latter. The first type of argument assumes not that people will actually practice what their positions justify, but only that consistency requires

3. Empirical beliefs are, roughly, those whose truth or falsity people try to determine through sense experience, either directly (by observation) or indirectly (by experimentation). They are often distinguished from conceptual beliefs (which are either definitions or claims whose truth or falsity depends on the meanings of words, as in "all bachelors are unmarried"), metaphysical beliefs (which go beyond sense experience or are presupposed by sense experience, as in "all events are caused" or "everything that exists has a sufficient reason for its existence"), and value beliefs (which are beliefs concerned with how the world ought or ought not to be or what is good or bad about the world rather than beliefs about the way the world is). There are philosophical difficulties with these definitions and with sharply distinguishing these types of beliefs, but it is often useful to distinguish debates involving mainly empirical beliefs from those involving, say, value beliefs. In the court case referred to in the previous footnote, for example, the judges can be interpreted as agreeing on the value belief that people ought to follow rules that will maximize good consequences but disagreeing over empirical predictions about the consequences of everybody's following a particular rule. When predictions are defended by appealing to history, sociology, or psychology, they can generally be classified as empirical beliefs. Many moral arguments can be reduced to differences over empirical predictions rather than differences over fundamental values, as the example in the previous footnote illustrates.

either accepting both (or neither) or changing the justification. Likewise, one cannot rebut the second argument—that voluntary euthanasia could lead to nonvoluntary—by pointing out that one can justify killing people when they request it without thereby justifying killing them without or against their request. This type of argument does not assume that a practice has to be thought justifiable before people will slide into it, so rebutting this argument requires evaluating the empirical evidence upon which it is founded. Both types of slippery-slope arguments are powerful tools for evaluating positions, but we must avoid the surprisingly common error of confusing the logical claims that support or rebut the one type with the empirical claims that support or rebut the other.

The consequences (of actions) to which utilitarians appeal are those that have to do with producing the greatest general good. But deontologists—the proponents of the other main moral tradition in Western ethics—deny that our fundamental moral task is to produce good, much less the greatest general good. They typically believe that we are required primarily to respect the good that already has been created. Insofar as they appeal to consequences of decisions or actions, they refer to the effects of those decisions or actions on the rights of those affected by them. During his ruling in the McFall-Shimp case, Judge Flaherty said, "Our society is based on the right and sanctity of the individual.... For a society which respects the right of one individual, to sink its teeth into the jugular vein or neck of one of its members, and suck from it sustenance for another member, is revolting." This sounds like a deontologist talking. He opposes the coerced giving of bone marrow and presumably even the coerced giving of blood, regardless of the impact of his opposition on the general good, because individuals have the right to control their own bodies. Inherent in the deontological viewpoint is the belief that persons have certain rights and duties that may not be violated in the pursuit of the greatest general good, the belief that even if finite agents could know enough about the future to be able to predict the consequences of their actions or rules,[4] people should not do a little evil that more good may come. People may not treat members of the body politic the way they treat parts of their own bodies—by cutting off an arm or pulling a tooth to maximize the good of the whole—because members of society are not just body parts. They also are individuals who are ends in themselves, with a uniqueness, a dignity, and an inherent worth that may not be aggregated into—and maybe sacrificed for—"the masses."

---

4. Since predictions about the consequences of actions or policies are highly debatable, one can claim that, although utilitarianism is simple in theory, it requires predictions that are too complicated for finite persons to make (Donagan, 199-209).

Like teleologists, deontologists have intramural debates that can yield vastly different advice. First, some believe that there is only one fundamental moral principle, whereas others believe that there are several of them. The most influential deontologist, eighteenth-century philosopher Immanuel Kant, thought there was only one basic principle,[5] although he presented it in different versions. Two of Kant's versions have become famous as separate principles.

One version states that our fundamental moral duty is to avoid acting in any way that we cannot "universalize"—that is, we must avoid any actions which we could not or would not allow everyone else in a morally similar circumstance to do. Thus we must be willing to be on the receiving end of our actions. Kant would say that Shimp may refuse to give bone marrow to McFall only if Shimp would be willing to have McFall refuse him a similar request. And Kant would say that McFall may try to coerce Shimp only if McFall would be willing to be coerced in a similar circumstance.

Kant's second version, which is often used in medical ethics, states that all persons must be treated as ends-in-themselves and not merely as means to others' ends. We may use others for our own ends, but only with their permission. This version is often translated into the principle of respecting autonomy, because treating others as ends-in-themselves involves respecting their rationality and their status as choice-makers. Medical professionals who use this imperative as their highest or only moral principle will often find themselves at odds with their colleagues, especially on the issue of informed consent. Many deontologists accept the principle of autonomy but believe that there are other basic principles as well, including the principle of beneficence (doing good for others). Of course, if a person holds more than one basic principle, those principles may come into conflict (in the sense that a person

5. Kant called this "the categorical imperative," conveying thereby that it applies unconditionally to all people, in distinction from those "hypothetical imperatives" that promise something if one follows them. "Never tell a lie" derives from the categorical imperative; "honesty is the best image" reduces to the prudential, hypothetical imperative that, if one is honest, one can expect a good reputation. Kant thought that the principle of "universalizing" (discussed in the chapter text) was necessary and sufficient for moral guidance. Today, many ethicists think of universalizability as just one of the defining marks that distinguish moral judgments from nonmoral judgments, such as judgments of taste and prudence. (*Nonmoral* judgments are not the same as *immoral* ones; the latter are bad moral judgments.) Other commonly cited defining marks of the moral realm are "overridingness" (moral considerations should have priority over all others), "prescriptivity" (moral claims prescribe rather than describe), and "taking a direct interest in the welfare of others." The meaning of *moral* is one of those much-debated meta-ethical issues that this book does not discuss in detail.

cannot fulfill all of them simultaneously). Medical people may experience this conflict, for example, when their patients' autonomous requests are not in their own best interests. Since it is very difficult to rank
principles in a way that tells us what to do in every conflict, many ethicists simply call them *prima facie* principles, by which they mean that
these principles are always relevant and important, but that sometimes
one of them has to override another (Ross, 19-36). And since there is no
algorithm or mechanical way of deciding which one overrides which,
moral agents are sometimes forced to make agonizing decisions that will
leave traces of regret, if not guilt, no matter what they do.

Debate over the basic moral principles is related to a second
major difference among deontologists. Just as utilitarians differ on the
nature of the intrinsic good, deontologists differ on the nature and range
of rights and duties. Most agree that rights and duties are correlated in
some way, so that if one person has a right, say, to be left alone, other
people have the duty not to interfere. But there is much disagreement
over what the basic rights and correlative duties are. Some deontologists restrict rights to "negative rights of noninterference"—rights not
to be harmed. This position can reduce itself to a narrow individualism,
in which nobody feels obligated to help anyone else except out of self-
interest. But negative rights can be interpreted as implying that, sometimes, not helping the helpless violates their negative rights. In other
words, not helping the helpless can be a way of harming them, especially when they are related to others through special roles created by
past events or actions: should parents refuse to nurture their children,
lifeguards refuse to save the drowning, or doctors refuse to continue
treating their patients, their refusals to help could actually be interpreted as inflictions of harm. Events, actions, roles, and relationships
that imply promises and create legitimate expectations can obligate one
to help others simply on the grounds that omitting to fulfill a legitimate
expectation can inflict as much harm as committing an action can. In
fact, McFall's lawyer argued ingeniously (though futilely) that Shimp's
undergoing the tissue-compatibility test created in McFall a legitimate
expectation of such a nature that Shimp's later refusal caused a critical
delay and thereby contributed to the acuteness of McFall's danger. This
argument may be a bit farfetched, but it does underscore the point that,
in some circumstances, harm can be caused by omissions as well as by
commissions. In Chapter Six we will notice that this point is sometimes
used to argue that everyone has a right to a minimal level of medical
care, not because providing it helps people but because not providing
it harms them.

Some deontologists go well beyond the "do not harm" principle

and claim that there are "entitlement rights," or positive rights to assistance. They claim that the rights to pursue education, legal advice, and
medical care, for example, go beyond the right not to be interfered with
and go beyond not being harmed; these rights imply that society has the
duty to provide these goods to anyone who needs them or at least to provide some minimum amount of them. In Chapter Six we will also notice
that "equal opportunity rights" can be used to argue for society's obligation to help those who need medical care, not because society would harm
them if it refused, but because society is obliged, at least to some extent,
to help its members achieve equal opportunity in meeting life's demands.

Related to deontological debates over rights and duties are differences over how we know them and how we justify our beliefs about
them. Appeals are made to divine revelation, to a "natural law" available to reason, to moral intuition, to the inherent demands of reason,[6] to
common sense, and to explicit or implicit contracts.

Appeals to contracts are especially common in a pluralist,
democratic society, because even those who deny that we can *discover*
our rights and duties (in revelation, intuition, or reason) agree that we
can *create* them by entering into contracts. To enter into a contract is to
perform a symbolic action—whether written, spoken, or otherwise gestured—that changes moral reality; it literally creates responsibilities and
privileges that did not exist before the interaction. But how many of our
moral or even legal rights and duties can be traced to our voluntarily entering into such contracts? Sometimes thinkers of a libertarian bent will
try to restrict our rights and duties only to the contracts we explicitly accept, but more often they will include contracts we implicitly accept,
such as the social contract we accept by using the privileges and resources of our society. The difficulty lies in specifying the rights and duties we have implicitly accepted. Pointing to an actual social contract,
such as a constitution, helps to specify only our legal rights and duties.
But even those who are tempted to reduce morality to legality are
troubled by the fact that legal constitutions can be and often should be
changed. If such changes—or, for that matter, the original writing of constitutions—are to avoid arbitrariness, we need some guidance about appropriate laws and obligations. Sometimes contract theorists rely for this
guidance simply on the enlightened self-interest of the contractors. In
the seventeenth century, Thomas Hobbes argued that self-interested
people should contract with an absolute sovereign, or else life would be

---

6. Both deontologists (Gewirth) and utilitarians (Hare) have argued that reason
itself demands their particular moral theories, theories that go well beyond those minimal
negative duties that others have argued are all that reason can provide.

nasty, brutish, and short. Today thinkers in Hobbes's tradition are more likely to be libertarians, arguing for a minimal state and for those minimal "side-constraints" (Nozick, 29), or negative rights and duties, that individuals would agree to so that they can pursue their own interests without bumping into each other's rights too hard.

The problem with relying on self-interested bargaining in establishing rights and duties is that the agreed-on rules are likely to favor those in the strongest bargaining position—namely, the powerful and the gifted. In his influential book *A Theory of Justice* (1971), John Rawls has developed an alternative—Kantian—version of social contract. He argues that principles of social justice are acceptable insofar as they can be unanimously accepted in a situation of fair choice, a situation in which no contractor has an unfair bargaining advantage. Assuming that people do not deserve the strengths or weaknesses they receive at birth, Rawls argues that, since these are the very advantages or disadvantages that put people in a strong or weak bargaining position, it would be unfair to choose principles when the contractors know each other's strengths and weaknesses. Principles chosen by self-interested contractors in such conditions would discriminate against the disadvantaged contractors. Since the latter do not deserve their disadvantages, such discrimination would be as morally arbitrary (and therefore as unjust) as discriminating against people on the basis of their color or caste.

Thus, Rawls argues, a situation of fair choice would be one in which "no one knows his place in society, his class position or social status, nor does anyone know his fortune in the distribution of natural assets and abilities, his intelligence, strength, and the like" (Rawls, 12). The contractors would know that various types of people—brilliant people and retarded people, healthy people and sickly people, religious fundamentalists and atheists, rich and poor, black and white, male and female, and so on—would be in the community, but a hypothetical "veil of ignorance" would prevent each of them from knowing which type of person he or she is. Thus the self-interested contractors would have to treat all other contractors as ends-in-themselves, because no contractor would know which type of person he or she was until after the contract was agreed on and the veil of ignorance lifted. McFall and Shimp would know that sometimes people would need bone marrow from others and that sometimes the needy would be tempted to coerce the others to give it, but they would have to agree on a policy about bone-marrow transplants (or, at least, principles on which the policy would be based) without knowing whether they would be donor or recipient or neither. Rawls argues that under these hypothetical but fair conditions, two basic principles would be unanimously chosen:

- First: each person is to have an equal right to the most extensive basic liberty compatible with a similar liberty for others.
- Second: social and economic inequalities are to be arranged so that they are both (a) reasonably expected to be to everyone's advantage and (b) attached to offices and positions open to all under conditions of fair equality of opportunity. (Rawls, 60)

These principles have become quite influential because they seem to avoid the difficulties of restricting our morality to self-interest, autonomy, or utility, basing it instead on a hypothetical contract that rational people can accept. The first (and primary) principle calls for strong liberty rights, or negative rights of noninterference. The second principle calls for a limit on how much advantaged people can exploit or ignore disadvantaged people; the latter have entitlement rights (or positive rights to be helped), especially to those community resources that give them a more equal opportunity to meet life's demands. This principle can be used to reinforce the claim of Chapter Six that all persons have the right to a minimum level of medical care.

Of course, not everyone agrees with Rawls. Libertarians think he emphasizes equality at the price of autonomy, while socialists think he allows too much inequality, and everyone wonders just how actual people can don his hypothetical veil of ignorance and how actual economic and social systems can approximate his hypothetical contract. Still, his theory is a good example of how the social-contract tradition can argue for hypothetical conditions in the contracting and thereby argue democratically for a quite broad and plausible deontological moral theory.

In concluding our brief summary of Western ethical thought, we should notice more than just the differences and the debates; we should also notice the possibilities for agreement. We noticed earlier that Judge Flaherty's decision in the McFall-Shimp case could be justified on both rule-utilitarian and deontological grounds. And a utilitarian and a deontologist have jointly written a helpful and influential textbook on medical ethics, a book in which there is solid agreement on the importance and implications of certain basic principles, even if there is disagreement over their grounding and ranking (Beauchamp and Childress). It is not unusual for medical professionals to agree that producing good consequences, avoiding the infliction of harm, and respecting autonomy are three important principles that should guide medical decision-making. Sometimes these principles are presented as a sort of neutral logic for moral-conflict resolution (Engelhardt), and at other times they're presented as a common-denominator morality (Beauchamp and Childress).

Sometimes they're presented from a utilitarian (Brandt) or deontological (Gewirth; Donagan) perspective; at other times they're presented as *prima facie* principles that are in tension with each other (Ross; Beauchamp and Childress; Engelhardt). The following section will suggest that many of the theories we have considered can be seen as one-sided developments of Christian covenantal ethics.

Covenantal Ethics

The previous chapter suggested that the biblical story of creation, fall, and redemption gives Christians a framework for understanding history and human nature, and that this framework in turn provides a perspective for cultivating appropriate moral virtues and understanding appropriate moral principles. For Christians, the central moral questions have to do with the appropriate responses to God's creative and redemptive activity and to the activities of those creatures who image God. The previous chapter also claimed that imaging God involves our being created in essential relationship with God, with our own selves, with other persons, and with the rest of creation.

As do many Christians, especially those in the Reformed tradition, we think that the idea of *covenant* best conveys the moral nature of these relationships.[7] Covenant is a central motif in the Bible. Indeed, the Bible's unifying theme is the covenants between God and God's people. Sometimes God covenanted with people simply by promising to do or not to do certain things. Thus God promised Noah and all living creatures not to destroy the world with another flood (Gen. 9:8-17), promised Abraham to make of him a great nation (Gen. 12:1-3), and promised David to establish his line forever (2 Sam. 7:11-17). These covenants did not specify the appropriate human responses, but in the covenant at Sinai (Exod. 19:1-9; Deut. 4:1-14) God reminded the people of past deliverance, promised that they would be God's holy people, and then stated the law that would shape them as a distinctive people. Whenever the law was treated as a commercial contract, as a way of earning salvation rather than as a way of being a responsive and holy people, the prophets had to remind Israel that multiplying the animal sacrifices and the rituals and

---

7. Joseph Allen's *Love and Conflict: A Covenantal Model of Christian Ethics* is an excellent discussion of covenantal ethics. See also G. Beach's "Covenantal Ethics." W. May's "Code and Covenant" and *Physician's Covenant*, R. Veatch's "Case for Contract" and *Theory of Medical Ethics*, B. Brody's "Legal Models," and D. Sturm's "Contextuality and Covenant" are important contributions to covenantal ethics as it applies to medical practice.

obeying the letter of the law while violating its spirit were no substitute for being loving, just, and merciful and living in a spirit of thanksgiving to God. These reminders did not prevent Israel from violating the Sinai covenant, and eventually Jeremiah prophesied that God would make a new covenant with his people, one in which the law would be written on their hearts, one in which God would forgive them their iniquity (Jer. 31:31-34). The New Testament (or New Covenant) specifies the establishing of this gracious covenant through the life, death, and resurrection of Jesus and teaches that Christians can participate in it by partaking of the Lord's Supper and becoming disciples of Christ. The apostle Paul constantly has to warn the church that discipleship is not a matter of obeying the letter of the law but of forming one's character out of gratitude to God and in accord with those virtues (especially charity) that mark a peaceful body of Christ. Thus the Bible portrays covenantal ethics as the appropriate response to God's creative and reconciling work, a response that involves accepting one's call to discipleship, to the rewards and responsibilities of being a member of God's body in the world.

Human covenants are not all-encompassing, as is the call to discipleship, and their origins are not as one-sided as is God's covenanting with us. But human covenants, such as those between husband and wife, parents and children, and teacher and student, share at least three features with God's covenants (Joseph Allen, 32; Beach, 113). First, they are rooted in events or actions, in gifts given or in mutual entrustments whereby persons become vulnerable to one another. Second, covenanting puts people in moral community with each other, a community in which both the common good and the good of each individual member are sought. Thus individuals' identities are shaped by their communities—they *are* their caring relationships—and communities' identities are shaped by the individuals the communities encompass. Third, covenants, with their identity-shaping privileges and responsibilities, tend to endure over time and are influenced by new developments in unspecifiable and open-ended ways. Moreover, the actions and events that affect the covenantal relationship are perceived and described differently than they would be without the covenant. Consider, for example, how spouses become vulnerable to each other in the identity-shaping covenant of marriage and how the sickness or success of one of them is perceived and responded to in ways influenced by the nature of the marriage. Of course, the entrusting in most covenants is not as intimate or wide ranging as that in marriages, but even the weaker covenant among citizens of a nation, for example, can affect how past and current events are perceived and how appropriate responses are determined.

These three features of covenants distinguish them from contracts or at least from the commercial contracts most familiar to us.[8] Notice that voluntariness plays a somewhat different role in covenants than it does in contracts. Covenanting with marriage vows, for example, is often perceived not as mere choice but as appropriate response to earlier shared experiences. And even if the vows are largely voluntary, the responsibilities they imply depend on the circumstances that future events and deeds produce. The implications of vowing fidelity in sickness and in health, for better or for worse, are largely beyond the knowledge and control of those so vowing. And parents who have heard the frustrated cry "I didn't ask to be born" know that the parent-child covenant is not completely voluntary either; it evolves as a response to events that not everyone asked for. Since how we respond to these events is not predetermined, the character of the covenant will be shaped by our freedom, but the demands that elicit the response are often outside our control. Thus the covenant model recognizes that responsibilities are not just voluntarily contracted between individual atoms, between autonomous selves that reach out to one another when it suits mutual self-interest. Rather, the corporate and historical dimensions of our existence cause some responsibilities to *bear down* on us, eliciting certain commitments that are seen as appropriate and demanded. We saw that rule utilitarians and deontologists sometimes try to underscore this aspect of morality by referring to the *role-relatedness* of responsibilities; "my station and its duties" are different when I'm a wife, when I'm a mother, and when I'm a stranger.

Contracts usually state explicitly the relevant rights and obligations of all parties involved, but anyone who has thought about writing up a marriage contract or a contract between a pastor and a congregation knows the difficulty of explicitly stating in contractual language what are really covenantal responsibilities. Some of them might be easily listed, such as who does the dishes or how many Sundays a pastor must be in the pulpit, but it is impossible and ludicrous to specify the meaning of "fidelity through sickness and health, for better or for worse," or the amount of time a pastor must spend with each bereaved family.

One of the reasons that those bonded in covenant cannot explic-

---

8. R. Veatch argues that covenants are contracts and tries to include within his contract model of ethics some of those features we claim are distinctly covenantal. W. May argues for a sharp distinction between contracts and covenants. The two concepts are open-ended enough that it would be difficult to legislate terminology, but we believe that our (and May's) distinction between the two types of relationships is socially and morally important regardless of how they are labeled. Notice that nothing we say implies that all contracts are written or that all covenants are unwritten.

itly list all the rights and duties of those in the covenant is that, since covenants generally involve elements of gift and indebtedness, there is often an incommensurability between the gift and any efforts to pay for it. William May cites an example from William Faulkner's novel entitled *Intruder in the Dust* (May, *Physician's Covenant*, 120): a black man saves a white boy's life, and the boy tries to compensate by giving him all his money—seventy cents. It is not the small amount that is ludicrous; what is ludicrous is the boy's trying to make money commensurate with the gift he received. Even saving the black man's life from racists, which the boy later feels obliged to do, is not so much a payment of the debt as a recognition that the gift established an ongoing covenant of mutual helping. If there are limits to the mutual privileges and responsibilities of those in covenant, they are more likely to be realized in a concrete situation than stated in a document.

Often the effort to calculate our covenantal responsibilities—to interpret them contractually—results in a paradoxical maximizing and minimizing of them. We noticed that the Old Testament prophets had to warn Israel repeatedly that maximizing the number of animal sacrifices and rituals was still to undervalue their debt to God for life and salvation. And the apostle Paul had to warn the Galatians that depending on law obedience (which certainly seemed an improvement over animal sacrifices and rituals) paradoxically undervalued both the gift and the debt. If salvation has to be paid for, then it is no longer a gift. Furthermore, even perfect obedience could not pay off the debt. The only appropriate response in the covenant of grace is to dedicate one's whole life, promptly and sincerely, out of gratitude and love. Of course, our covenants with each other are not as all-embracing as our covenant with God, but they are analogous. Parents, for example, might be almost as insulted by a child that tries infinitely hard to earn their love through perfect obedience as they would be by one who tries to substitute conniving ritualistic flattery for obedience. Parents would say of both children that they are trying to prove the wrong thing, that they should think of themselves as beloved children in grateful covenant, not as hired servants under calculated contract. Of course, children and parents have responsibilities toward each other, as do spouses and friends. But when these responsibilities have to be addressed in terms of legalistically stated rights and duties—as they sometimes do — we know that something has gone wrong with the covenant and that it is being reduced to a contract.

Implicit in what was earlier listed as the third feature of covenants is another reason why it is difficult to reduce covenantal responsibilities to explicit contractual obligations: since many covenantal relationships endure over time, they have a changing character, depending on events, decisions, and developments. To contradict a line from Shakespeare, love is not love which alters *not* when it alteration finds. At least the expression of love must change—as a child grows, for example, or as a friendship develops. In a covenantal union, the question is not what are the child's, parent's, spouse's, friend's, or patient's eternally valid rights; the question is what are his or her temporally changing needs and gifts, and how can I appropriately respond with help, love, respect, or discipline? So covenantal living shapes responsibilities, and responsibilities shape covenantal living, and both are shaped by events that impinge on them, but it is extremely difficult to legalistically list the ways in which this happens.

We saw that parties to a contract can be treated as ends-in-themselves and not merely as means to others' ends. Since they voluntarily enter the contract, they are respected as givers and hearers of reasons; their decisions as stated in the contract are respected even when others think that violating their decisions would be in the best interests of those who made them. We saw that it is this feature of contracts that leads some moral theorists to use the contract as an appropriate model for moral relationships in a pluralistic society which democratically assumes all persons are equal. Covenantal partners are also respected as givers and hearers of reasons and as ends-in-themselves. However, covenantal thinking does not base this respect on the assumption that those in covenant are always equal partners. Equality may be a goal in covenants, but it is not always a starting point, because conditions such as illness, immaturity, and differing expertise can make covenanted people quite unequal. Perhaps they are equal in dignity and worth, but they are not always equal in their ability to express that dignity and worth. So the inequality of people is as relevant to covenantal responsibilities as is their equality. The increased vulnerability of one partner automatically implies greater responsibility on the part of the other. Therefore, covenanting can be very different from the sort of bargaining for a contract that exploits the vulnerability of the other party.

Thus professionals who have a covenant model for their relationships with their clients or patients can respect the latter's autonomy, even when it is diminished, by caring about their clients' or patients' vulnerability rather than exploiting it. Moreover, such professionals will recognize that individuals are in covenantal solidarity with others and will sometimes use that solidarity to pursue an individual's best interests when that individual's choice-making is impaired. That covenantal solidarity can be an avenue to an individual's best interest is simply a recognition of the communal dimension of personal existence. Deep, caring relationships are not just a secondary feature of individual atoms; "no man is an island," and we *are* our caring relationships. They shape us and help give us our identity. So covenantal ethics recognizes both that we are essentially social beings and that all of us are unique individuals with a worth and a dignity of our own. And, in a Christian context, it recognizes that the appropriate response to each unique individual includes both the disposition toward nurturing love and the disposition to stand back and respect an individual giver and hearer of reasons as one created in God's image.

Not all covenants are the same. It is useful to distinguish between "the inclusive covenant" and "special covenants" (Joseph Allen, 39). Christians believe that they are in covenant with God and with all of creation. From this *inclusive* covenant flow the responsibilities and privileges of being a child of God, a neighbor to anyone we meet, and a steward over the rest of creation. This covenant is formed solely by God's gifts of creation and redemption, although we must use our freedom in responding to these gifts. God provides guidance but also takes the risk of not forcing the obedience that is the fulfillment of our freedom. Membership in *special* covenants is more limited than that of the inclusive covenant. Many special covenants arise out of voluntary agreements between people, although, as with the inclusive covenant, we are born into some special covenants that we did not originally make. Thus the membership of some covenantal communities, including those of family, congregation, and even a physician's family practice, can be enlarged or reduced by birth, adoption, or death without everyone's so choosing.

The privileges and responsibilities of special covenants are sometimes solely a matter of mutual agreement, but often they are dictated by the inherent nature of the relationship and the needs and opportunities that arise as the covenant endures across time. Health professionals, for example, have the responsibility for deciding and announcing the goals of their practice and the guidelines they will follow. But the previous chapter noted that the nature of their relationship with ill or dying persons dictates that their goals and guidelines must also be shaped by the distinctive situation and needs caused by illness, as well as by the progress of their patients through their life spans. And Chapter Ten will argue that if the medical profession fails to serve the distinctive needs of the dying by deciding that curing is its only goal, it neglects its responsibility by not appropriately responding to events.

We can now notice how the main currents of Western ethics, summarized in the previous section, incorporate important aspects of covenantal ethics, even if they do so in one-sided ways. First, covenantal ethics has an idea about the natural end of human existence and about the virtues appropriate to that end, an idea we also see in the ethics of the ancient Greeks (who held the first version of teleological ethics we summarized).

Of course, in covenantal ethics the end is not an Aristotelian ideal of rational contemplation, as it was for the Greeks. Although reasoning is important to how we image God, it serves more as a *means to caring* than as an intrinsic good. The virtues of a thoughtful steward must conduce to more than just the life of the mind. Second, covenantal ethics is interested in doing good, an emphasis reflected in utilitarianism. Of course, to do unto others as you would have them do unto you is not simply to maximize preference satisfaction, but it certainly is more than a morality of side constraints that merely respects others' negative rights. And "love your neighbors" does not imply that love is an intrinsic good the production of which must be maximized, but it certainly does imply a concern for our neighbors' happiness and welfare that goes beyond simply not treading on them. Moreover, covenantal ethics recognizes the inherently social nature of persons, another emphasis we see in utilitarianism. Although it does not reduce an individual to an expendable part of the whole, it does see that a person's welfare is often best sought in conjunction with the welfare of those whose deep, caring relationships help constitute that person's identity. Although it does not find it expedient that one person should die for the people (because it avoids doing evil that good may come), it does allow numbers to count when considering a just distribution of basic goods, as we will argue in Chapter Six. Third, the deontological viewpoint has an affinity with covenantal ethics. Members of a covenant are valued as unique individuals. Being reverenced as imagers of God, they are respected as ends-in-themselves. This means that their autonomous choice-making can count for more than others' ideas of what is good for them, that what deontologists call their *rights* must be respected, although covenantal ethics is more likely to talk about reverence, respect, dispositions, and responsibilities than about contractual rights and duties.

Although covenantal responsibilities derive from gifts and mutual entrusting and cannot be reduced to contractual duties, contracts can have at least two important subsidiary roles. First, many of our interactions are meant to be carefully limited to certain privileges and obligations. When we buy a car, we want a very explicit statement about what is covered by the warranty and what we must do to keep the warranty valid. We do not necessarily expect or desire to begin a vague covenant of mutual entrustment with the dealer. Limited contractual negotiations are perfectly acceptable, even when mistrust is not an issue, because they help all participating parties to be very clear about the details of strictly limited interactions. Probably some professional and therapeutic relationships should be limited in a tightly contractual way, but it is sad when all professional and human interactions are so treated.

The second subsidiary role that contracts can play derives from the fallen character of human entrustments. The most important and well-intentioned of covenants can break down because of sin, ignorance, or incompetence. As we will note later in this chapter, when breakdowns occur, we should think first of restoration and reconciliation rather than compensation and punishment. But sometimes the rupture cannot be healed, and people begin talking through third parties—malpractice or divorce lawyers. At such a point, the bare bones of the covenant must be examined—not for resuscitation but for guidance about the minimal duties and privileges implied in the earlier entrustment. Even when the covenant does not rupture, fallen spouses, preoccupied parents, overly busy professionals, confused clients, and rebellious children sometimes need to be reminded of the minimal claims that can be made, claims that can be asserted as rights rather than requested as charity. Thus a covenantal model for the moral life recognizes that contractual-rights-and-duties thinking, even of a minimalist sort, plays several legitimate roles in our social and moral life, though it will never imply that these minimal rights and duties are sufficient for the moral life.

Precisely what are the basic Christian covenantal dispositions and responsibilities? There is no easy way to classify or even list them. Christians have always felt that the list of cardinal virtues inherited from the Greeks — prudence, justice, courage, and temperance — was incomplete, and they have added the theological virtues of faith, hope, and love. But patience, piety, reverence, humility, gratefulness, trustworthiness, and fidelity also seem to be important Christian virtues, and it is not clear that any of them is simply implicit in any of the other virtues just cited. Moreover, prudence can be in tension with love, and patience with justice (and so on), so a list of virtues or principles—even a complete list—would not yet be a ranking of them. But only a ranking of them would enable one to avoid the moral perplexity that occurs when one's virtues or principles come into conflict. And, of course, the meanings of such terms as "prudence," "humility," and "love" can be quite unclear and can vary quite widely. These difficulties imply that Christians probably would find it impossible to agree on an ethical system that would provide a clear-cut answer to all moral problems.

But Christians are not without biblical guidance. First, Jesus reaffirmed the old covenant's assertion that love is fundamental (Deut. 6:5). Moreover, he emphasized that love for God cannot be isolated from love for neighbor (Matt. 22:37-40; Mark 12:29-31). Second, by linking this injunction with the parable of the good Samaritan, Jesus made it clear that love is a responsibility of the inclusive covenant and is not to be restricted to special covenants. The scope of a Christian's love must extend to strangers and not just to family and friends. Third, the apostle Paul reasserts the primacy of love but also notes that faith and hope are important Christian dispositions (1 Cor. 13:13). This addition is important because it underscores the points that what persons believe love (or morality) requires of them will depend on what they believe is happening in the world and that the latter belief is decisively influenced by their religious faith and hope. As we suggested in the previous chapter, the belief that those whom we love are imagers of God will condition how we love them; in particular, we will discern the relevance of respect and humility in our caring for others.

This point can be generalized: covenantal ethics is loving response to those with whom we are in caring relationships, and the appropriateness of our responses (responsibilities) is discerned in the context of our religiously influenced beliefs about human nature and history. As we will notice in later chapters, distinctive beliefs about creation, fall, redemption, and resurrection can condition our decision about what is appropriate caring. People without these beliefs can care for others, of course, but determining the appropriate caring response can be greatly affected by whether one's ultimate hope is in God or in, say, science.

Are there any rights and responsibilities that ought to be recognized by all people, regardless of their theological beliefs? Yes; we have already seen that some covenantal privileges and responsibilities coincide with the minimal rights and duties recognized by the narrowest of contractual traditions. They can be thought of as inalienable rights and strict duties, such as the right to life and the duty not to inflict harm on others. Perhaps things have gone wrong when we need to *claim* rights or duties or when we need to *coerce* others to recognize them, but things do go wrong. Moreover, there are certain covenantal elements so fundamental to persons and societies that everyone recognizes them. For example, the basic elements of the inclusive covenant—rights and duties concerning life and liberty—are listed in almost all national constitutions. In the Western world, the most easily agreed-on rights and duties tend to be the negative ones of noninterference and not inflicting harm. Perhaps this agreement reflects a one-sided individualism that posits the individual as prior to community rather than in relationship with it. It may also reflect the view that in a peaceable pluralist society, liberty should be impinged upon and harm should be inflicted only to protect the innocent from being harmed. As we noted earlier, this view can extend the notions of liberty and harm enough to recognize that sometimes a failure to help the helpless is an infliction of harm,[9] as when

9. But confusion can result when the fierce Western defense of rights and freedoms is combined with a very broad Marxist notion of what those rights and freedoms are.

parents fail to nurture children or professionals fail to abide by a contract. Thus the most basic covenantal privileges and responsibilities often overlap constitutionally recognized rights and obligations. But, of course, most of the responsibilities that covenantal people would discern as appropriate in a given situation could not even be listed in a constitution, much less enforced by the state.

Probably the best way to think of covenantal responsibilities is to picture them on a spectrum, with minimal, legally enforceable ones at one end of the spectrum and, at the other end, those requiring heroic sacrifice for the sake of another's well-being. In the middle will be responsibilities such as truthfulness and civility that are morally mandated but not legally enforceable unless they are part of special roles or contracts. Throughout the spectrum, both the awesome respect appropriate toward imagers of God and the nurturing compassion appropriate toward the vulnerable should be sufficient motives for covenanted people. But at one end the state's sword power (its right and duty to use coercion, including its power to tax) provides added motivation, whereas at the other end the power of gratitude and the inspiring stories of good Samaritans and shepherds who lay down their lives for their sheep must be sufficient incentives. To coerce all covenantal responsibilities would be not only unworkable (imagine trying to strap down David Shimp for a bone-marrow transplant) but also destructive to the covenantal responsibility and disposition to freely nurture and respect others out of gratitude, love, and awe. To equate covenantal responsibilities with legal duties or even moral duties would constrict moral character and risk substituting law for grace and gratitude.

A few weeks after Shimp refused to give him bone marrow, Robert McFall died. (Whether the bone-marrow transplant would have saved McFall was uncertain.) His last request was that his family forgive Shimp. When Shimp heard about McFall's death, he said, "I could throw up right now. I feel terrible about Robert dying, but he asked me for something I couldn't give. That's all I can say now. I feel sick" (Beauchamp and Childress, 316). We may infer that, although not all was well

---

This can be seen in certain United Nations documents, such as the Universal Declaration of Human Rights, which combines Western notions of equality before the law and prohibition of torture and arbitrary arrest (Articles 5 and 9) with full-blown positive rights to leisure and holidays with pay (Article 24), and the Constitution of the World Health Organization, which in its preamble claims that "complete physical, mental, and social well-being" is "one of the fundamental rights of every human being." A covenantal model of individuals in community will certainly recognize that the leisure and well-being of everyone is part of our inclusive covenantal responsibilities but will avoid collapsing all those responsibilities into strict rights and duties enforceable by the sword-power of the state.

in the McFall-Shimp extended family, in both Shimp and McFall there remained a sense of covenanted relationship and the discerning of appropriate responses to each other's needs. One may wonder what might have happened if, instead of using the strong but limited arm of the law (for which he should perhaps have sought forgiveness from Shimp), McFall had appealed to covenantal considerations. If so, McFall might have come to recognize that Shimp was in caring relationship not just with McFall but also with Shimp's mother and his wife (who reportedly was upset that Shimp underwent the initial tissue-compatibility test without asking her). The task of reconciliation, then, would have been perceived as more subtle and much wider than the task of aiming the law at Shimp alone. Of course, including Shimp's mother and wife in an effort at reconciliation might not have resulted in a favorable outcome, but then neither did the lawsuit. At least a less legalistic appeal could have highlighted the fact that people both show and shape their characters and self-identities as well as influence their futures by their responses when others' lives and needs impact upon their own. When it is really a gift that is being requested (and not a refraining from harming), appeal to covenantal discernment rather than a legalistic reinterpretation (that would allow coercion) is not only more appropriate; it is also less likely to leave a bad taste.

　　Christians, of course, use the Bible to think through the responsibilities not only of the inclusive covenant but also of the most important of the special covenants, such as those between parents and children, wife and husband, and even physician and patient. The Bible guides us in appropriate response to God's actions as well as in obedience to God's commands and in imitation of God's example. So when we consider God's covenantal caring, we consider it as an example we are commanded to imitate, and we also consider the appropriate response to it. We see not only that God's love is an inclusive love that binds us together in community but also that it is an individuating love that is affectionate toward each of us in our uniqueness. It is portrayed as a mother's love: "Can a woman forget her sucking child, that she should have no compassion on the son of her womb?" (Isa. 49:15). Now, a mother's love cannot be reduced either to a self-giving, self-sacrificing love *(agape)* or to a love that is drawn out by and takes delight in its object *(eros)*. So, too, a covenantal relationship that is all philanthropic self-sacrifice, that is all noble pity without empathy or liking for the other, is not as godlike as it is sometimes thought to be. Another point is that just as a mother loves each child as an individual who, in an important sense, is irreplaceable, so the divine shepherd is portrayed as being concerned about the one lamb that is lost and not just about the ninety-nine that are safe in the sheepfold.

Moreover, God's love endures over time, failing not even when we are unfaithful. Isaiah portrays God as our husband, who is definitely hurt by our unfaithfulness but whose instinct for reconciliation heals the rupture: "For a brief moment I forsook you, but with great compassion I will gather you" (54:7). When contracts are broken, we think first about justice, compensation, and punishment; when covenants are ruptured, we think first about restoration, reconciliation, and healing. Reconciliation, of course, is not mere indulgence, and healing can involve the painful resetting of broken bones or the traumatic excising of cancerous growth.

Finally, God's love seeks to meet our fundamental needs, especially when we are most vulnerable. The parable of the good Samaritan is just one example of the biblical bias toward those who need care, including medical care. God does help those who help themselves, and he does not condone laziness, but his care is especially for those who cannot help themselves.

Two cautions are in order when we use the divine covenant as a model for human covenants. The first is that we are neither gods nor messiahs, and a relationship in which one finite person is expected to be or tries to be the lord and savior of another is doomed to idolatry, exhaustion, and disappointment. The next chapter will apply this warning especially to medical professionals. The second caution is that the divine covenant is not simply a model; it expresses a reality that motivates and conditions all other covenants. To lose this transcendent context for our human covenants is to lose an important motivation for living up to the responsibilities of the inclusive covenant and an important restriction on our special covenants. Children of God—and disciples of Christ—have a motive for loving and respecting one another and also a locus for ultimate loyalty and fidelity that avoids the pitfalls of giving ultimate allegiance to finite creatures, who cannot carry such weight.

Many people, including many patients and colleagues of Christian medical professionals, will not base their morality on covenantal ethics, much less use the divine covenant as a model for human covenants. Given what we have said about the affinities between covenantal ethics and its main alternatives, it should not surprise us that sometimes those using an alternative outlook will simply reach a similar decision by a different route. But given what we have said about the differences between outlooks, we can expect some important disagreements. The next section discusses how to respond to disagreement in a pluralist society.

Respect, Tolerance, and Cooperation

Diversity and the contradiction of basic convictions have been with us from the dawn of human history, but the effort to include such diversity within one political boundary—to avoid making martyrs out of those thought to be wrong—is quite recent and, even today, far from universal. A good, workable pluralist society not only contains diversity but also seeks to handle disagreement in a civilized way—by appealing to the rationality of the disputants, to their respect for alternative viewpoints, and to the complexity of value systems and value-laden issues (Newman, 70). We must now ask when Christians can respect alternatives, when they can tolerate them, and when they can cooperate with them. We begin with the attitude of respect.

Engaging in public debate forces us to recognize standards for the respectability of positions, standards that apply to the way a belief is arrived at and defended as well as to its content. These standards may vary somewhat among individuals, but they are likely to include such common-sense criteria as consistency, clarity, comprehensiveness, plausibility, and practicability — criteria that are largely intellectual but not without a moral bite as well.[10] Thus we can respect many alternative positions without falling into the traps of thinking that everybody is right (relativism) or that nobody is right (nihilism) or that nobody knows who is right (skepticism) or that, at bottom, everybody is saying the same thing. When a position meets the common-sense criteria to a sufficient degree and the holder of the position is willing to publicly defend it, taking objections seriously and appealing to reasonable standards of adequacy, we can see it as a respectable position, even if we are convinced it is wrong. We can endorse its adequacy without endorsing its truth (Rescher, 243); we can agree that an intelligent person of goodwill can argue for it, though we ourselves argue against it. Thus an attitude of respect toward a position one thinks is wrong is the willingness to say, "I disagree with your position, but your defense of it convinces me that it is reasonable."

If we combine this definition with the belief that, when they are being reasonable, people should follow their own consciences, we can also think that people should try to do what they think is right even though we think they are wrong.[11] As explained later in this section, this

---

10. Can a position simultaneously be intellectually impeccable and morally reprehensible? Not according to those who believe that reason itself demands a substantive morality. But if they are wrong, then the criteria for "respectability" must include something about minimal moral plausibility in addition to intellectual acceptability.

11. Can we believe that other people are wrong and simultaneously tell them that they ought to try to do what they think is right? ("Try to" must be included because,

attitude is compatible with our trying to prevent them from doing what they think is right, a fact which underscores the point that half-truths can be perceived as dangerous even when they are also perceived as respectable. For example, a Christian physician can respect the position of Jehovah's Witnesses who refuse to allow their children blood transfusions and at the same time be intolerant of their position by seeking a court order to override their decision.

Of course, many positions must be perceived as disrespectable. This fact does not entail necessarily perceiving the persons who hold these positions as disrespectable any more than holding a respectable position entails a generalization about the intellect or character of the person holding that position. It is true that holding many disrespectable positions will imply something bad about a person, but it is quite possible to think that intelligent and well-intentioned persons occasionally hold positions which they are unwilling or unable to rationally defend or which seem blatantly inconsistent, implausible, or just plain silly. Of course, not all foolish positions are dangerous; they can even be part of a charming idiosyncrasy. So we can sometimes tolerate and even cooperate with conclusions that we think were arrived at in an intellectually deficient way.

Distinguishing between positions that we regard as dangerous and those we regard as disrespectable helps us recognize that we can vigorously oppose and refuse to cooperate with positions that we see can be rationally defended. Sometimes what divides people is not an intellectual failure or some gross, culpable ignorance or a corrupted consciousness,[12] but a belief or perspective on which intelligent and well-intentioned people may well differ. Thus we can combine our opposition to a position with sincere regard for it and with polite civility toward those who hold it. As the earlier example concerning Jehovah's Witnesses illustrates, understanding this point enables committed people in a pluralist society to forcefully oppose a decision that they respect.

---

if we think their position is respectable but dangerous, we may have to be intolerant of it. The psychological dynamics of such a situation would be analogous to thinking that your opponents should try to win while you are trying to prevent them from winning.) E. Langerak ("Teaching How to Disagree") argues that we can. If he is wrong, then the attitude of respect implies only that the other's position is understandable and plausible but not that the other ought to try to act on it.

12. Sometimes people who are otherwise perfectly decent seem to have been raised in a way that infects them with moral blindness concerning a particular issue—for example, certain slave owners in the antebellum South, Nazis, and racists. The term "corrupted consciousness" might be applied to them, but this category must be used carefully; otherwise most moral disagreements will degenerate into name-calling.

Respect or disrespect for a position is primarily a mental attitude. Tolerance, intolerance, cooperation, and uncooperation are largely behavioral responses to a position or, more precisely, to others' behavior when they are acting in accordance with that position.

A tolerant attitude in effect says, "I disagree with your decision on this matter that I care about, but I will not attempt, directly or indirectly, to interfere with your behavior." Intolerance, of course, does try to interfere with behavior — either directly, through personal force or threat, or indirectly, by trying to make the behavior illegal or proscribed in some way. As the Latin root *tolerare* indicates, tolerance is the *enduring* of something disagreeable, which implies that tolerance concerns something one cares about. So tolerance is neither indifference to nor broad-minded delight in diversity, although the resultant behaviors can sometimes coincide. Religious tolerance, for example, is compatible with taking religion extremely seriously, and to equate it with religious indifference or broad-mindedness is a mistake. Another point is that tolerance, strictly speaking, implies that we think we could proscribe the behavior, so it is not simply resignation at the latter's inevitability. Of course, we might decide that coercion, though possible, would come at too high a price; this decision might elicit a begrudging tolerance, but it would still be tolerance.

Tolerance should not be confused either with the refusal to blame or with forgiveness of the blameworthy; we saw that we can be intolerant of the behavior of Jehovah's Witnesses who refuse to give their young children blood transfusions, yet be very understanding and respectful of their position and refuse to blame them. And we can find blameworthy—even be unforgiving toward—unrepentant rock singers who debase human sexuality, and, at the same time, we should be at least somewhat tolerant of their behavior on the grounds that not everything that is wrong should be made illegal.[13]

A cooperative attitude goes beyond tolerance and says, in effect, "I may disagree with you on this matter, but I will help you do what you think is right." An uncooperative attitude, says, in effect, "My disagree-

13. Tolerance is logically independent of relativism, skepticism, nihilism, and uncertainty (G. Harrison). Indeed, if being tolerant of a certain behavior implies that you think that behavior is wrong, it is incompatible with these views. Our definition states only that one must disagree with the action if one says he or she tolerates it, and disagreement can involve mere disapproval or disliking. In short, it can involve matters of taste. A relativist (who asserts that another person is *right* whenever the other's society thinks so) can find another's behavior obnoxious, as can a skeptic (who thinks no one can know what is right), a nihilist (who thinks there is no right or wrong), or one who is uncertain about a particular issue. So these views are compatible with tolerance. But they are also compatible with intolerance. In fact, the view that nobody knows what is right or wrong on moral

ment with you is such that I refuse to help you do what you think is right."
An uncooperative attitude can range from passive lack of help, such as
that of some conscientious objectors or some nurses who refuse to assist
during abortion, to rather active dissociation, such as public resignation
or whistle-blowing. Even the latter, however, is not necessarily intolerance, which takes steps to coercively interfere with another's behavior.
So cooperation goes beyond tolerance, and intolerance goes beyond an
uncooperative attitude, though there may be borderline cases, such as
when someone threatens to resign or to publicly expose a bad policy.

Cooperation and tolerance should not be confused with compromising one's principles or integrity. There are people who are so
eager to please or to avoid controversy that they go along with actions
they find reprehensible. They become alienated from themselves to
avoid being alienated from others.[14] There are opportunists who sacrifice whatever principles they have in order to get ahead. And there are
moral cowards who cannot resist any significant pressure to conform.
All of these tolerate and cooperate with views they disagree with, but
they do so in an unprincipled way.

Principled tolerance and cooperation are closer to, but not necessarily the same as, pragmatic or utilitarian compromise. In the spirit of
"politics as the art of compromise," we may sometimes agree to a less reprehensible policy in order to avoid the more reprehensible policy that
would result without the compromise. We tolerate the evil of hands getting dirty—perhaps even cooperatively getting our own dirty—to prevent even more evil. People can do this with integrity if they accept some
sort of utilitarian principle that requires them to minimize evil. And non-
utilitarians can do so by appealing to *prima facie* obligations to promote
solidarity, to avoid undermining a basically legitimate institution, or to
use temporary and pragmatic strategy in the pursuit of eventual righteousness.

Christians can respect certain arguments for the latter sort of
compromise, but to evaluate them would require another book (Benjamin). Here we want simply to observe that free, finite, and fallen hearers
and givers of reasons—even redeemed ones—will disagree over the

---

matters can be combined with a strong argument for intolerance toward certain behaviors
(even between consenting adults) on the grounds that only a fragile social consensus holds
society together (Devlin). Whatever historical correlation there may be between relativism,
skepticism, or the loss of moral confidence on the one hand, and, on the other hand, behavior that is similar to behavior elicited by tolerance, the former are logically distinct from
tolerance, and none of them is either necessary or sufficient for it.

14. This paragraph and the next are indebted to conversations with Martin Benjamin and to his manuscript entitled "Compromise and Integrity in Ethics and Politics."

details of covenantal responsibilities involved in both the inclusive and the special covenants. That is why Christians have reason to recognize the appropriateness of various combinations of respect, disrespect, tolerance, intolerance, cooperation, and uncooperation toward those with whom we disagree. If we never respect, cooperate with, or tolerate views that differ from ours on the details, we will alienate ourselves from community and will end up with almost as many states, denominations, and other institutions as we have people. On the other hand, if we always respect, tolerate, and cooperate, no matter how great the disagreement, we will become alienated from ourselves and our God. Sometimes our own integrity will require intolerance of views we respect. Sometimes, especially for professionals, it may require tolerance but uncooperation. Sometimes, when others do the right thing for very wrong reasons, we will find it appropriate to cooperate with views we disrespect.

We noted earlier that the standards for respect have largely to do with intellectual adequacy. The implicit standards for tolerance and cooperation have more to do with the morally relevant effects of the action or policy being proposed. When a certain action or policy puts innocent people not only at risk of not being helped but also at risk of being significantly and irreversibly harmed, only very powerful counterconsiderations should override our responsibility to be uncooperative and intolerant.[15] The position we called *paternalism* in the previous chapter would be intolerant of an action or policy even when only the agent of the action is at risk of such harm. Nonpaternalists would be tolerant in such a case, though perhaps uncooperative. When Jesus said "He who is not with me is against me" (Matt. 12:30), he was referring to those who charged him with devilry; he would not tolerate false accusations against the innocent (even when such accusations were, from a Mosaic perspective, theologically understandable). When he said "He that is not against us is for us" (Mark 9:40), he was referring to the unauthorized and opportunistic casting out of devils in his own name; he would cooperate with, or at least tolerate, another's opposition to evil even when the motivation was suspicious.

The implication of this section is that, in general, we should be uncooperative and intolerant whenever there is significant impingement on basic human rights (those correlated with what we called the minimal-basic-duties side of the covenantal responsibilities spectrum, such as life and basic liberties). We should be uncooperative and intolerant whether

---

15. In such a case one's responsibility to be uncooperative and intolerant can be thought of as a *prima facie* responsibility, one that could be overridden only by stronger moral duties such as the duty not to inflict harm on even more innocent people.

the impingement is motivated by respectable considerations, such as when Jehovah's Witnesses refuse to allow blood transfusions for their children, or by disrespectable ones, such as those sometimes motivating child abuse. On the other hand, we should disagree with (and argue against) but regretfully tolerate some refusals to help others. In such cases we should be tolerant, whether the refusal is motivated by religious principle, such as when a pregnant Jehovah's Witness refuses a blood transfusion for herself (one that would also save the fetus's life), or by less noble motives, such as when Shimp refused to give life-saving bone marrow to McFall. And sometimes we should tolerate but refuse to cooperate with what we regard as violations of what we earlier called the moral mandates in the middle of the spectrum of covenantal responsibility. Conscientious objectors to all violence do this, and many of us do it with respect to those who commit slow suicide through chain smoking or are fanatically addicted to otherwise healthful activities such as music and sports. Sometimes special role obligations and covenantal obligations require intolerance toward activities that others can tolerate or even cooperate with. Thus parents must correct children for even minor violations, and medical professionals must be intolerant of colleagues' gossiping about or deceiving their patients even when such gossip or deception can be tolerated outside the special covenant. Professional ethics often makes strict, legally enforceable duties out of behaviors that the inclusive covenant encourages but regulates only through persuasion.

The question of cooperating with a position with which one disagrees arises most poignantly when one is part of a hierarchical professional team; it arises, for example, when nurses are told to do something they think is wrong. If they are quite uncertain about their own view or if they perceive the resultant harm as minor and reversible or if the person they perceive as harmed requests that the action be done, then their commitment to team solidarity and respect for autonomy can call for cooperation. When professionals cooperate with or tolerate an action or policy that makes them very uncomfortable, they may have the responsibility to act collectively to change the policy that pressures such cooperation. We will notice in the next chapter that professionals accept a collective responsibility to collectively oppose some policies that an individual professional cannot be expected to risk his or her livelihood in opposing alone. In general, the question of cooperation and tolerance calls for a weighing of many types of considerations — personal identity and integrity, professional identity and values, uncertainty surrounding the decision, the limits on opposing givers and hearers of reasons who have their own identities and responsibilities before God, the need for social harmony and professional solidarity, and the obligations to those affected by the decision.

Even when we decide to be personally intolerant of a position, we must ask whether our reasons imply that we should work toward legal intolerance. The latter involves the sword power of the state, which is both powerful and double edged. When we try to use it to convert people to a viewpoint that has well-reasoned opposition—and perhaps sometimes we must—we should recognize that it can turn on us. In general, we should avoid using it unless there is widespread agreement that the evil being outlawed is indeed the intolerable evil that the law says it is. When we criminalize actions not just to prevent clear-cut and intolerable evils (like theft) but also to nurture a distinctive moral character (like the values of monogamy), we need consensus. Otherwise we undermine respect for the law and create chaos, as the American experiment with prohibition showed. Even when we have consensus, we must recognize a *prima facie* responsibility not to impinge on the God-given responsibility for moral choice. And, generally, when our willingness to imprison someone derives from a distinctive theological or religious belief, we must be sure that only an intolerably corrupt consciousness could fail to appreciate that belief; otherwise our holy war may dishonor God by harming those who image God in their choice-making capacities.[16]

Tolerance and cooperation, like fire and secrecy, are as necessary to civilized society as they can be dangerous to it (Bok, *Secrets,* 18; Benjamin, 6). Covenanted people must think hard and pray hard about guidance for appropriate responses to those with whom they disagree, because these decisions are as important as they are difficult. Throughout this volume we give suggestions about appropriate combinations of respect, tolerance, cooperation, and their opposites, but we recognize that some of the most debatable points involve not what one's own view is on some moral issue but how to respond appropriately to those who disagree.

This chapter has attempted to provide a conceptual framework for the remainder of the book. Its overview of current ethical theories, of covenantal ethics, of affinities and differences among them, and of appropriate responses to alternative viewpoints has been lengthy yet has often been concise to the point of being abstract. Our remaining task is to consider the nature of the medical profession and how professionals and others might use this conceptual framework in thinking through some of the problems they confront today.

---

16. A Christian covenantal approach to legislating morality is discussed more fully in A. Verhey's "In Defense of Theocracy." Various combinations of respect, tolerance, cooperation, and their opposites are discussed more fully in E. Langerak's "Teaching How to Disagree" and "Tolerance, Cooperation, and Respect for Wrong Views."

4. *The Character of Medicine*

Medical professionals have every right to be confused about society's ambivalence toward them. In spite of—or, perhaps, because of—their being revered as the high priests in control of the technological mysteries that bring salvation, they are sued as soon as something goes wrong and often accused of incompetence, arrogance, or greed. This chapter argues that an understanding of the character of the medical profession and the privileges and responsibilities inherent in the special covenant it has with society can help us understand public ambivalence toward medical professionals. We will discuss the character of medicine as a practice, as a profession, and as a calling, hoping to illuminate not just the character of medicine but also the character of the relationships medical professionals have with their patients and with one another.

Medicine as a Practice

What do we mean when we call medicine a practice? Alasdair MacIntyre provides a definition of a practice that has received much attention from those writing about the medical profession. Although it is very complicated, we will give his definition and then try to show how attention to its details provides insight into the character of medical practice: "By a 'practice' I am going to mean any coherent and complex form of socially established cooperative human activity through which goods internal to that form of activity are realized in the course of trying to achieve those standards of excellence which are appropriate to, and partially definitive of, that form of human activity, with the result that human powers to achieve excellence, and human conceptions of the ends and goods involved, are systematically extended" (*After Virtue*, 187). Under this definition, not every human activity can be termed a practice because not all human activities are complex and cooperative, nor do all of them have internal goods, and not all of them systematically extend human powers to achieve excellence. MacIntyre says, for example, that tic-tac-toe and planting tulips are not practices, whereas chess and farming are. Of course, there is room for debate about precisely which activities are practices, and probably there are many borderline cases. But we believe that medicine clearly is a practice as defined by MacIntyre and that discussing medicine in terms of the main elements of his definition can help us focus on important aspects of its character.

First, medicine is a *human* activity, subject to all the limitations that mark human beings. Insofar as medicine is a science, it is subject to the limitations of human knowledge. Presently the amount of knowledge encompassed by disciplines such as biology, chemistry, and physics is vast, but it is still limited—perhaps even minute—in comparison with what remains to be learned. So, too, with medicine. Even if physicians could master all that is currently known in medical science, some of the diagnostic and therapeutic decisions they make based upon today's knowledge will no doubt prove to be "wrong" when judged by tomorrow's discoveries. And, of course, no one human being (or, for that matter, no group of human beings like physicians) can know more than a small fraction of the available scientific knowledge, even with the help of data stored on computers. Consequently, we can expect some decisions that can be deemed "wrong" even in the light of currently available knowledge. Such ignorance is not necessarily or even usually the result of sloth, negligence, or ineptitude; it is a consequence of human finitude.

Moreover, medicine is as much an art as a science. Human beings and their illnesses are so complex that physicians generally cannot simply apply scientific generalizations to them, not even generalizations of a refined statistical sort, because particular individuals with their idiosyncratic histories and behaviors can elude classifications. Perhaps medical research tries to deal with universal phenomena, but the practice of medicine must apply that knowledge to particular individuals, who may or may not respond predictably according to any laws of medical science. MacIntyre and Samuel Gorovitz refer to the gap between medical generalizations and individual cases as the "necessary fallibility" (p. 62) of the predictive powers of physicians with regard to an individual patient. Thus, whereas medical science may tell us that female breast cancer has a 20 percent cure rate, the physician must treat a unique individual for whom that cancer has either a 0 percent or a 100 percent chance of cure. This uncertainty pervades medical practice. Different people will respond differently to the same medication. What helps some will not help others. The pertussis vaccine will effectively protect nearly all children from whooping cough, but it will cause severe neurological damage in one out of every million children. There is presently no way to know whether a particular child before a particular physician will be that one-in-a-million child.

Medicine cannot be the exact science which many think it to be. It is a probabilistic effort: the physician can do only what is *probably* the best thing for a given patient and then make adjustments based upon the individual's unique response. As an enterprise inherently bound to unique individuals in a fallen world, medicine will remain a fallible discipline marked by ambiguity and uncertainty. Poor results will sometimes occur, often not the consequence of any person's mistake but rather a manifestation of the unexpected or the unusual.

The inherent uncertainties in human medicine seem so obvious that one wonders why so many people hold unrealistic expectations about medical expertise and why they search for blame and call on malpractice lawyers whenever something goes wrong. Part of the reason for the latter, of course, is that genuine incompetence is sometimes exhibited by medical professionals. However, even when there is no evidence of malpractice, many patients are still the victims of a bad outcome. This fact often moves a victim's sympathetic peers on the jury of a malpractice suit to compensate the victim in the only way currently available—namely, by finding a person or institution at fault and by giving a large award to the victim. One result of this tendency is a malpractice crisis in which compensation to victims is not only very erratic but also very costly, because it promotes high insurance rates and expensive defensive medicine. Perhaps better professional discipline could lower the incidence of genuine malpractice and perhaps a "no-fault" compensation fund could provide a fairer and less expensive procedure than lawsuits for helping victims cope with bad outcomes. But such steps will not in themselves reduce the gap between medical uncertainty and unrealistically high expectations about what medicine can provide.

There is some evidence that the medical profession itself fosters an unjustified sense of medical infallibility. Medical students often seem to be "trained for certainty" both in making decisions and in reassuring patients (Katz, 185). Physicians' confidence, it is often thought, produces a "placebo effect," inspiring patients toward cures that might not occur if patients thought their physicians really did not know exactly what to do (Katz, 189-99). The difficulty for medicine as a human practice is that it must retain a patient's confidence and at the same time recognize medicine's fallibility and educate the patient to recognize it as well. We believe that proper use of "informed consent" (Chapter Two, pp. 57-66) can help medicine walk this tightrope, but we also appreciate the complexity of the problem.[1]

The second element to notice in MacIntyre's definition of a practice is that a practice seeks internal goods. Any practice can share external goods—such as fame and fortune—with other practices and activities, but it also seeks its own internal goods. The character of medicine as a practice depends on the goods sought by that practice. If the primary goal of medicine is the happiness of those who can afford its services, then its character will be different than it will be if medicine's goal is to relieve suffering or fight disease. The goals of medicine have been variously defined, and it is probably futile to insist that all medical professionals have precisely the same aim. Relief of suffering, prolongation of life, assault on disease, restoration of autonomy, and promotion of well-being are all traditional goals. However, we believe that clarity about the character of medicine is enhanced if these goals are understood primarily as ways to restore or maintain the health of patients or, when that is impossible, to provide the palliative care that reduces the suffering of the dying.

In Chapter Two we defined human health as the well-functioning of human beings in their particular physical and social environments. This definition implies that health is a matter of degree and is relative both to individuals' goals and to their environments. For example, a person whose knee aches while running can be called unhealthy if that person's normal functioning includes running. Individuals who have no desire or need to run, however, can hardly be said to be unhealthy by virtue of knowing that their knees would get sore if they did run. Another example can be seen in the presence of the sickle-cell trait, which is the inherited condition of those black people who have a particular "abnormal" hemoglobin molecule. For blacks living in malarial regions the sickle-cell trait is advantageous because the abnormal hemoglobin molecule protects such persons from infection by the malarial parasite. Individuals with the trait experience no symptoms or adverse effects except at very high altitudes. Thus the sickle-cell trait helps

---

1. The article we cited by S. Gorovitz and A. MacIntyre on medical fallibility has elicited much discussion. See M. Bayles and A. Caplan's "Medical Fallibility and Malpractice," a reply by Gorovitz ("Medical Fallibility: A Rejoinder"), and the response by Caplan and Bayles ("A Response to Professor Gorovitz"). See also R. Munson's "Why Medicine Cannot Be a Science," B. Minogio's "Error, Malpractice, and the Problem of Universals," and M. Martin's "On a New Theory of Medical Fallibility." In addition to J. Katz's book, the books by H. Bursztain et al. *(Medical Choices, Medical Chances)* and D. Hilfiker *(Healing the Wounds)* address the problem of physicians and patients sharing and coping with uncertainty.

to maintain a state of health in those who live in malarial regions. In American and European blacks, however, the sickle-cell trait may constitute an unhealthy condition. Since malaria rarely strikes in these regions, the trait loses its adaptive value and can in fact be life-threatening to those who travel by plane. The risk of cabin depressurization at high altitudes has even been used to discourage blacks with this condition from becoming airline pilots or attendants (Kopelman, 144). The degree to which health is relative can be clarified by distinguishing between two aspects of unhealth—disease and illness.[2]

Disease may be thought of as the anatomic, physiologic, or biochemical fact of malfunctioning. It represents a state of deterioration, degeneration, or disturbance of normal life processes. Disease is characterized by the measurable malfunction of anatomical, biochemical, or physiological processes. These are called *malfunctions* because they are of disvalue to the organism under consideration. Although the notion of disease thus involves value judgments, agreement on them requires only a shared view of normal organic functioning. There is enough agreement here that, by and large, diseases are thought to be objectively detectable by any observer who performs the appropriate physical examination, laboratory test, radiologic examination, or diagnostic procedure (Kopelman, 147).

Illness, on the other hand, is the psychosocial perception of being unwell. It is the subjective, personal experience of lost wholeness in which we feel alienated from ourselves. We experience our bodies as other than our own. Illness is characterized by a sense of disorder and loss of control. It is rooted in the subjective human experience of one's existence and may exist in the absence of disease. While defined primarily by the individual, illness may in part be defined socially and culturally. Our sense of being ill is related to our perception that some aspect of our functioning has become impaired. The culture within which one normally functions will thus play a role in defining whether or not a given individual defines himself or herself as ill. Furthermore, many cultures recognize the "sick role" as being a special one in which the individual is exempted from certain responsibilities and obligations.

Illness and disease are two distinct yet interrelated aspects of the state of unhealth. In many cases the patient's sense of being ill represents the manifestation of disease. However, this may not always be the case. Many patients present themselves to physicians with illness complaints

2. Several authors have explored the differences between disease and illness, as well as the influence of culture on the understanding of disease and illness. These include —in addition to L. Kopelman—A. Kleinman et al. and O. Temkin.

for which no disease can be found. It may be the case that an organic cause exists but cannot be perceived by the clinician. On the other hand, the illness may not have a ready biochemical, anatomical, or physiological explanation (Temkin; Kleinman et al.). It is clear that a man incapacitated by headaches for which no organic cause can be found nonetheless experiences dis-ease, even if he is not diseased. Disease may also exist without any concurrent illness, as in the case of asymptomatic sickle-cell anemia and high blood pressure.

Disease and illness are both important aspects of the phenomenon of unhealth. Therefore, to be concerned with health requires attention to both aspects. Just as we must avoid the temptation of reducing the embodied person to either a body or a spirit, we must also avoid reducing the state of unhealth to either disease or illness. It is as embodied persons that human beings experience illness and contract disease. To be concerned with health and unhealth is to be concerned with both disease and illness.

This point has implications for the focus of medicine, which has been the subject of much disagreement and confusion. Most often illness brings patients to seek the help of physicians. Patients seek the help of others precisely because they sense that something is awry and lack the knowledge to deal with that sense of dis-ease. As many as half of these patients have no organic disease (Stoeckle et al.). However, physicians are trained mainly to deal with disease, not with illness. The four years of medical school prepare them to diagnose and treat biochemical and physiological disorders, but often they have little training in addressing patients' experiences of illness. Consequently, while patients focus their attention on the illnesses they experience, physicians often focus on the search for organic disease, becoming frustrated if no measurable abnormality can be found. This communication gap has recently been characterized by Richard Baron's phrase "I can't hear you while I'm listening," referring to physicians' temptation to ignore what patients are telling them in their spirited search for some objective evidence of disease. They may fail to hear the patients' words as they listen intently for abnormal heart sounds. While physicians focus their attention on the cure of disease, they often ignore or forget their patients' experience of disease and the needs entailed by illness. An important remedy for this problem is indicated by our discussion: physicians should remember that, although the distinctive expertise of physicians is the diagnosis and treatment of disease, the basic aim of medicine is health, and that the maintenance and restoration of health require attending to illness as well as to disease.

Two further observations are relevant at this point. The first is that health can be better served by preventive measures than by curative measures. One source suggests that environment, lifestyle, social context, and genetics may contribute up to 94 percent of what constitutes good health, while medical care contributes as little as 6 percent (Childress, "Priorities," 562). Yet 90 percent of the health-care dollar in the United States goes toward medical care. It is time for us to recognize in our spending that the internal good of medicine may be best promoted by measures other than therapeutic intervention. The second observation is that death will inevitably defeat efforts to maintain and restore health; therefore, as we noted in Chapter Two, medical care for the dying must aim not just at maintaining as high a degree of well-functioning as possible but also at comforting those beyond cure. Perhaps physicians should be trained primarily for the cure of diseases, but they should also be trained to recognize when caring requires something other than curing.[3]

Medicine, then, is a human and therefore fallible practice that seeks the good called *health*. MacIntyre's definition of a practice, quoted at the beginning of this section, speaks of standards of excellence appropriate to and partly definitive of a practice. We will discuss the standards of medical practice in the next section, but here we should notice the final dimension of the definition — that the result of a practice is to extend human powers for achieving excellence and to extend human conceptions of the ends and goods involved in achieving human excellence. Achieving human excellence in this broad sense involves cultivating the conditions conducive to human flourishing. In an earlier chapter we defined human flourishing in terms of imaging God; that established, we believe it is important to notice that the good of medicine, like the good of any human practice, is not an end in itself but is subordinate to our calling to be God's representatives and to everything that involves. Health, the good sought by medicine, plays a crucial role in the capacity for human flourishing, and therefore medicine is very important. But health may and must sometimes be risked out of loyalty to God's kingdom, and those who allow the pursuit of health (in themselves or others) to override all their other responsibilities have turned a human practice that should serve other ends into an idol—an idol, moreover, with clay feet.

---

3. That dying people have distinctive medical needs is perhaps the strongest argument that the internal good of medicine is the relief of suffering rather than or in addition to the pursuit of health. Although we worry that such a view is susceptible to some of the same dangers involved in expanding the notion of health to mean "well-being" rather than "well-functioning" (discussed in Chapter Two), we agree that perhaps medicine's main role for dying people is to provide as much comfort as is possible and consistent with a well-functioning coping with dying. We believe that dying is not primarily a medical problem and that medicine's role at the deathbed is important but limited.

Medicine as a Profession

It is perhaps impossible to give a precise definition of a profession,[4] but professions tend to be characterized by requiring extensive training that has a significant intellectual component, by providing service with potential for important good or harm, by licensing and organization, by having a legal monopoly on a service, and especially by having a significant amount of autonomy in deciding what services to provide and how to provide them (Bayles, 7-11). Paul Starr's widely discussed book entitled *The Social Transformation of American Medicine* bears the subtitle *The Rise of a Sovereign Profession and the Making of a Vast Industry*. This phrase is a somewhat tendentious way of calling attention both to what is characteristic of medicine as a profession and to medicine's developing relationship with other organizations. As Starr's book suggests, medicine acquired—especially after its insistence on scientific training—a great deal of autonomy in deciding on its own standards of excellence. Traditionally it also had a great deal of autonomy in deciding on its relationship with the organizations—such as hospitals and nursing homes—that society subsidizes in order to facilitate the providing of medical services. Lately, of course, public suspicions and cost-cutting measures are forcing medicine into institutional relationships that restrict its autonomy and threaten to turn it into a vast industrial complex (Whol) in which corporations, business administrators, insurance companies, and government reimbursement categories influence medical decision-making.

There is a complicated interplay between the medical profession's internal goods—and the standards of excellence appropriate to them—and such external goods as the money received for service provided. Particular payment methods—fee for service rendered, salary level, per-capita prepayment plans—can affect how medical professionals pursue health care. This fact should be a source of concern for both medical professionals and the general public.

For guidance in thinking about the direction in which the medi-

---

4. E. Freidson suggests that the problem of defining professions "is created by attempting to treat profession as if it were a generic concept rather than a changing historic concept, with particular roots in an industrial notion strongly influenced by Anglo-American institutions" (p. 22). H. Wilensky argues that "professionalization" (a process) is the basic category and that the process involves doing something full-time, establishing specialized schools (and associating them with universities), forming an organization, developing a code of ethics, and obtaining legal protection of the organization's licensing privileges. Differences between the scholarly professions (teaching, science) and the consulting professions (law, medicine) complicate efforts to generalize about professions and their relation to other institutions.

cal profession should go, it is useful to recall why medicine is such a socially important profession and why it has a moral dimension. As Stanley Hauerwas argues, an important role of medicine is "to bind the suffering and the nonsuffering into the same community" (*Suffering Presence*, 26):

> What an extraordinary gesture it is for a society to set aside some to dedicate their lives to the cure of the ill. That we do so, I think, is not primarily because we are self-interested and thus want to guarantee that when we are ill we will not be abandoned, but because we are unwilling to abandon others who need help. Therefore medicine as a moral practice draws its substance from the extraordinary moral commitment of a society to care for the ill. Medicine, as many of its critics like to point out, may have little significance for insuring the health of a population. (Effective sanitation is much more important for the health of a population than medicine.) But the care we provide to individuals through the office of medicine is no less morally significant for that. (*Suffering Presence*, 13)

A simple market model for medicine—which claims that medicine is a commodity for sale—implies that the public has a stake in medical ethics only because the public should have something to say about the sort of services provided by those who have been given a legal monopoly over those services. And a social-contract model for medicine—which claims that society contracts with the profession to provide services and to make decisions that may have a moral dimension—implies that the public has a stake in medical ethics whenever the profession's activities impinge on autonomy or other socially important values. But Hauerwas points toward a third reason why the public is interested in what medical professionals think is appropriate or inappropriate in medical decision-making: through the medical profession society is able to express its covenantal relationships with those who are especially vulnerable because of illness and suffering. When there is consensus within the profession, within society, and between the profession and society about the internal goods of medicine, and when the providing of those internal goods is not significantly influenced by demands related to external goods such as payment and efficiency, society can perhaps trust the profession by itself to determine the standards of excellence that characterize sound medical practice. But if that consensus breaks down or if the services that can be provided must be rationed by external constraints, it should not surprise us that the profession will come under external scrutiny and that the potential for mistrust and misunderstanding will rise. The debates over "Baby Doe" regulations and reimbursement schemes, which impose legal and economic considerations on medical decision-making, are just two examples of what happens when consensus about our covenant with the vulnerable breaks down or when external goods become a constraint on internal medical goods.

In these times of mistrust, the medical profession has both a problem and an opportunity. The problem, of course, is that its autonomy is being challenged. The good old days, when people simply trusted medical professionals to do the right thing, are gone. The opportunity is the chance for the profession to exercise leadership in educating the public and the legislators about the goods as well as the limitations of medicine. To do so, medical professionals must be willing to enter the often frustrating debates over economic policy, health-care legislation, and the rights, privileges, and responsibilities of both medical professionals and the public. Probably the time is past when medical professionals can simply strive for excellence in their own work, leaving politics and policy to others. There is too much confusion over what that excellence is or implies, and there are too many external constraints impinging upon medical professionals.

In the dialogue between medical professionals and society, the testimony of individual professionals can be extremely important, as is demonstrated by the writings of Edmund Pellegrino (*Humanism and the Physician* and *A Philosophical Basis of Medical Practice* [with David Thomasma]), Eric Cassell (*Healer's Art*), David Hilfiker (*Healing the Wounds*), Lewis Thomas (*The Youngest Science*), and Peggy Anderson (*Nurse*). But also required is a sense of collective responsibility, the responsibility which cannot be attributed to individual professionals but which pertains to the profession as a whole.[5] It may be argued that professional organizations such as the American Medical Association and the American Nurses' Association have concentrated their energies on the external goods of medicine, such as payment and protecting pro-

---

5. The notion of *corporate* responsibility is ambiguous, falling somewhere between *group* responsibility and *collective* responsibility. Members of a group practice each have individual responsibility for their separate contributions to the activities of the group. Each individual shares a part of the group responsibility. But in complex organizations like a profession or a bureaucracy, there can develop states of affairs or accepted "ways of life" that are undesirable but that cannot be located as the responsibility of any particular individual; the profession or group as a whole is responsible. It is as easy for individuals to duck this sort of collective responsibility as it is important for some individuals to exercise leadership in forcing the collective to confront it. Because there are limits to how much one can expect individuals to risk in trying to change the accepted practices of a collective, it is important for groups of individuals who share a calling or vision about what those activities should be to help each other in confronting the collective. G. Mellema discusses group responsibility in *Individuals, Groups, and Shared Moral Responsibility*. For an analysis of collective responsibility as applied to a medical profession, see J. Muyskens' *Moral Problems in Nursing* (158-67).

fessional turf, but we earlier implied that concern for these issues can often be justified in terms of their indirect relationship to the internal goods of medical practice—to healing and health. For that reason, organizations of medical professionals can be expected to participate in public debate, using the traditional standards of excellence to generate and evaluate proposals for higher standards, deeper obligations, and fairer policies than are currently in place and to resist political and economic pressures that undermine traditional ideals.

Some physicians, for example, have been too accepting of practices—such as certain types of cosmetic surgery and certain uses of medicine in sports—that go *beyond* concern for health as well-functioning. But the American Medical Association has consistently opposed some of the practices that go *against* its traditional ideals. For example, it consistently rejects mercy killing, arguing that even when healers cannot heal, they ought not to relieve suffering by intentionally eliminating the sufferer. And it has insisted that healers not be the hired killers the state uses to carry out legal executions.[6]

Today other issues also deserve the attention of medical professionals rising to meet their collective responsibility. For example, the education of physicians can be cruel and abusive in its demands and not conducive to producing humane and caring practitioners. The problem goes beyond the curriculum revisions that have lately received attention: too often the teachers in charge of developing physicians during medical school and residency years have more research and publishing skills than clinical skills, more skills for scientifically analyzing and diagnosing patients than for compassionately caring for patients and developing healing relationships. Consequently, many emerging physicians have not had ideal role models. Another issue for collective concern is access to medical care for all those who need it. Individual medical professionals and groups of them can provide some "pro bono" services for the needy in their neighborhoods and can even donate time to travel to parts of the world that have overwhelming needs, but it is unfair for all the burden to be on those that have the needed skills, and it is also the case that "charity services" will miss many of the needy who are not in the right place at the right time. Effective pursuit of its internal goods requires that the medical profession also consider collective and systematic organizational ways for a society to bond itself with its suffering members.

A final issue in need of collective effort is the pursuit of local

6. Participation in an execution is explicitly forbidden by the AMA Principles of Medical Ethics, adopted 20 June 1980 (Sargent).

and international policies that enhance rather than ruin people's health. Just as fluoride policies are naturally the concern of the dental profession because of their impact on that profession's internal good, any policies that significantly affect health are naturally the concern of the medical profession. Although medical practitioners may be primarily concerned with their own patients, they should not avoid the collective responsibility to work for measures that enhance the health of the population as a whole. Therefore, medical professionals should be encouraged to take collective stands on sanitation, vaccinations, pollution, seat belts, smoking, chemical abuse, nuclear war, health-care legislation, and any other issues of policy, public health, or lifestyle that have significant impact on the good these professionals publicly profess to pursue. Of course, as we noted earlier, health is not the only good, and a society cannot allow any profession to make its good into a god. Medical professionals who have wisdom and vision will be careful to avoid this pitfall.

Medicine as a Calling

Where do the wisdom and motivation to set and pursue priorities come from? The resources of one's own profession—its internal goods, its inherent standards of excellence, and the integrity and loyalty of one's colleagues—are certainly one source. But when a profession codifies these resources into an explicit statement that can gain professional consensus in a pluralist society, the result is often a list of rather vague and minimal considerations like those found in the latest professional codes (see Appendix D).

Christians believe that the idea of vocation, or God's calling to each of his children, provides the vision and motivation that avoid the dangers of idolatry, fanaticism, and narrowly focused interests. The idea of *calling* is probably inherently a religious idea (Hoitenga, 309). All Christians are called to discipleship in whatever occupations they engage. The elements of calling — reconciliation, celebration, service, caring, and stewardship—are not confined just to certain professions, though it may be that certain professions can more easily than others integrate the inherent values of the profession with the vision, guidance, and motivation intrinsic to Christian calling. The tradition of thinking of Jesus as "the great physician" suggests that the medical profession, perhaps along with the teaching and ministerial professions, is one of these. To claim that the Christian calling is an excellent vision for medi-

cal professionals is not to claim that non-Christians lack all sense of calling. Perhaps they can also find an ennobling principle—such as the appeal to posterity or to the formation of a classless utopia—that may provide them with vision and motivation to set and pursue worthy
priorities in medicine. The challenge is to have a vision that motivates
without falling into idolatry and fanaticism.

We will not here repeat our discussions about the motivation
and guidance provided by a view of others as imagers of God; by the
idea of covenantal ethics; by the Christian understanding of tragedy; by
such Christian virtues as watchfulness, truthfulness, humility, gratitude,
courage, prayerfulness, and altruism; and by the God-like willingness
to share another's suffering by being present and compassionate and by
refusing to abandon the sufferer. The question we address here is
whether these elements of the Christian calling apply in medical practice only to what Robert Veatch calls "sectarian" medicine ("Against
Virtue," 338) or whether they also apply in what he calls "stranger" medicine and to broader professional concerns.

As medicine has become more complex and more expensive, the
care of patients has moved from the private, home-based setting to the
public, hospital-based setting. Much of the medical care previously received from a familiar family physician is now delivered by strangers in
the strange and mysterious world of the hospital. Furthermore, expanding transportation capabilities have increased mobility, shifted the population from rural to urban areas, and reduced the opportunity for many
people to develop a lifelong relationship with a single familiar physician. Perhaps more than half of today's medical encounters are between
strangers (Veatch, "The Physician," 196). Not only may patients encounter an unfamiliar physician when they are likely to be at their most
vulnerable, but they may encounter in that unfamiliar physician a person who holds a set of values quite unlike their own. As a result, suspicion and explicit contract have threatened to replace trust and unspoken
commitment in the physician-patient relationship.

One way for Christians to avoid the latter problem is to establish institutions explicitly committed to the Christian calling. Not only
would patients and physicians be more likely to develop long-term relationships in such a setting, but, even when the medical encounter was
with strangers, both sides could assume shared values and a common
calling. Having such institutions is a good idea even though economies
of scale, government regulation on nondiscriminatory hiring policies,
and other problems make it difficult for them to achieve their ideals.
But most Christian professionals do not work in such "sectarian"
(Veatch, "Against Virtue," 338) institutions; their work regularly brings

them into intimate contact with patients and colleagues who are "strangers" and who may be ignorant of or hostile toward Christian convictions.

When they encounter strangers in huge organizations, Christian professionals should let their convictions inform their conversation and conduct in a way that not only provides guidance for themselves but also provides models for others. As we suggested in the previous chapter, Christian professionals in secular settings are likely to confront the issue of when to respect, tolerate, and cooperate with positions they disagree with. This issue is complicated when one has trouble understanding alternative positions without stereotyping them and when one feels a professional and Christian loyalty to help (within limits) others be loyal to their own convictions. While maintaining one's own integrity, one must nurture the integrity of others and not use their vulnerability to influence them unduly. Still, one of the most important ways Christian medical professionals can serve God's cause is by striving, as individuals, to integrate their professional identities and services with their Christian calling (Hoitenga).

However, for a Christian medical practitioner to be content with being a model of Christian vocation at work in the medical profession —as important and difficult as that is—would be for him or her to ignore the structural and political dimensions of the problems that society and the medical profession face (DeVries, 155). Christian vision and motivation are also needed by those individuals and groups who assume the collective responsibilities of the profession. It is true that individuals are not necessarily responsible for undesirable aspects of the ethics, ethos, and way of life of their profession, but as Albert Flores and Deborah Johnson remind us (542-43), individuals do voluntarily assume professional roles, and there is "space" within role obligations for individuals to challenge either the status quo of a profession or its drifting in an undesirable direction. If, for example, external constraints are pushing medicine toward a commercial-commodity model of its services and if that model is at odds with both professional ideals and Christian calling, then Christian professionals can and should challenge this change. They can do so as individuals and, more effectively, as organized groups within the profession. The concerted efforts of professionals in the Luke Society, the Christian Medical Society, Christian Community Health Fellowship, and the Christian Nurses Association can make a difference. Not only can they sponsor projects that exemplify Christian professionalism in action; they can also be an organized part of the debate within the profession and between the profession and society about what medicine is and should be.

The Character of Relationships in Medicine

Much of the debate over what medicine is and should be amounts to a debate over the nature of the relationships that are part of medical practice. This debate, in turn, has often become a debate about the models or metaphors used for these relationships. Relationships are often *shaped* by language we mean to use only to *describe*. For example, compare the concept of family life expressed by language that pictures the family relationship as a hierarchy with the concept of family life expressed by language that pictures it as a partnership. There is already an abundance of literature on the models that describe and shape the relationships in medical practice, especially those among physicians, nurses, and patients.[7] Sometimes medical professionals are portrayed as fighters of diseases, a metaphor in which the patient's body becomes a battleground, the physician becomes a general, and the nurses become the infantry. Combine this model with the notion that medicine is a commodity, and medical professionals get pictured as hired assassins who are scientifically trained to locate and destroy the enemy (invasive diseases) without seriously wounding the clients who hire them.

A second influential way of thinking about medicine is the engineering model, which is often combined with the biomedical model (Engel, 43). This way of thinking tends to approach medicine in the mechanistic and reductionistic manner of scientific inquiry. Under the assumption that the best way to understand patients is to understand their component parts, the physician is pictured as an engineer, a technician, or a plumber of the body, whose role it is to discover which parts are broken or corroded and to fix them. The danger with this model is not only that it ignores the wholeness of the patient but also that it risks reducing the value-laden dimension of medical decisions to technical questions about how to minimize disease and maximize prolongation of biological life.

A third model pictures physicians as priests who are in control of the mysteries that are beyond patients' understanding. The priestly model recognizes the value-laden character of medical decisions but

7. A number of writers have described models that characterize some of the more prevalent modes in which patients and physicians interact. R. Veatch, having suggested an engineering model, a priestly model, and a collegial model, finally settles upon a contractual model as the most responsible ("Models"). W. May considers a covenantal model to be a better alternative to the contractual model ("Code and Covenant"; *Physician's Covenant*). K. D. Clouser has argued that models are unnecessary and only serve to blur the fact that physicians have the same moral obligations toward their patients that all humans have toward each other.

leaves them entirely up to physicians, who, it is assumed, know what is best for patients and will act in the patients' best interests. Physicians take control for patients and protect them from bad news or difficult decisions that, supposedly, patients cannot and need not participate in. What we said in Chapter Two about paternalism applies to the priestly model, which risks treating patients as something other than imagers of God; it fails to see them as givers and hearers of reasons, as choicemakers with whom physicians must converse before they intervene.

Lately, medicine has been moving toward a contract model. This movement may be part of a general trend in a society that loves negotiating contracts—even marriage contracts—and tends to communicate through its burgeoning number of lawyers, substituting signatures for handshakes and, when things go wrong, the swift suit for the old-fashioned quick draw. But it also reflects the "stranger" character of medicine and the fact that many medical contacts are for health assessment rather than therapy (Dickman, 201). When a person goes to a stranger for a checkup required by an employer, it is easy to think of the medical service rendered as a commodity and the relationship between giver and receiver as limited to commercial concerns of competence, explicit disclosure, confidentiality, and reimbursement.

The contract model does avoid some of the condescension and other dangers of alternative models: it views the patient and the physician as equal partners in an agreement that exchanges services for appropriate compensation; it insists that expectations and obligations are made explicit from the beginning and that the patient be consulted before any changes are made in the treatment plan; and it encourages dialogue and possibly compromise between patient and physician with regard to diagnosis and treatment plans. This model serves to check the paternalism of the priestly model by raising the patient to the level of a contract partner who must be consulted regarding all decisions, and this model seeks to guarantee patients a more active and equal role in their own cases, providing even vulnerable patients with a means of control over professionals, including those professionals who are strangers but in whom patients have placed their (conditional) trust.

Models and the metaphors that describe them have also been used to understand the nursing profession. Perhaps because the patron saint of nursing, Florence Nightingale, was a military nurse or perhaps because of the tendency to think of medicine as a war on disease, the metaphor that first shaped the nursing profession was that of loyal soldier. Nightingale herself tended to think in terms of "understanding and obeying orders," and a typical turn-of-the-century nursing text spoke of the "implicit, unquestioning obedience" that must characterize nurses

(Winslow, 34). Even when the military connotations were toned down, the nurse was thought of as the physician's handmaiden, and loyalty to the physician was considered a nurse's chief virtue. Her relationship with the patient was modeled in various ways, depending on the situation. Nurses in emergency rooms or intensive-care units were thought of as biomedical technicians, and those in other contexts often were thought of as surrogate mothers who, under the priestly and paternal eye of the physician, would maternally tend to the patient's needs.

But already in 1929 nurses discovered that they were legally liable if they followed physicians' orders without questioning,[8] and the increasing professionalization of nursing—which called for a nurse's use of discretionary judgment and for stricter educational requirements— has yielded a model for nursing in which nurses have an independent contract with patients. No longer does nurses' loyalty to their patients reside in their primary loyalty to physicians. Nurses now direct their primary loyalty toward patients. Whereas a 1953 nurses' code emphasized loyally following physicians' orders and maintaining confidence in physicians, the 1976 American Nurses' Association code emphasizes a nurse's primary commitment to the patient (now called "client," in accord with a contract model). The Interpretive Statement lays out the implication: "Hence, in the role of client advocate, the nurse must be alert to and take appropriate action regarding any instances of incompetent, unethical, or illegal practice by any member of the health care team" (American Nurses' Association, *Code*, 8). Here we have the patient-advocate model, which is recommended in many nursing schools as the professional alternative to being a loyal handmaiden to physicians and a surrogate mother to patients. Of course, physicians also consider themselves to be patient advocates. But if advocacy implies suspicions about other professionals, we may be trading a hierarchical model for one that fosters conflict rather than cooperation. This would be a loss, because there is good evidence that the most important factor for hospital patients' recovery is not the latest technology or the lowest nurse-patient ratio, but a spirit of respectful cooperation between physicians and nurses ("MD, Nurse Teamwork," 24).

Probably the important question is not whether health professionals are advocates for their patients but how that advocacy works in relation to patients and other professionals. And here we have some

8. In 1929 Lorenza Somera followed a physician's order which mistakenly called for her to prepare cocaine rather than procaine injections (Winslow, 35). The patient receiving the injections subsequently died as a direct result of the mistake. Somera was found guilty of manslaughter because of her failure to question the order.

worries about modeling the therapeutic relationship in terms of legal contracts and patients' rights. The advantage of the contract model is that it treats all parties as givers and hearers of reasons: patients are not to be treated merely as bodies, and professionals are not merely animated tools (either of patients or of other professionals).

Yet, when narrowly or legalistically conceived, contract thinking in medicine can create problems. First, the assumed equality of the contracting parties is often unrealistic. However equal they are in dignity and worth, the competence of persons who are ill is often severely diminished, and even clearheaded patients depend on health professionals to explain what is wrong and what can be done about it. Of course, inequality of knowledge is a factor in many contract relationships, such as when our cars or television sets need fixing. In illness, however, not only do we generally lack the opportunity to "shop around for competent medical care," but we also have something at stake that is central to our identity and well-being. Second, the element of unpredictability and the inherent uncertainty of diagnosis and prognosis make it impossible to spell out explicitly the nature and limits of a medical contract. Many times what may be needed can be only vaguely stated—like the "for better or worse" clause in marriage vows, not like the fine print of a warranty. Our third worry, related to the inherent unpredictability of what patients and medical professionals may require of each other, is the paradoxical tendency toward both minimalism and maximalism that we observed earlier about contracts (Chapter Three, p. 86). Physicians may order every test that a lawyer with twenty-twenty hindsight might argue in court was relevant to a particular patient's care, yet they may avoid any time-consuming bedside dialogue—because nothing in the contract requires it. Thus the costs and limitations of "defensive medicine" may be a dangerous part of a contract model.

Our fourth and final consideration[9] involves the "mutual gift" element in medicine, which, because of their ahistorical nature, contracts cannot adequately convey. The gift that medical professionals give their patients is obvious; it was mentioned by the first code of medical ethics adopted by the American Medical Association in 1847: "A patient should, after his recovery, entertain a just and enduring sense of the value of the services rendered him by his physician; for these are of such a character, that no mere pecuniary acknowledgment can repay or cancel

9. See W. May ("Code and Covenant") and R. Masters ("Is Contract an Adequate Basis for Medical Ethics?") for considerations against the contract model. See R. Veatch (*A Theory of Medical Ethics*) for a sensitive and knowledgeable defense of a contract model that is not legalistically or narrowly construed.

them." This part of the code was later dropped, perhaps because it seemed a bit self-serving, but it is true that when one person is God's means for saving the life or restoring the health of another, a gift relationship is established that money cannot express. Perhaps less obvious than the gift that physicians give their patients are the gifts that patients give their health professionals. The 1847 code did not mention these, but William May ("Code and Covenant") has called attention to a number of ways in which physicians are in debt to society, which includes their patients. Physicians' debts to society derive not only from their heavily subsidized education and the monopoly on much-needed and quite lucrative services which they enjoy, but also from the suffering and death of countless patients, including those literally "practiced upon" and all those in history who have suffered and died while medicine was accumulating the fund of knowledge and expertise that professionals now have at their disposal. This, too, is a debt that money cannot express.

The preceding considerations lead us to believe that by and large the language of covenant is the best model of the relationship between medical professionals and their patients as well as between medical professionals themselves. Of course, as we noted when discussing covenantal ethics in the previous chapter, sometimes encounters with others are purely and appropriately contractual, and probably this is also sometimes true for medical interactions, especially when mutual expectations are precisely definable, both parties are in full control of themselves, and nothing significant is at stake. But when the encounter is with an ill and vulnerable patient, when life itself may be at stake, and when it is impossible to predict what will happen and what demands may be placed on both parties, then a strictly contractual model of the relationship misconstrues what is happening and can warp what ought to happen. A covenantal model does a better job both of describing the relationship and of prescribing the implicit responsibilities. The three elements of covenants that we noted in the previous chapter—that they are rooted in gifts, or mutual entrustments, whereby people become vulnerable to one another; that they put people in moral community with one another; and that they endure over time and are influenced by new developments in unspecifiable and open-ended ways—seem to characterize most clinical relationships.

It is interesting that as early as the Hippocratic oath (see Appendix D) medical people recognized that their relationships with one another have more of a covenantal than a contractual character. The oath recognizes as gifts the knowledge and skill bestowed on the practitioners by their teachers, and practitioners swear, therefore, to treat their teachers like their parents and their teachers' families like their own families, ministering to their needs as to their own. This is a classic example of a covenant as opposed to a contract. Today's practitioners may have difficulty feeling that way about their teachers, but the collegiality and professional courtesy that permeate the medical professions can hardly be reduced to legalistic contract. This covenant does, however, have its dark side, as laypeople sometimes discover when they try to get professionals to testify against one another.

One difficulty with extending this covenantal thinking to include the relationship of medical professionals with their patients is that it may seem to imply a bottomless pit of time-consuming obligations with patients, whose needs can often be overwhelming. In Appendix A, Kurt Kooyer addresses an important aspect of this problem by asking how one can balance emotional investment with clinical detachment. Here we will call attention to two other points. The first is to recall a caution noted in the previous chapter—that, when one finite person is expected to be or tries to be the lord and savior of another, the situation is ripe for idolatry, exhaustion, and disappointment. Setting oneself up as the sole savior of another may be an occupational hazard of the medical profession; if so, medical professionals must be careful not to allow the covenant model to baptize this tendency. Christian medical people who are familiar with both the beauty and the pitfalls of covenantal thinking in their own lives can be helpful to their profession by teaching and exemplifying both the depth and the limitations of human covenants.

The second point is that medical people are involved in many covenants and roles. As members of the inclusive covenant with God and all God's children and creation, they have stewardship responsibilities that impinge on their laudable tendency to move heaven and earth for the sake of their patients. Medical people are also spouses, parents, children, friends, teachers, and so forth. These roles may impose important responsibilities that conflict with the special responsibilities of the physician's role, but these other roles must not be neglected. God calls his children to service in many areas of life. Neglecting responsibilities in one area of life for the sake of achieving excellence in another must be avoided. The calling of parent or spouse carries obligations and responsibilities that many have neglected for the sake of career, profession, or patients. If we add to these covenantal responsibilities the usual ones deriving from relationships with country, state, church, civic, charitable, cultural, environmental, and international organizations, we can see the potential for vast and conflicting responsibilities that seem impossible to fulfill. Moreover, medical professionals need time for themselves and their own projects, or they cannot be persons to whom others can confidently entrust themselves. If they can never read good literature— other than hastily perused professional literature—or attend plays or enjoy nature's beauty, they will become very one-sided individuals. Fortunate are the professionals with the wisdom and vision to set priorities; they need and deserve the support of a society and of patients who understand and appreciate the many difficult covenantal responsibilities demanding their attention as well as the need for nourishment in their private, individual lives.

One reason that a covenantal model of medical relationships is appropriate is that the medical profession is constantly involved in tragedy. Its pursuit of health and healing combined with human frailty and mortality ensures that its decision-making will take place where evils gather and goods collide. The next chapter addresses itself to that dimension of medicine.

5. Technology, Tragedy, and Christianity

The stethoscope dangling from the pocket of a lab coat has replaced the serpent coiling on the staff of Aesculapius as the most readily identifiable symbol of medicine. The most familiar images of modern medicine are its tools, and if we would understand modern medicine, then we must come to terms with its technology.

To visit any hospital or clinic is to encounter a fascinating and terrifying collection of tools. In any intensive-care unit, pumps make strange, soft noises, other machines command attention with little bleeping sounds, and the blinking lights of still others demand notice. Even those who are uninitiated in such mysteries and who cannot decipher any meaning in the sounds and the lights find it difficult to turn from them or to look past them. With sweet and silent awe, people are driven to admire, trust, and envy those who know how to read and use these machines with technological grace.

The tools of medicine are ubiquitous, from the stethoscope and blood-pressure band to the neonatal intensive-care unit. Technology provides the images for modern medicine, so in this chapter we will try to understand the meaning of this technology—the human significance of these tools—and thereby to understand something of the meaning of medicine as well.

In our last chapter we noted the importance of metaphor to an understanding of medicine. In this chapter we will use a story, which is a kind of extended metaphor, to understand medical technology and the medicine it images. The story we have chosen is the tragic story. We will try to understand technology in terms of tragedy (Hauerwas, "Medicine," 184-202; MacIntyre, "How Virtues Become Vices," 110-11). That is not an arbitrary or whimsical choice, for to visit any hospital or clinic is to encounter not only technology but tragedy. The machines both point us toward tragedy and hide it from us, but anyone with eyes to see and ears to hear will finally see tragedy beyond the blinking lights and hear its sighs above the bleeping sounds. It is not an arbitrary or whimsical choice, but it is also not an altogether unambiguous choice, for the eyes of faith are finally not content with the tragic vision. Christianity knows and tells a story that is beyond tragedy, and we will want finally to understand medical technology and the medicine it images in terms of the Christian story.

Tragedy

Technology and "The Sad Story"

There is more than one sort of tragedy, of course, and more than one sort of tragedy is encountered in hospitals and clinics. The simplest form of tragedy—and the one first encountered—is "the sad story," the narrative of disaster or catastrophe, the story of massive heart attack, metastasized cancer, scarred and blocked fallopian tubes, broken bodies, and the like. Perhaps there are as many tragic stories of this sort as there are patients.

The appropriate human and Christian response to this sort of tragedy has always been sympathy and care. For centuries, however, such sympathy and care were almost helpless in the face of such tragedy. The nurse's duty was just to care when there was no cure; the doctor's duty was sometimes simply to tell the patient "to provide for his soul's health, as that of his body was in dangerous condition," as Don Quixote's physician put it to him (quoted by Aries, 4). Everyone acknowledged the tragedy, but what could be done? Some were simply "overmastered by their diseases," to quote an ancient Hippocratic treatise (Hippocrates, 317). Then Francis Bacon (1561-1626) made an innovative suggestion: he urged the rejection of that old category of being "overmastered" by a disease and insisted that to pronounce any disease incurable "gives a legal sanction as it were to neglect and inattention, and exempts ignorance from discredit" (quoted by Amundsen, 28). This innovative perspective gradually shaped the medical profession and finally prompted in our own age the development of a medical science and technology that no longer leave us quite so helpless and hopeless in the face of the sad stories of human suffering and premature dying.

That's the first thing to be said of intensive-care technology and the medicine it images: it is born of sympathy with people in the midst of tragedy; it is motivated by compassion for those who suffer; it expresses care for embodied persons who are threatened; and these and the development of this technology are appropriate human and Christian responses to the sad stories people tell with and of their bodies.

Technology, in this view—Bacon's view—is simply knowledge put to work for human well-being, simply the set of tools we develop and use to help us make and achieve what we want. Knowledge is power, Bacon said, and that power is linked to new possibilities for human flourishing. You care, and technology is the tool by which you learn to care—if not more intensely, then at least more effectively. You want to restore health; you want to preserve life; you want to conquer infertility; and—recently at least, sometimes at least—medical interventions utilizing the developing technologies have been remarkably successful. Until recently, medical interventions probably took more lives than they saved, but in the last few decades Bacon's project for medicine has seen astonishing successes. Knowledge is power, and gains in knowledge have led to increased powers to intervene purposefully to forestall death and to restore health, to seek and to serve human well-being.

This, then, is the second thing to be said of medical technology: the motive of compassion is matched—sometimes, at least—by outcomes of health and flourishing. Sometimes the sad stories, with the help of these machines, with the help of medicine, have a happy ending after all. Some patients do recover with the help of these machines and sometimes learn to celebrate life and their measure of health in ways they had not before. It's a good story, and technology—and the medicine of which it is an image—must be understood in terms of that good story if we are to understand technology and medicine at all. The heroes of this story, of course, are the doctors and nurses and other medical professionals— enlisted on the side of human life and health, battling against the evil empire of death and disease. Their courage is their refusal to call any disease incurable; their strength, weapons forged in study and research; their allies, the universities and laboratories. It's a good story, and medicine plays a good role in it. Doctors and nurses are heroic characters; it's folly to deny their heroism.

Technology and "The Flawed Hero"

But the heroic character can be tragic, too. The tragedies one encounters in intensive-care units are not just the sad stories of patients. There is an older view of tragedy, Aristotle's view, that the tragic story is the story of a hero with a tragic flaw of character.[1] The heroes in the stories of intensive caring are doctors and nurses. Their characters are shaped by the tradition and the communities to which they belong—and by the tools they use. *Doctor* or *nurse* describes who a person is as well as what he or she does; it is an identity as well as a title, a character as well as a role. It is a good identity, a good character, enlisted on the side of life and health, fighting a messy—and losing—but heroic battle against death and disease. Life is a good, and even if it is not the only good, it is a good prerequisite for valuing other goods. God intends life for people; God's creative and redemptive will chooses life; the signs of it are a rainbow and a commandment and an empty tomb. A character formed to protect and sustain life is a commendable character, a virtuous character.

But this character can also be flawed. The military images we have just used to commend the commitment to human life and health also hint at the possibility of a tragic flaw. The doctor and the nurse can be crusaders. Their passion for a certain good end can blind them to the injustice of certain means. And the very technology that makes them heroes in our stories increases the possibilities of their becoming tragic heroes. This is the third thing to be said of technology in critical-care units and the medicine of which it is the image: technology *is* power, and not ever just the power of humanity over nature but also always the power of some people over others (C. S. Lewis, 69). Technology is power, and in the hands of a doctor or nurse technology is not joined just to good motives and good ends but is, willy-nilly, also always power over the patient. It is not that the tragic hero necessarily cares less; the virtue he or she lacks is not love or care but justice. The crusader, the tragic hero of critical-care units, is prepared to override patients' wills, to dominate them when they will not cooperate, to take advantage of their relative powerlessness in order to achieve the good of life or health.

Note that we are not claiming that every physician and nurse lacks the virtue of justice or that the character of doctor and nurse is essentially flawed. On the contrary, we have said that the character of phy-

---

1. Aristotle's notion of *hamartia* or "tragic error" has been much discussed. See a review of the literature in J. Barbour's *Tragedy* (pp. 2-6). There is a developing consensus that by *hamartia* Aristotle did not mean "moral guilt" but rather an act that was at least partly excusable, whether by ignorance or some compulsion, and partly culpable, bringing about the hero's downfall. Aristotle's view of the unity of the virtues—that they do not conflict—prevents him from seeing the conflict of goods in Sophoclean tragedy. And his view that a superbly good man would necessarily prosper prevents him from admitting to the possibility of a tragic downfall without *hamartia*. To the degree that our presentation of the tragic flaw acknowledges that *virtues* as well as ignorance and powerful passions can lead to "tragic error," it is probably closer to Sophoclean tragedy itself than to Aristotle's reading of it.

sician and nurse is essentially virtuous, formed by its compassion for human life and health. The point is simply that technology is power, and power creates possibilities both for heroism and for tragedy.

But more can and must be said, because technology involves a perspective on the patient that can affect the medicine of which it is an image. Doctors and nurses with only a technological perspective on the patient see and treat the patient as manipulable nature, as nature that can be understood—and treated—only as the sum total of the chemical and physical mechanisms that operate on it and in it according to universal principles and scientific laws. Seen from the technological perspective, nature, including human nature, is determined by scientific laws, has no exceptions—or only predictable exceptions, exceptions understandable according to the same universal principles and, therefore, not really exceptions at all (Gorovitz and MacIntyre, 51-71; Hauerwas, "Medicine," 197-99). The doctor or nurse who uses medical technology in the heroic attempt to give a patient's sad story a happy ending adopts and must adopt that technological perspective on his or her patients.

But our traditional moral and religious understanding of human nature has emphasized the individuality and the exceptionality of the human species. Indeed, our regard for persons, our respect for them *as* persons, is in no small measure related to our conviction of their individuality and exceptionality, their difference both from other creatures and from each other. We have thought men and women worthy of our love, our intensive caring, our fidelity, because we have seen them as different from one another, as individual, as exceptional.

The point is this: there is a tension between the technological perspective on human nature and the traditional moral and religious perspective on human nature (Jenson). And this is the fourth thing to be said about technology and the medicine it images: certain mental habits can be formed by the use of technology, and the character of our heroes can be formed by the tools they use. Technology can seduce doctors and nurses into a perspective on human nature which weakens their capacity to overcome and vanquish the temptation to be crusaders, the tragic heroes of intensive care

Let the point not be misunderstood. The point is not that taking this technological perspective on the patient is bad. We have already said that technology—and the medicine it images and the perspective it requires and supports—is good, that it is folly to deny it. And the point is not that adopting this perspective makes it impossible for a care-giver to see and treat the patient as an agent, or to see and treat this passive and manipulable nature as a person, or to see and treat the one who suffers the technological diagnostic and therapeutic procedures as an exceptional and individual character whose story involves values besides his life and goods besides his health. But adopting this technological perspective does make it more difficult and can subtly wear down the capacities of doctors and nurses to see the patient as one whose individuality and exceptionality are not to be trampled upon, even for the sake of a good end.

The story of the tragic hero helps to clarify, perhaps, why so much of the literature in medical ethics and so much of the public discourse about medical care focus on the rights of patients—and it can also help us to understand both what is good and what is bad about this focus. The crusader must be restrained for his own sake as well as for the patient's. The crusader may not be permitted arbitrary dominance. And the language of rights is the most compelling language we have to constrain and restrain the powerful.

Consider, for example, a scene from the movie *Whose Life Is It, Anyway?* Harrison, the sculptor whose sad story includes an automobile accident that leaves him a quadriplegic, refuses the Valium prescribed to calm him after he first begins to question the wisdom of continuing life. Dr. Emerson takes advantage of Harrison's quadriplegia and injects Harrison with a narcotic against his will. It is a violent, unjust act—well-intentioned, well-motivated, but unjust all the same. Dr. Emerson is not a villain, however, but a tragic hero, a crusader. Ironically, this powerful act against the powerless quadriplegic seems to determine Harrison's course. The injection and his inability to resist it so repel him that he begins to investigate and then to assert his legal power to stop the doctor and to render him powerless to "save" him. He asserts his right to die, his right to autonomy. The doctor's response, in turn, is to crusade to have his patient declared "incompetent," to render him finally powerless and without options, so that the doctor can achieve his good cause.

The same dynamics are at work in the current public discussion of patient rights and in the legal assertions of patient autonomy and the right to refuse treatment. They are prompted and sustained by a public perception of medical professionals not as villains but as tragic heroes, as heroes flawed tragically by their tendency to crusade for the good they serve. And the movement for patient rights can be appreciated as an appropriate restraint on the crusader and welcomed by medical professionals as an occasion to review the sort of story that is their own and as a reminder of the legitimacy and moral necessity of seeing their patient as individual and exceptional. But the movement stands in danger of its own crusade, of using its power to render the doctor and the nurse powerless in this relationship, of making them simply "animated tools" of the medical consumer's wishes. ("Animated tool," of course, is Aristotle's definition of a slave.) The movement threatens to merge the doctor and the nurse with their own technology, another "tool" in that fascinating and terrifying collection. And, of course, neither slave nor tool is a role medical professionals should wish to call their own.

The current focus on patient rights protects patients against the arbitrary dominance of a crusader. That is what's good about it. But it leaves only two options for doctors and nurses. They can choose the role of tragic hero, the powerful crusader, attempting to render the patient powerless and choiceless, so that they can achieve the good they publicly profess, or they can choose the role of slave, machine, "animated tool," no longer a heroic character at all, simply doing as they are told, choiceless themselves.[2] But a focus on story may provide another option for the tragic hero. Our heroes may learn to tell a different story about their work, to take a different narrative as their own. Medicine may be reformed by stories as well as restrained by rights. People may choose to tell a story of collaboration and cooperation rather than a story of either arbitrary dominance or confrontation. Of course, genuine collaboration, at least between persons who are individual and exceptional, will always risk confrontation. But in the story we want to tell, no one

2. Perhaps Paul Ramsey has seen most clearly and expressed most eloquently both what's good about this focus on patients and what's wrong with it. In Aristotelian fashion he has "leaned against" first one defect in the ethos of society and then another. In *The Patient as Person* he "leaned against" not only the "research imperative" but also the therapeutic imperative, insisting with Kantian rigor on "informed consent": "The sanctity of human life prevents ultimate trespass upon him *even for the sake of treating his bodily life*" (p. xii, italics added). Again: "Medical ethics is not solely a benefit-producing ethics even in regard to the individual patient, since he should not always be helped without his will" (p. 2). Informed consent is the "chief *canon of loyalty*" (p. 2), the "cardinal *canon of loyalty*" (p. 5). Again: "Man's capacity to become joint adventurers in a common cause makes the consensual relation possible; man's propensity to over reach his joint adventurer even in a good cause makes consent necessary" (p. 6). "No man is good enough to cure another without his consent" (p. 7). And, finally, Ramsey urges the doctor to "lean against his understanding of the medical imperative in order to keep it optional for his patients; and . . . as a man who happens also to be a doctor, he should make room for the primacy of human moral judgment on the part of the men who are his patients, the relatives of his patients, and their spiritual counselors to elect life-sustaining remedies or to elect them not" (p. 124).

Eight years later, still seeking to protect individuals, especially the voiceless, Ramsey wrote *Ethics at the Edges of Life*, in which he leans against the "atomistic individualism" of our society, calling attention to what's bad about the Kantian emphasis on autonomy, insisting that "treatment refusal is a relative right, contrary to what is believed today by those who would reduce medical ethics to patient autonomy and a right to die" (p. 156). Now Ramsey leans against Robert Veatch, accusing his emphasis on patient rights of moving "too far in the direction of subjective voluntarism and automated physicians" (pp. 159, 161-71).

Ramsey evidently wants to protect both the patient from being mistreated by the crusader and the physician from being reduced to an "animated tool" (*Ethics at the Edges of Life*, 158).

should rush to the sort of confrontation which leaves one person powerful and in charge and the other powerless and optionless. We should want to preserve the possibility of renewed collaboration.

Too much contemporary moral philosophy and public policy is too ready to invoke the category of rights and to disenfranchise one or another of those joined together on the project of the patient's well-being, one or another of the partners in dialogue (and confrontation) about what the patient's well-being really involves and requires. Currently the role of the law is too often simply to put an end to the conversation, to decide "who should decide," and so to allocate choice-making power clearly and finally. We suggest a different role for the law: to foster and even to provoke prolonged conversation between the parties to the dispute about the patient's well-being (following Burt, 124-43). Of course, such discussion may yield no final agreement. The confrontation may not yield renewed collaboration, and so a procedural solution—a solution in terms of who should decide rather than in terms of what should be decided—may, in the end, be unavoidable. In that event, let the competent patient's decision be trump.

Let the competent patient's decision be trump—but note that it is the patient's integrity which must be honored and respected, not merely some arbitrary choice the patient voices. To demand respect, to be trump finally in the conversation about her well-being, her choice must be intelligible in terms of the narrative she has created for herself in the past. Even the patient's freedom, we would suggest, must be understood in a narrative context.[3] Patients come to their decisions from a variety of narratives and communities. A Jehovah's Witness refuses a necessary blood transfusion; a burn victim refuses a painful bath therapy; a sculptor rendered a quadriplegic refuses dialysis; an elderly physician suffering cancer and heart disease writes "do not resuscitate" on his own medical record; a multiple sclerosis victim, after fifteen years of coping with the disease, attempts suicide and refuses medical help. All of these refuse treatment. But care-givers should know a good deal more about each of them, about their narratives and communities, before honoring their refusal. Why? Because autonomy is not simply the arbi-

---

3. It may be worth observing that it seems to be only in academic journals that the calls to respect autonomy and the assertions of a right to refuse treatment are supported by the impartial principles and perspective of contemporary moral philosophy. Such an account is terribly important, but ordinary people tend to support their own right to refuse treatment by telling stories, stories of Aunt Mary's being powerless and at the mercy of machines and of the people who know how to use them, stories of Uncle Henry's being violated by a crusader. The doctors and nurses in such stories are not usually so much villains as tragic heroes whose tragic flaw is that they are crusaders.

trary freedom to will whatever one will. Arbitrary freedom of the patient is not a sufficient basis for restraining the medical crusader (if only because the very arbitrariness of such autonomy makes it possible that the decision will be different tomorrow). When care-givers learn, however, that the Jehovah's Witness is serious in her commitments, then they should be prepared to honor her decision. When care-givers learn that the victim of multiple sclerosis is depressed because of his family's recent lack of attention to him due to the illness of his mother-in-law, then they should be prepared to override his decision. When care-givers learn that the burn victim is perhaps primarily concerned to assert some power over against his own experience of powerlessness, then they should try to provide him with some other access to the experience of power even as they continue the treatment. Integrity must be respected, the faithfulness of the patient to his or her own identity and character, the exercise of freedom to create one unified life within which his or her choices are quite predictable (but no less free). We need not applaud all those who make decisions consistent with their identities, but we must honor choices compelled by a person's integrity.

In the end, as a last resort, we must let the competent patient's decision be trump, but we must also let doctors and nurses tell a story true to their character, formed by a history and a community and even their tools, disposed to preserve life, to sustain health, to relieve pain. They should not own a story of "animated tool," simply doing the bidding of the medical consumer. And they should not own the story of the crusader, however much their tools tempt them to it. They should not render the patient passive, powerless, and choiceless in order to accomplish the good they pursue because of their moral passions and projects as doctors and nurses.

A focus on the importance of the story that doctors and nurses would tell of and for themselves makes it possible not only to constrain the powerful crusader but also to form and reform medical professionals, to make them less susceptible to that tragic flaw of character. It allows one to call attention, for example, to the importance of little things, because little things, as we all know from reading good stories, can reveal a character and shape it. To refer to a patient as, say, "the cardiac arrest down the hall" is a little thing indeed, but it can reveal a character whose perspective on the patient is limited to the technological. Such references are dangerous not only because the patient may overhear them but because they form character, because they nurture and reinforce a disposition toward the patient that tempts the character to become a crusader. To call the patient by name—to say "Dan Fisher" or "Jan Gallagher"—is to acknowledge the patient's particularity and exceptionality; it is also to take a simple but precious opportunity to form a character less susceptible to the tragic flaw.

The little things—including concern and respect for a patient's reticence about nakedness, or insight into his embarrassment over bathroom functions, or the human touch that signifies compassion—are important precisely because in them care-givers tell their story, create a narrative that they call their own. As in any good story, the actions of a character in moments of crisis will be predictable, for they will have integrity with the character that has been revealed and formed in the little things that have gone before.

So the story that doctors and nurses tell of themselves allows us to call attention again to that moment of crisis, to that moment when their help has been refused, when the confrontation with a patient has not yielded renewed collaboration, when in the end the patient's word is trump. At that moment and beyond it doctors and nurses must still care. They must learn to tell a story that they care not only when they cannot cure but also when they may not cure, not only when it is impossible to cure but also when they are not permitted to cure. That may be a harder and more heroic task still, but it may in the end yield not just a set of restraints against medicine but the reform and renewal of medicine as a genuinely heroic profession.

Technology and "The Gathering of Evils"

The genuine disputes about a patient's well-being and what it requires of medical professionals introduce a still older notion of tragedy. In the view of Sophocles, the great Greek dramatist (5th century B.C.), the tragic story is not simply the sad story and not simply the story of a hero with a tragic flaw of character. For Sophocles the tragic story is a story in which goods collide and evils gather so that any choice is a "tragic" choice. Because goods collide, to choose one good is to choose against another good, and, of course, we should never choose against the good. Because evils gather, they cannot all be avoided, but, of course, we should never choose the evil.[4] Such tragedies are also—and often—encountered in medical care.

They are often encountered in allocation decisions (Calabresi

4. Although Aristotle's account of tragedy makes use of Sophoclean stories, Aristotle's assumptions about the unity and harmony of the good foreclose the possibility of his accepting this portrayal of human existence by the great tragedian. See J. Barbour, A. MacIntyre (*After Virtue*, 157-58), and S. Hauerwas ("Medicine," 184-202).

and Bobbitt; Ramsey, *Patient*, 239-75; Verhey, "Organs"). What nurse has not experienced the tragic finitude of her own resources for helping? To whom will she give her care when a dying patient needs someone to talk to, a patient who has had a heart attack needs constant monitoring, and too many others need more care than can be provided? What doctor has not put off one patient for the sake of another? What hospital administrator has not faced hard and sometimes tragic decisions about the allocation of resources? Society itself faces hard choices about how great a share of its resources to devote to medicine and about how to distribute those medical resources justly. Some of these decisions are tragic choices, because goods collide and evils gather.

Tragic choices, however, are encountered not only when a caregiver is forced to choose between patients but also when he or she must choose concerning the care of an individual patient. To resuscitate patients may preserve their lives, but it may also prolong their suffering. Medical technology may preserve a bundle of distorted and needlessly pained nerves and tissues or—sometimes against all probability calculations—a human person, as imperfect as any, more disfigured and handicapped than most, perhaps, but a person nonetheless, whose humility and heroism suggest to the rest of us what human life ought to be like (Hauerwas, "Medicine," 193; MacIntyre, "How Virtues Become Vices," 109). Some of these decisions are tragic choices, where goods collide and evils gather. Tragic choices are always a consequence of our finitude, of the fact that we are not gods, that our power and resources, while considerable, are still finite, and that our mortality cannot be annulled.

Thinking about technology in the light of Sophocles's notion of tragedy leads us, therefore, to make a fifth observation about technology and the medical care it images: technology does not and cannot eliminate tragedy of the Sophoclean sort; technology does not provide an escape either from the finitude of our resources or from our mortality. This is obvious, it may be said, but we have not been disposed to acknowledge the obvious. Perhaps our enthusiasm for technology as a response to the sad story has blinded us to the limits of technology. Perhaps because medicine reminds us so vividly of tragedy, we have used it ironically to hide and deny the tragic limits of our resources and our mortality (Hauerwas, "Medicine," 190). With respect to medical technology, we have been disposed to promise "everything for everyone"— but our resources, while considerable, *are* limited. We have been disposed to fight against our own mortality, but finally all of us are "overmastered by our diseases"—in spite of Sir Francis Bacon.

For all of its benefits, for all of its significance as a response to the sad stories people tell with and of their bodies, technology has yet to deliver us, and will not deliver us, from our finitude or to our flourishing. It is God who brings a new heaven and a new earth, not technology. The final victory over disease and death is a divine victory, not a technological one. If we acknowledge the obvious—that technology provides no escape either from the finitude of our resources or from our mortality—then it may be possible also to lower our expectations and demands of medical technology, once again to admit, however sadly, that sometimes some people are overmastered by their diseases, and to respond in other than technological ways to these threats to human life and flourishing, to care even when we cannot cure and, indeed, even to limit care-less technological meddling in a patient's living of his or her final days.

The technological imperative that "if we can, we must" is a techno-logic that should have no validity in human logic or in a critical-care unit which acknowledges that technology provides no escape from limited resources or from our own mortality. Physicians and nurses may not deny this tragic truth about technology, either to themselves or to their patients. They should intend life and its flourishing, and they should use their tools to nurture and sustain life and its flourishing. But sometimes to preserve life is *not* to serve the cause of life *and* its flourishing. The medical service rendered to the cause of human flourishing is the restoration of health; sometimes, in a world like this one, that service can only be the minimal one of the restoration or preservation of a capacity for human relationships and/or the relief of pain. When goods collide—when it is possible to preserve life but not, even minimally, to serve human flourishing—then the choice is a tragic one. The tragic choice is not settled by the techno-logic of "if we can, we must." The physician will not intend death, will not practice hospitality toward it, but neither will the physician intend the absence of human flourishing in an irreversible coma, nor will he or she practice hospitality toward suffering. When resisting death holds no promise of either the restoration of a capacity for human relationships or the relief of pain, then the physician may allow death its apparent and inevitable victory.

Before the physician faces that Sophoclean choice, the patient may confront tragic choices of his own. The patient's survival and ease may be the law of the physician's being, but they are not necessarily (or even commendably) the law of the patient's own being. The patient may know goods and have duties that can tragically conflict with the sustaining of either his life or his ease or both. The tasks of reconciliation and forgiveness and joy with family and friends and enemies may lead to decisions about medical care that foreseeably shorten his life or risk adding to his suffering. The patient may not intend his death, but he may weigh other goods against the good of his own survival and discern that he has duties for which life and ease may and must be risked. These goods and duties, which determined how he lived, must yet determine how he lives even while he is dying, and they may lead to tragic decisions to forego the medical care recommended by a doctor committed to this patient's survival and ease.

When goods collide and evils gather, as they do in such cases, a sixth observation is required concerning technology: the use of technology — and the refusal to use it — can be irremediably ambiguous morally. Any claim to "solve" these problems will provide only comic relief in a tragic story and demonstrate that we do not understand either the limits of medical technology or the limits of philosophy and theology (MacIntyre, "How Virtues Become Vices," 110-11). When medical technology is used to preserve a life engaged only in suffering a lingering dying, it may be appropriate (and we think it *is* appropriate) to withdraw the technology—but doing so is not good. It is a tragic choice—an irremediably ambiguous choice. To attempt to solve it with a rule is comic, but not to attempt to solve it is morally irresponsible.[5] In such a case, any rule that releases medicine from the burden of uselessly extending suffering imposes on it the burden of ending innocent human life (MacIntyre, "How Virtues Become Vices," 109). One should not choose either death or a lingering dying for another person—but choose one must. The choice is not right or wrong but right and wrong, not good or bad but good and bad; the choice is tragic in the Sophoclean sense.

It should not surprise us that we face such choices in medicine; in much of our life together we are confronted with such trade-offs and ambiguities. If we accept the good that medical technology — and the medicine it images—has to offer, then we must learn to accept the ambiguities and tragedy as well (Hauerwas, "Medicine," 201). There are hard choices to be made, hard losses to be accepted, but the choices and the losses can be endured. They become destructive when we refuse to recognize them for what they are—when, for example, we call death a good or another's suffering a good. They become destructive when we refuse to acknowledge ourselves for what we are — finite and mortal, tragic figures in need finally of God's grace and God's future. They become destructive when we refuse to acknowledge medicine for what it is —a tragic profession that does not finally free people from their finitude or their mortality but extends care to people in the midst of tragedy.

5. Even if the ability of reason to solve dilemmas is questioned, there remains the danger of intellectual sloth. Ambiguity sometimes has to be acknowledged at the end of our best attempts to discern what ought to be done, not at the beginning as an excuse for neglecting our best intellectual effort.

If medicine is recognized as a profession fraught with tragedy, then physicians and nurses will be less tempted to be crusaders, less ready to violate patients' integrity for the sake of some good end of medicine, and less tempted to a proud pretense of overcoming tragedy by denying the limits of our resources and our mortality. The acknowledgment of tragedy may require truthfulness and humility, but it will also sustain such virtues. It will inspire an old story of medicine, a story of care-giving in the midst of tragedy. If limits are not acknowledged, if there is not an appropriate sense of the tragic, then medical professionals may not be able to sustain the capacity and the responsibility to care (and to care intensively) even when they cannot or may not cure. And intensive care, it will be recalled, is what inspired and justified medical technology in the first place.

Thus far we have tried to understand and respond to medical technology—and the medicine it images—in the context of a particular sort of story, a story particularly appropriate to medical care: tragedy. We may delight in technology (and medicine) because of the power they give to intervene in a sad story and (sometimes) to give it a happy ending. We must be wary of technology (and medicine) because of the occasion and temptation they provide to exercise power over the patient unjustly, to become a crusader, a tragic hero of critical care. And, finally, we must accept the limits of technology (and medicine), the limits of our finite resources, and our inevitable mortality. We should accept medical technology (and medicine) not as a way to overcome tragedy but as a way to express care for one another in the midst of tragedy.

Tragedy and the Christian Tradition

The choice of tragedy as a narrative within which to understand technology and the medicine it images is not self-evidently coherent for those who own the Christian story and the Christian tradition, for the Christian tradition has usually been ambivalent about tragedy.[6]

There is a sense, of course, in which Christianity rejects tragedy as a final account of things and points beyond it. The Christian story is a glad story, not a sad story. It is good news, glad tidings,

---

6. There is a long-standing dispute, for example, about whether "the tragic vision" is compatible with "the Christian perspective." There is a fine discussion of this issue in D. Raphael (pp. 187-88 *et passim*).

a story one may love to tell. The Christian story is a story of an un-flawed hero, Jesus of Nazareth, the perfect man, tempted in all things as we are, but without sin, without the tragic flaw. And the Christian story is the story of one God, the God of our Lord Jesus Christ, who in grace and goodness creates, sustains, and redeems the world and humanity. Such grace is not fate to be resisted (or acknowledged) but a gift to be received and celebrated. Such goodness is the source of every good, and every good is coherent and harmonious—not con-flicting and cacophonous—in it. The Christian story is not a tragedy, and the Christian perspective is finally not a tragic vision. So one may and must ask whether the story of tragedy is an appropriate story for Christians to use when they try to understand technology and the medicine it images. But while Christianity points us *beyond* tragedy, we must remember that it is beyond *tragedy* that it points us.

The Christian faith does not make liars of us. It does not require or permit us to deny the tragic truth about our world. Disease and death, the power of sin and the sins of those in power, scarcity and mortality—that's the tragic truth about our world. The truth about our world hangs on a cross. And the cross is no lie—neither as a revelation of human evil nor as a revelation of divine love. The cross sustains the truthfulness nec-essary for us to acknowledge the tragic even while it sustains the hope necessary for us to look beyond it to the triumph of God.

The Sad Story and the Christian Tradition

The Christian tradition does not deny the sad story people tell with and of their bodies. The position of Mary Baker Eddy, which says that sick-ness is an illusion, is not science, and neither is it Christian (Barth, 365). Sickness and death are real. Not only are they real; they are real evils. They are not the covenant promise of God. God promises and intends life and its flourishing in health, not death and sickness, its "forerunner and messenger" (Barth, 366).

The Christian tradition has always been troubled by the reality of evil. And reflection about evil has sometimes been tempted in two directions. One direction is simply the agonized acknowledgment of the reality of evil. This may be heroic, but it frequently tears meaning from life. The Christian tradition has wanted to point *beyond* tragedy. The other direction is to hold fast to meaning, but too frequently and too facilely this direction has denied or ignored the reality of evil. The Chris-tian tradition knew that it had to point beyond *tragedy*. Theologically, then, these two directions may be identified with two generalizations: if evil is real, God is not good; and if God is good, evil is not real. But the Christian tradition has not wanted to take either of these directions, to accept either of these generalizations. The Christian tradition both affirms that the one covenant God is good and acknowledges that evil is real. And, indeed, in the Christian story of the cross the world's worst evil is seen, and God's goodness is discovered and announced. And by this story the Christian community continues to direct the people of God to a faithful response to the reality of evil: patient love.

To those who suffer, the story of the cross of Jesus is a glad story indeed, but a glad story that does not deny the sad story. The good news does not announce an end to our pain or an avoidance of our death, but it provides an unshakable assurance that we do not suffer alone, that we are not and will not be abandoned, that Jesus suffers with us, that God cares. The glad story is indeed a hard reminder that in a world like this one, however righteous or repentant we are, we cannot expect to be spared pain and sorrow. Certainly health and life are goods that we may and should seek, but we cannot expect to be spared pain, sorrow, and death; as Jesus said, "a disciple is not above his teacher" (Matt. 10:24). In our sad stories, we keep good company. That's a part of the good news, and then there is this: beyond the cross, beyond the sad story, is the resurrection, the triumph of God, a new age in which there is neither pain nor death anymore.

The story of the cross is good news to the suffering and a call to those who would follow Jesus to minister to the suffering, to love the sick, to have compassion on the suffering, to care for the dying, to grieve with those who grieve. Such a calling can nurture and sustain the vocation of medicine to heal and to care, to intervene—if possible—against the evils of suffering and premature dying, but never to abandon the patient even if and when the intervention does not provide a happy ending to the sad story.

Christians acknowledge the sad story and out of Christian integrity respond to it with care and compassion. So Christians, too, may delight in technology as a gift of God that bestows the power to intervene in a sad story and to give it (sometimes) a happy ending. But Christians are also pointed beyond the sad story to the good news, and so Christians are freed from relying finally on technology to provide the glad story or to sustain them in the face of their suffering and dying. So Christians may delight in technology without having extravagant expectations of it. It is God who suffers for us and with us—not technology. It is God—not technology—who will bring in the new age, when pain and death will be no more. Those are convictions that can sustain and nurture care not only in the face of the sad stories of an individual's pain and suffering but also in the face of the failure of technological intervention; those are convictions that neither technology itself nor even an appropriate sense of the tragic can provide.[7]

The Flawed Hero and the Christian Tradition

The Christian tradition knows an unflawed hero, Jesus of Nazareth, but it also knows the reality of sin. It knows the power of sin and the temptations to sin that exist in power. So, while it sees *beyond* tragedy in the story of Jesus, it also sees *tragedy* in acknowledging that all are sinners. When it says that Jesus was like us in all things, sin excepted, it points not only to an unflawed hero but also realistically to the continuing power of sin over each of the rest of us and to the reality of the temptations in anyone's power over another.

Thus the Christian tradition recognizes the tragic hero of critical care in the crusader who is prepared to violate a patient's integrity for the sake of the good of medicine. It acknowledges that the power of medicine for good is always, willy-nilly, power over the patient. It worries that a technological perspective on the patient is a temptation to see and treat the patient simply as manipulable nature and not as an individual and exceptional exemplar of God's image.

The good news of the gospel has to do, of course, with an unflawed hero. It has to do, of course, with the forgiveness of sins. But it also has to do with the conversion, the *metanoia*, of following this Jesus, the renewal of life under the lordship of this Jesus, the repentance and renewal of the tragic hero.

The glad story gives a curious account of power. It turns conventional judgments about power upside down. The story of the unflawed hero is a story of a wounded healer, a suffering son of man who will come on clouds of glory, who is "lifted up" on a cross, whose kingdom, power, and glory are revealed and established in his weakness. This Jesus was the agent of a kingdom where "many that are first will be last, and the last first" (Mark 10:31), where "every one who exalts himself will be humbled, and he who humbles himself will be exalted" (Luke 14:11). To follow Jesus,

7. E. Becker (p. 18) talks about the problem of "a new theodicy" since the Newtonian revolution: "If the new nature was so regular and beautiful, then why was there evil in the world?" The scientific and technical mind still needed a "theodicy" but "couldn't put the burden on God. Man had to settle for a new limited explanation, an anthropodicy which would cover only those evils that allow for human remedy." When science and technology are the final hope, extravagant expectations are unavoidable, and any failure to provide "a happy ending" equals a failure of care.

to welcome already the kingdom he promised, does not mean to become powerless, but it does require us to construe power as a call to humble service. In conventional perspective the one in power "lords it over" those who are powerless, but "it shall not be so among you" (Mark 10:43).

The medical professional whose disposition is shaped by this glad story, whose character is formed by this unflawed hero, will have resources of character to resist the temptations in power, to turn from the story of the crusader to the story of the humble servant, resources that are simply not provided by the tradition and tools of the medical community. The medical professional who owns this story will recognize that she is not the Messiah, that she images her Lord not only in the power to heal but also in the disposition to patiently serve, and that her patients image her Lord in their very weakness and suffering. By the grace of the glad story, she will see in the powerlessness of her patients not only manipulable nature but also the Lord who calls her to care.

The patient who owns Jesus as Lord will be content neither with the passivity of the so-called sick role, to which the crusader would assign him, nor with the assertions of autonomy some are urging as a check against the crusader. The patient who acknowledges Jesus (or anyone) as *Lord* can hardly claim to be autonomous, at least in the sense of being "a law unto oneself." And one who acknowledges *Jesus* as Lord can hardly claim that sickness or suffering or even dying relieves him of responsibility.

So the medical professional is neither the "animated tool" nor the "Lord" of the patient. And the patient is neither "manipulable nature" nor "manipulative consumer" to the medical professional. They confront each other as neither "Lord" nor "slave" of the other but as servants of the one Lord, the wounded healer, in their respective roles.[8] The confrontation of medical professional and patient will not suddenly and

---

8. A parallel could be drawn to the so-called *Haustafeln* of the New Testament and other exhortations to "be subject." Wives, slaves, children, citizens, church members —all are told to "be subject." This emphasis on subjection seems to accept and baptize conventional role assignments in the first century, and so it has frequently been an embarrassment to the church. But the church did not simply borrow conventional morality; it transformed it by the new vision of power. The role obligations were *reciprocal*. The duty of submission was *mutual*. The background of intelligibility for these passages is supplied not by conventional class and role distinctions but by Christ, the one Lord, the great sufferer. So one's attention is drawn not to one's own place and role but to the other *as neighbor*. See further A. Verhey's *Great Reversal* (67-69). Christian advice to the patient in the twentieth century might well be, "Be subject to your physician." This advice might be a little embarrassing today, but, put in the same context of reciprocal obligations, mutual submission, the conviction that Jesus is Lord, and attention to the neighbor, it might also lead to a transformation of existing role assignments without the excess and sacrifices of asserting autonomy.

miraculously become collaboration and agreement, but where the story of this unflawed hero is told and owned, there will not be any rush to the "last resort" of a procedural solution, which simply decides who should decide (rather than what should be decided) and which leaves either patient or physician powerless and optionless. A follower of this unflawed hero will not be disposed to exercise her power or to assert her rights in order to leave the other powerless in the confrontation and optionless in the decision.

The Christian acknowledges the reality of sin and human susceptibility to its continuing power. So the Christian, too, may well be wary of being tempted by technology to be a crusader, the tragic hero of intensive care. But the Christian is also pointed beyond the tragic hero to an unflawed hero, and so the Christian is freed to tell and live a story of relationships (even relationships between the so-called powerful and the so-called powerless) that are renewed by the curious power of the cross and marked by mutual submission and neighborly love, by patient attempts at renewed collaboration, and by common recognition of the one Lord before whom both are servants and of the one Servant who commands them both. And in this story there are resources and convictions to sustain and nurture the conversation about what ought to be done when others have given up and have invoked a procedural solution, simply deciding who should decide. Beyond the point at which an ethic that focuses only on autonomy would have happily rendered the physician powerless and optionless, the "animated tool" of the medical consumer, and beyond the point at which a purely technological perspective would have happily reduced the patient to "manipulable nature" and left him powerless and optionless, the Christian story still invites patient and physician—and all other parties to the dispute about what ought to be done—to reason together and to pray together and to discern together the shape of Christian integrity.

The Gathering of Evils and the Christian Tradition

Again the possibility of a genuine dispute about what a patient's well-being requires points us toward Sophoclean tragedy, the gathering of evils and the conflict of goods, so that any choice is a tragic choice and irremediably ambiguous.

The Christian tradition points us beyond the tragic vision of an ultimate heterogeneity and incommensurability of goods to one God in whom goodness is also one. If God is sovereign, then good is one. But the Christian tradition also reminds us that God's cosmic sovereignty is "not yet." The enemy forces of pain and tears and death and hunger and the whole legion of evils have not yet laid down their arms and admitted defeat. When God raised Jesus from the dead in victory over the powers of death and sin, God disclosed and established God's own final reign, but we still await the future of that victory. Here and now our world and our medicine are *not yet* God's reign. Here and now, even as we welcome God's cause and serve it, we face many and diverse evils, death and suffering among them. Here and now, even as we seek to consent to God's sovereignty, part of what we know to be God's cause comes into conflict with another part of what we know to be God's cause. In allocating funds, for example, should we feed the hungry or protect the powerless or heal the sick? In making decisions about the care of one person, should we preserve his life or minimize his suffering? Here and now there is moral ambiguity; it is not yet a kingdom of shalom even among the goods which all belong to God's reign.

Christian realism about the fact that our world and our medicine are "not yet" God's cosmic sovereignty can nurture and sustain our capacity to acknowledge that medicine is a tragic profession, providing no escape from either our finitude or our mortality, and that it is sometimes irremediably ambiguous morally. It is God who brings in the new age, not us, not even if we have magnificent tools. The final triumph over disease and death and suffering is a divine victory, not a technological one. But for now the legion of evils attack on every side, so that to defend God's cause on one front may be to leave it open to attack on another. Medicine is a tragic profession.

But the Christian tradition again points us *beyond* tragedy to God's grace and future. When out of the conflicting goods life is not chosen, when out of the gathering evils death is not avoided, then Christian physicians and Christian patients and Christian clerics point beyond tragedy, testifying confidently to God's final triumph. A medicine that points beyond tragedy to the final triumph of God is a watchful profession. A watchful profession does not deny the not-yet character of our life and medicine. It does not claim to inaugurate God's reign. It looks to God. While we wait and watch for God's final triumph, looking to God can sustain and nurture *truthfulness* about our finitude, about the limits imposed by our mortality and by the limitations of our resources. Looking to God can sustain and nurture *humility,* the readiness to acknowledge that we are not gods but the creatures of God, cherished by God, and in need finally of God's grace and God's future, the readiness to acknowledge that our causes are not exhaustive of God's cause: Looking to God can sustain and nurture *gratitude* for the opportunities within our limitations—perhaps not to usher in a new heaven and a new earth but perhaps to save a life or to remove someone's pain or to ease someone's suffering or to relieve the bitterness of someone's tears or at least to wipe those tears away with compassion. Looking to God can sustain and nurture *care,* care even for those who are least, for those who don't amount to much according to other stories. Looking to God can sustain and nurture *respect* for the integrity of embodied persons made in God's image. Looking to God can sustain and nurture the sense of God's forgiveness in the midst of moral ambiguity and so, finally, the *courage* to make the ambiguous choice in the confidence of God's grace and future.

Medicine as a watchful profession remains a tragic profession—but capable of care in the midst of tragedy and able to point *beyond* tragedy to God's victory and future.[9]

9. Another draft of this chapter is forthcoming in a festschrift, edited by Kenneth Vaux, for the (late) eminent Christian moral theologian Paul Ramsey.

6. Scarcity and Health Care: Personal, Public, and Professional Responsibilities

Crisis is commonplace in medicine. Coping with tragedy comes with the territory. But, as we have seen, crises and tragedies come in different forms. The form of crisis routinely handled by medicine is the medical emergency; the form of tragedy most familiar to medicine is the sad story that people tell with and about their bodies. A remarkable assortment of technologies can be brought to bear quickly and skillfully in response to such crises and tragedies.

Today, however, a new crisis confronts medicine and the societies that sponsor it. This crisis, caused in part by the very success of medicine, is not medical but financial: societies simply do not have the resources to do all that medicine can do or all that it may want to do for all whose health might be served. In this financial crisis, medicine and the societies that sponsor it face tough choices and sometimes tragic choices —choices tragic according to Sophocles's definition, choices made when goods collide and cannot all be chosen and when evils gather and cannot all be avoided. This crisis requires three things: first, that individuals take responsibility for their own health, acknowledging that their responsibility to others includes their own discerning use of health-care resources for themselves; second, that societies attempt both to contain spiraling medical costs and to allocate limited resources equitably; and third, that medical professionals be true to their profession while being truthful with themselves and their patients about the limits of their resources.

These personal, social, and professional responsibilities —and the way they are shaped and underscored by the recognition of limited resources —are the subject of this chapter. In the context of scarce resources, individuals can and should do a great deal to protect and nurture their own health, and societies can and should do a great deal to diminish wasteful use of medical resources and to secure justice in the access to health care. But neither personal responsibility nor public policy will eliminate either scarcity or the tragic choices born of scarcity. As Sophocles knew, the crucial issues in tragic circumstances are issues of identity, character, and virtue. It is not too much to say that the financial crisis in medicine is an identity crisis for medicine and an occasion for asking and determining what sorts of societies sponsor it. The public-policy questions of cost containment and equitable access to medical care are important, and societies must deal with them, but no public-policy solution will substitute for professional integrity or personal responsibility. Genuine tragedies, after all, do not admit of ready solutions —by public policy or any other human means. They can, however, be endured by strength of character and virtue. Thus the future of medicine may yet be one in which we may take human and public delight as well as technological pride.

The Financial Crisis: Scarcity and Sanctity

It is hardly necessary to pause to demonstrate the financial crisis in medicine. The media have been full of accounts of spiraling medical costs and of plans to contain them. The total expenditure for medical care[1] in the United States for 1984 was 387.4 billion dollars, or about $1,500 per person (Schroeder, 12). The United States now spends more than 10 percent of its gross national product on medical care, compared to less than 5 percent in 1950. And medical-care spending continues to increase more rapidly than other spending.

There is nothing magical about 10 percent; it is not written in Scripture that a society should spend less than 10 percent of its gross national product on medical care. It is far from obvious how much of a country's resources should be spent on health. Perhaps the United States can and should spend still more on medical care—and thus less on missiles. But there is a limit to how much a society should spend on health care, and many people say the United States and other Western coun-

---

1. Health care must be distinguished from medical care. Medical care is that part of health care which medical professionals do. Health care is a broader category; it includes what individuals do for themselves—exercise, watch their diet, make wise lifestyle choices, and so on—and what communities do—provide safe drinking water, impose public health measures, and so on. The two are obviously sometimes related—for example, a physician providing medical care may give advice about nutrition or smoking, advice that is then acted upon in personal health care or in public-welfare measures and regulations.

tries have reached it. They argue that a society should value things besides health—education, human services for the poor and elderly, a clean environment, safe cities, entertainment, and, yes, national security. There is a health-care spending limit for both rich nations and poor, and if a society is to establish and to enforce that limit, it will need to develop cost-containment strategies and make decisions about the allocation of public funds.

There was a time when affordable insurance programs, public and private, could and would guarantee payment for whatever medical services medicine could provide and an insured patient needed. Now medicine can do more—a good deal more—as a result of the advances in medical research and technology. So the patient "needs" more—transplant surgery or dialysis or in vitro fertilization or. . . . And now insurance programs are no longer affordable.

There are many causes for the escalating costs of medical care, but we have already mentioned the two things most often cited as responsible for increasing medical costs: private insurance programs and the recent successes of medicine.

It is often argued that the insurance programs have created a situation in which none of those who control costs have any incentive to contain them. Physicians, customarily paid by insurance companies for services rendered, stand to make more money by delivering more services. Those services, of course, can often be justified in terms of the patient's good. Thus physicians dealing with insurance programs have little reason to control costs. Patients, protected from the direct costs of medical care by insurance programs, are able to demand the best of medical care; "more" seems better. Thus patients dealing with insurance companies have little incentive to control costs. Private insurance companies themselves have based their premiums on a percentage of their total reimbursements. As reimbursements increase, so do premiums and profits. Thus insurance companies, too, have little incentive to control health-care costs.

There is no doubt that conventional insurance programs did nothing to check spiraling costs, but the successes of medicine are at least as responsible for causing them. The success of medicine has contributed to spiraling costs in at least two ways. In the first place, technology—including medical technology — provides a way of satisfying human wants, but successful technologies—including successful medical technologies—never *only* satisfy human wants; they stimulate them as well. People want to live, they want to be healthy, and medical technology has recently become remarkably successful in forestalling death and restoring health. But people are not satisfied. They want to live longer still;

they want to be healthier still. They want never to die—but if they must, then they want to live until that final moment with the same vigor, appetite, and attractiveness that they had when they were twenty. The successes of medicine have led to rising expectations of it, increasing demands upon it, and broader applications for it. It all costs money, of course—and there is a limit to how much a society can and should spend on medical care.

In the second place, the successes of medicine have kept sick people alive. People suffering the effects of chronic disease—heart attack, stroke, cancer, and so on—though often not cured of the disease, are enabled by the successes of medicine to live and sometimes even to flourish or at least often to function. There are, for example, more people with severe kidney disease in the United States today than there were twenty years ago because technology is keeping them alive. The curious and paradoxical consequence of good medical care is sometimes an increase in morbidity. To be sure, some of medicine's most dramatic successes have produced cures for diseases. Immunizations against diphtheria, whooping cough, and other childhood diseases and the use of antibiotics against bacterial infections have made stunning and very cost-effective contributions to our health. But people eventually die of something, and as infections become less threatening, cardiovascular, degenerative, and malignant diseases become more prevalent. Predictably, medical successes against chronic diseases tend to be costly and to establish a costly dependence upon continuing medical care. Perhaps as much as 80 percent of medical-care resources in the United States is now devoted to chronic disease. Many people are urging that society limit the amount spent on the treatment of chronic diseases in order to have more resources available for the preventive measures that may forestall chronic disease and for the research that may lead to more effective and inexpensive treatment.

However a society decides to limit the total amount it spends on health care, it will face subsequent decisions about how to allocate those funds among competing claims *within* health care: education, prevention, research, acute care, primary care, chronic care, and so on. Making these decisions means answering hard questions. For example, should we fund the continuing development of the artificial heart at great expense when the nutritional needs of many in our society are not met? There are limits on how a society can and should spend *within* health care, but to establish and to enforce those limits will require hard and tragic choices in situations where goods collide and cannot all be chosen, where evils gather and cannot all be avoided.

These decisions about allocating funds to health care—some-

times called "macro-allocation" decisions—eventually lead to and necessitate decisions within medical care that are sometimes called "micro-
allocation" decisions—who is going to receive the scarce vaccine, the
scarce organ, the scarce intensive-care bed. The recognition and enforcement of limits on health care will finally require decisions about who
shall live when not all can live.

It is scarcity of resources that makes allocation decisions necessary. There are limits. No society can afford to do all that medicine can
do or all that it wants to do for all patients (or all prospective patients).
It is the sanctity of God's image bearers that makes allocation decisions
tragic. When the goods and services to be allocated are goods and services upon which life and health depend, and when the life and health
that are contingent upon allocative choices are the life and health of
those who image God, who are objects of the unbounded love of God,
and who therefore may rightfully invoke the respect and care of others,
then allocation decisions are necessarily tragic. The appropriate human
and Christian response to the sad stories people tell with and about
their bodies has always been sympathy and care. All persons, after all,
even (or especially) those whose stories are sad stories, are the objects
of God's unbounded love. All persons, even those who misuse their
freedom, bear the image of God. Therefore, when scarcity makes allocation decisions necessary, the decision to let anyone die because not
all can live, to let anyone suffer because not all can be spared, or to let
the health of anyone go unnurtured because the health of all cannot be
served is a tragic decision.

Some people have made it their business—no, more than their
business, their *profession,* their avowed public identity—to respond to
the sad stories of heart attacks, tumors growing slowly but surely, and
medical emergencies caused by disaster or catastrophe with the sympathy and care appropriate to the sanctity of the individual. Medicine
has learned to care, if not more intensely, at least more effectively. Sometimes the sad story can be given a happy ending, but to do so costs money
—and once again limits loom, as do tragic decisions.

In allocation decisions there have been two strategies for denying tragedy: one is to deny sanctity, and the other is to deny scarcity. Both
strategies can be seen in the response to kidney dialysis in the United
States.

In 1961 a committee was formed at the Seattle Artificial Kidney
Center to select those patients who would receive kidney dialysis when
not all could. This committee allocated the scarce resource to those
whom they considered the most valuable to society. In using social worth
as their criterion for selection, they denied the equal sanctity of each of

the medically acceptable candidates whose lives were at stake. Many people quite properly protested. Paul Freund, for example, argued that "in a matter of choosing for life or death, not involving specific wrong-doing, no one should assume the responsibility of judging *comparative* worthiness to live on the basis of unfocused criteria of virtue and social worthiness" (p. xiii). *Life* magazine christened the committee "the Seattle God Committee" (Alexander, 102). Their sanctity-denying strategy was deemed morally unacceptable then, and it remains so.

The other strategy was to deny scarcity, to provide almost universal funding for kidney dialysis in order to acknowledge and affirm sanctity. In 1972 the U.S. Congress voted to fund kidney dialysis for everyone who suffered from end-stage renal disease. Kidney dialysis would be provided to all who needed it. The program proved far more expensive than Congress originally intended. But, more significantly, the strategy of denying scarcity was self-deceptive from the beginning, because a policy promising kidney dialysis for everyone still distinguishes those dying of end-stage renal disease from those dying from other equally grave diseases, placing the needs of some above the needs of others. There are limits, and the tragedy of allocation decisions cannot be hidden or denied for long.

It is possible for a society to face limits honestly and to attempt to allocate limited resources responsibly. In Great Britain, for example, although physicians would like to utilize more resources, they recognize that the country is not wealthy enough to provide all possible medical care to all patients (Schwartz and Aaron, 53). One British physician said of intensive care, "It has to be appropriate to the surroundings. Now, what we have by your standards is way short of the mark. It would be too small in America, but if you took this unit and put it down in the middle of Sri Lanka or India, it would stick out like a sore thumb. It would be an obscene waste of money" (Schwartz and Aaron, 54). In Britain, evidently, both citizens and physicians have learned to accept the limitations upon health care and to live within those limits, but, as Henry Aaron and William Schwartz suggest, citizens in the United States are much less likely to accept such limits. The British strategy is not to deny scarcity or to deny sanctity but to rely on the judgment of clinical practitioners to allocate limited resources in ways that provide the greatest overall health benefit for the most people. In treatment of patients with kidney disease, for example, there are limits, and a physician knows that to grant dialysis to one patient is to deprive another, but the criterion for selection is not "social worth" but "clinical judgment" (Calabresi and Bobbitt, 230). Such "clinical judgments" can themselves mask tragedy—as when young children are excluded as poorer medical risks because they are less likely to adhere to the strict regimen of hemodialysis (Calabresi and Bobbitt, 185), or those older than fifty are excluded as "a bit crumbly" (Aaron and Schwartz, 35), or laborers are excluded because physical strain makes treatment less likely to be successful for them than, say, academics (Calabresi and Bobbitt, 185).

The British system does not resolve such tragedy or even always face it honestly—but its readiness to acknowledge scarcity and its reluctance to violate sanctity stand as a model for this chapter. The acknowledgment of scarcity requires a renewed emphasis on personal responsibility for health. The acknowledgment of sanctity as well as scarcity requires a readiness to question the subtle "rationing" of health care that occurs in budget cuts to social programs, social policies that make medical care inaccessible to the uninsured, and the development of expensive technologies that will benefit only a few.[2] The acknowledgment of scarcity and sanctity should cause us to question the wisdom of a health-care reimbursement system that rewards expensive technological interventions far more generously than it rewards primary care or preventive medicine and to question the justice of a reimbursement system that places physicians in the uncomfortable position of either seeing the uninsured without remuneration or not seeing them at all (Daniels, "Why Saying No to Patients in the United States Is So Hard"). Thus scarcity and sanctity make it important for us to consider individual responsibility, stewardship of resources, and justice and care for the poor, but they also lead inescapably to tragedy and will require costly integrity from medical professionals.

Personal Responsibility for Health

The recognition of scarcity has had the wholesome effect of reminding people of what they can do to nurture and sustain their own health— and it is considerable. Moreover, the recognition of scarcity has underscored the fact that one's personal responsibility for one's own health is also a responsibility to others. And Christians may welcome this renewed emphasis on personal responsibility for health because they acknowledge it to be part of their response of gratitude to God for the good

2. A case in point: over the past twenty years the U.S. government has invested $250 million to develop an artificial heart (Preston, 6), which led Harmon Smith, a moral theologian at Duke University, to comment, "I don't understand the fascination with these absurd, bizarre experiments when we have babies born every day in the U.S. who are brain-damaged because of malnutrition. It is a serious indictment of our society" (Friedrich, 73).

gifts God gives, including the good gifts of life and health. That response of gratitude to God nurtures the care Christians take of their own health; their responsibility to God makes them ready to assume responsibility for their own health.

Of course, Christians will not make idols of human life and health. Life and health are good gifts of God the creator and provider and the intention of God the redeemer, so they are goods Christians may and must sustain. But they are not gods, nor even the greatest goods; accordingly, other responsibilities to God sometimes take precedence over care for one's own health and life, other goods for which one may be and must be prepared to risk and sacrifice health and even life. The martyrs knew this well, of course, and all Christians are witness bearers to the Christian confidence in God's final triumph when they are willing to suffer and even to die for the sake of the greater good of faithfulness to God, who intends the neighbor's good as well. In dying, then, Christians may have duties that weigh against sustaining their lives for another day or week or month or year. Christians who are dying may choose to live in ways that enable fellowship with friends and reconciliation with enemies and even fun with their families, even if it means foregoing some hospital-based care and the technology that could extend the time they have left. In living, too, Christians may risk their health and even their lives for the sake of a neighbor's good and may not pursue health with an all-consuming passion that pushes all else aside.

But even if health and life are not gods, it bears repeating that they are good gifts of God and that as image bearers of God people have been made stewards of these gifts. People are responsible to God for caring for the measure of health and life they have been given.

Christians can call people to responsible stewardship of their health simply on the basis of prudence. It is simply not prudent to engage in behaviors or to continue in habits that in the end are likely to lead to chronic diseases that are both oppressive and expensive. And many of the chronic diseases that afflict people today do result from behavior that can be avoided. Heart disease, cancer, peptic ulcers, AIDS, and strokes often appear to be related to avoidable personal behavior. Smoking, obesity, excessive use of alcohol, the recreational use of drugs, excessive stress, poor diet, sexual promiscuity, and exposure to environmental and occupational hazards and pollutants—not to mention automobile accidents and violent crimes — account for an incredible number of pressing health problems (Knowles, 62-65)—problems that are avoidable, for the most part, if healthy behaviors are adopted. It is prudent to do what every grandmother has always said was good for you and is now confirmed by the scientific study of Nedra Belloc and

Lester Breslow. Grandmothers and scientists give these seven rules for health: Get a good night's sleep. Eat three meals a day and limit snacks. Be sure to eat breakfast. Keep your weight under control. Don't drink too much alcohol. Exercise regularly. Don't smoke.

One should ask whether it is prudent to smoke when smoking is a primary cause of lung cancer and heart disease and plays a role in nearly one-fifth of all deaths in the United States (Ravenholt, "Addiction Mortality"). Every person who smokes risks serious disease involving the heart, lungs, kidneys, bladder, and other organs. Smoking has been linked to the increased risk of lung cancer, heart disease, cervical cancer, stroke, laryngeal cancer, peripheral artery disease, oral cancer, esophogeal cancer, bladder cancer, pancreatic cancer, chronic obstructive lung disease, peptic ulcer disease, and other diseases. In addition, pregnant women who smoke suffer an increased risk of neonatal death and are twice as likely to give birth to infants with low birth weight. The estimated annual mortality from cigarette smoking in the United States is more than 350,000. Thirty percent of all deaths due to cancer and coronary heart disease are attributable to smoking. Such horror stories, one would think, would be enough to move a prudent person to stop.

Horror stories can be told about the effects of failing to keep any one of the seven rules for health. The strange thing is that the horror stories—the barrage of scientific studies calling attention to the costs, both personal and financial, of certain behaviors and lifestyles—apparently are no better at changing behavior than Grandmother was. True, the number of smokers is down, but people persist in unhealthful behaviors. A 1982 public-opinion survey by the American Medical Association indicated that Americans are very aware of the relationship between lifestyle and health, yet they persist in choosing unhealthful lifestyles. The motivation to live healthy lives simply seems to be missing (AMA, "Report," 116). Prudence seems to be lacking or loafing. Perhaps idolatrous expectations of medical technology, the extravagant confidence that it will deliver us from our sins to our flourishing, lead us to think that we may do what feels good now and figure that medicine will fix us up when our bodies begin to break down. Perhaps, as John Knowles thinks (p. 75), the contemporary focus on rights and liberties and the pursuit of self-fulfillment have left us with little capacity for a sense of personal responsibility.

When prudence fails, scarcity may yet teach people that the appropriate maintenance of their own health is part of their responsibility to others. The seven rules for staying healthy, for example, can be thought of not only as guidelines for personal prudence but also as part of our responsibility to and for others, as the stewardly preservation of health-care resources. Smoking may be thought of not only in terms of its effect on the smoker's health but also in terms of its effects on non-smokers. There is evidence that anyone regularly exposed to smoke runs an increased risk of lung cancer, and children whose parents smoke have an increased incidence of respiratory disease (Chandler, 148; Fielding and Phenow, 1452-60). The costs to others are not only increased health risks. It is estimated that employers pay $300 to $800 per year in excess costs for each smoking employee. The health-care costs associated with smoking are over $16 billion a year. The nonsmoker pays about $100 a year through taxes and health-insurance premiums to support health care for smoking-related illnesses (Fielding).

Similar accounts could be given of the effect of other poor personal health habits on others. Utah, for example, spends considerably less per capita on health care than Nevada. Not surprisingly, although these states are remarkably similar in geography, climate, and population density, by every measure of health the residents of Utah are a good deal healthier than the residents of Nevada. Part of the explanation is surely the contrast between the abstention and stability of the lifestyle of the Mormons in Utah and the indulgent and stressful lifestyle of their neighbors in Las Vegas and Reno, where the odds favor getting sick (V. Fuchs, 52-55). Care for one's own health is a part of the minimal responsibility not to burden others.

Thus both prudence and responsibility to others should prompt people to take responsibility for their own health—but so should piety. Surely, fear can motivate people, and guilt and anxiety for others, but the Christian church can and must proclaim a "more excellent way," a vision of humanity restored to a responsible dominion over that which God created good, including our own bodies. People are responsible to God for God's gifts of life and health. So piety as well as prudence may move Christians to care for their bodies, to nurture their health, to sustain their life. They can say yes to God's intentions in as simple an action as walking or bicycling instead of driving sometimes. They can say amen to God's purposes in so difficult a thing as saying no to a cigarette, a drug, a drink. They can delight in God's creative, provident, and redemptive cause simply by following their grandmothers' advice about living sensibly.

Of course, God's cause cannot be reduced to our health and life, nor can faithfulness to God be reduced to the seven commandments of healthy living. Nevertheless, piety will not disown a personal responsibility for health but will instead delight in it as a part of grateful stewardship.

A great deal can and should be done by people taking responsibility for their own health. Nurturing that responsibility would be a far greater contribution to the health of a society than developing a totally implantable artificial heart. And physicians and society can do a great deal to enable and encourage people to take responsibility for their own health.

Physicians have an important role as teachers, a role too little rewarded by insurance systems, which compensate them only for discrete, piecework services to the sick (May, *Physician's Covenant,* 147). Physicians can provide information that people can use to maintain their health, but physicians also may and must engage in the delicate but deliberate business of transforming the habits of their patients. Such interference in patients' lives is risky because it can turn into a puritanical paternalism, but in situations in which physicians have a covenant with patients, not merely a contract, patients may expect some transformations as well as transactions. And where teaching is the instrument of such transformations, the intellect and will of such patients are not violated or left uninvolved. Indeed, good teachers do not transform students against their will or without appealing to their intellect but enable their students to "see their lives and their habits in a new light and thereby aid them in unlocking a freedom to perform in new ways" (May, *Physician's Covenant,* 150).

And society itself can help people take responsibility for their own health. Government, for example, can sponsor research programs and educational programs on the effect that food, drugs, activities, lifestyles, and environment have on our health. By exploring ways to provide adequate housing and shelter, clean water sources, sanitary methods of waste disposal, and education about the techniques and importance of personal hygiene, a government can make it possible for many people to be better able to take responsibility for their own health, and many sources of disease can be significantly reduced.

Much can and should be done by people taking responsibility for their own health and by physicians and society in nurturing that responsibility—but the problem of scarcity will remain. If everyone took his or her personal responsibility seriously, society would almost certainly be much healthier, but it still would not have unlimited medical resources. Indeed, the claim here is not that personal responsibility will make allocation decisions unnecessary but that those professional services and public programs that nurture and sustain personal responsibility—educational and preventive services and programs—deserve a priority in allocation decisions that they have not yet received.

The emphasis on personal responsibility is sometimes suggested as a solution to the choices scarcity requires. Specifically, there are some people who argue that no funds should be provided for those who "deserve" their illness, that society should not have to bear the financial burden of anyone's irresponsibility. But that some shirk personal responsibility should not be used to justify disowning our responsibility for one another, whether sick or well. It is appropriate and important to emphasize our personal responsibility to God for our own health and life, but it is dangerous and destructive when that emphasis is used to justify the neglect of our responsibilities to God and to our neighbors for maintaining and restoring our neighbors' health.

It is sometimes the case that the sick may reasonably be blamed for becoming sick — but only sometimes; seldom does the entire responsibility belong to the patient. The irresponsibility of the person who is sick—even when that irresponsibility is clear—may not be used to condemn the sick or to deny public accountability and the need for public remedies.

Our reason for emphasizing personal responsibility is not to assign blame but to encourage people to cherish and nurture God's gifts of health and life. Perhaps this point can be protected against misunderstanding if we emphasize that staying well is not easy and that it can be made easier or harder by the community within which one lives. Staying healthy has been made a good deal easier for most of us in the United States, for example, by public sanitation, immunization measures, fluoridated water, and other public provisions. But staying healthy is not easy for a poor, pregnant black woman in Washington, D.C. Nor is it easy for villagers in the Sudan, where the water supply harbors a debilitating and deadly parasite, or for the 35,000 children throughout the world who will die today of diarrhea and malnutrition. The emphasis on personal responsibility does not warrant blaming the victims. Even the responsibility for the diseases linked to smoking cigarettes has to be considered in social context. The smoker may begin smoking because he is enticed by advertisements or pressured by peers, may find it difficult to stop because nicotine is addictive, and may get cancer because of exposure to asbestos or radiation. Meanwhile, tobacco manufacturers use package warnings to disown their responsibility, and the government subsidizes tobacco growers (Lappe). Our point is not to deny personal responsibility but to prevent putting all the blame on the victims of illness or disease. We are sometimes inclined to do so in order that we may—by distancing ourselves from the "irresponsible sick," by denying our solidarity with and obligations toward the suffering—feel justified in refusing to use our resources against their sickness.

Jesus did not use the connection of sin and sickness to condemn the sick. Indeed, he broke the connection of sin and sickness when it was used to blame the blind man or his parents. Instead, he pointed to the power of God to forgive and to heal, and he made that power felt. Those who follow Jesus will watch and work for a world where the sick and the outcast and the poor get well, not blamed. Faithfulness to God will acknowledge our responsibility to and for others. It will compel us to initiate and maintain public policies and preventive programs that make it possible and increasingly easy for others to be responsible for their own health; it will nurture and sustain a social and medical response to the sick that is ready not to condemn but to care and to cure if possible, and that is also ready to reflect the suffering presence of God when our powers and resources to cure are too limited to express the triumph of God.

Stewardship and Cost Containment

In any context of scarce resources, the efficient use of those resources is an important consideration; waste should not be tolerated. Cost effectiveness must play a role in deciding whether to adopt a new technology or to discard an old one. It is necessary to nurture responsibility for the efficient use of resources in both health-care providers and health-care consumers. All of this is relatively uncontroversial today—but also relatively novel, having become a primary concern in medical care only in the last decade.

Following World War II, medical research and services expanded rapidly. Postwar prosperity made expansion possible, and the postwar confidence in science (which had produced not only an atomic bomb but also radar and penicillin) made expansion of medical research and medical facilities a national priority (Starr, 335-63).

In the 1960s the confidence in further growth and expansion of medical research and facilities began to be challenged by the recognition of deficiencies in the distribution of medical goods and services. Great temples of modern science, equipped with the latest advances in diagnostic and therapeutic equipment, stood next to "medically abandoned" neighborhoods where even primary care was absent (Starr, 363). American medicine, a symbol of scientific progress since World War II, became a symbol of social injustice during the 1960s. The observation that abundance and absence of medical care stood side by side prompted legislative action directed at securing access to medical care for all Americans (Starr, 363-78).

During this time Canada progressively established a national health-care system that guaranteed health care for all Canadians. The United States also took action. Medicaid and Medicare, government-funded insurance plans for the poor and elderly, were perhaps the major legislative accomplishments of this period, but community health centers and programs to provide physicians for rural and inner-city locations were also established. These legislative initiatives significantly increased the access of the poor to health care (Starr, 373; for a survey of programs and their effectiveness, see C. E. Lewis et al.).

The financial crisis began in the 1970s; the spiraling costs of medicine and the government's increasing share of those costs made cost containment of medical care part of the public agenda. Initially the spiraling costs made public efforts to improve access to medical care in the United States seem all the more urgent. In 1974 both President Nixon (Rep.) and Senator Ted Kennedy (Dem.) were urging a national health-insurance program that would have assured access for the entire population. Establishment of some such program looked certain, but Watergate and a serious recession worked against immediate approval, and the legislation was delayed—and finally forgotten (Starr, 393-405). Since that time the legislative focus in the United States has increasingly shifted from securing access to cost containment alone. The concern for efficiency is, as we have said, not controverted, and some costs can be reduced without compromising the quality of care or access to it. For example, one study indicates that costs could be cut by 10 percent at no risk to patients if they would be admitted to the hospital the day of coronary-artery bypass surgery rather than two days before (Loop). Another study demonstrates that more definite criteria for admission to cardiac-care units for patients with known or suspected myocardial infarction could reduce costs without any additional risk to the "low risk" patients admitted to routine nursing-care units instead (Fuchs and Scheidt). Such research on cost-containment strategies must be continued,[3] new and current technologies must be rigorously assessed for their cost effectiveness, and those technological interven-

---

3. Of course, such research must meet the standards for any medical research involving human subjects. These standards include a prior assessment of the risks and potential benefits of the experiment, assessment of the research design and the scientific competence of the researchers, and, crucially, the free and informed consent of the patient-subject. This requirement of informed consent may not be relaxed in experimentation designed to provide knowledge concerning the cost effectiveness of therapies; indeed, the patient-subject should be told candidly that the purpose of the experimental protocol is to assess the cost effectiveness of a new or conventional therapy. We recognize the difficulties as well as the importance of the informed consent standard among captive and vulnerable populations, including the sick and the poor, and would condemn morally questionable protocols that involve only the poor. Those who are both poor and sick should not be the first to be recruited for cost-effectiveness research, and if the wealthy sick, including sick physicians, refuse participation in such experiments, then the poor sick should not be recruited at all (see H. Jonas, "Philosophical Reflections").

tions that are costly but of marginal benefit or of benefit to too few must be rejected (Relman, "The Future"; Leaf). Such measures alone, however, are unlikely to provide sufficient savings to resolve the financial crisis of medicine.

And some cost-containment measures have clearly threatened access to health care. In federal cost-cutting measures, hundreds of community health centers, which formerly met the needs of many of those people not covered under the Medicaid program, have been closed (Mundinger). Programs like WIC (Women, Infants, and Children Supplemental Food Program), a nutritional program for pregnant women and children, have been cut; now WIC, at least, has only enough funding to serve one-third of those pregnant women who are eligible (*Final Report*, 26), despite the fact that the program has been shown to decrease the incidence of low birth weight by as much as 75 percent (*Fiscal Imperative*, 14). Programs directed at placing physicians in rural and inner-city locations have also been dismantled. Most serious of all, perhaps, are the cost-cutting measures that have tightened eligibility requirements for Medicaid; currently only 50 percent of the nation's poor are covered. Some states cover as few as 20 percent (U.S. DHHS, *Health— United States: 1984*). About 40 percent of the nation's poor are children, but currently Medicaid covers only a third of them.

These cutbacks, touted as necessary to reduce federal and state expenditures on health care, may in the long run prove very costly. For example, the poor in the United States suffer a high incidence of low birth weight and neonatal mortality, both of which can be ameliorated through proper prenatal care and nutrition. Cutbacks in programs like WIC will almost certainly result in an enormous expenditure of funds in other areas. It has been estimated that every dollar saved by not providing prenatal care will eventually cost two dollars in neonatal intensive care, not to mention the costs of special education. Again, the incidence of measles rises as federal expenditures on vaccination fall (Blendon and Rogers). Because the poor lack the resources to pay, many of them postpone seeking treatment or find themselves unable to get needed care, and the health status of the poor has suffered as a result of this neglect. There is a direct relationship between low income and the prevalence of serious chronic disease (Blendon and Rogers). The increased use of basic health-care services has been shown to result in improved health (Blendon and Rogers), and insurance coverage appears to be the key factor that determines the use of health-care services (Martin, Dolkart, and Freko; Wilensky and Berk). A recent study in California sought to examine the effect that eliminating the state's medical benefits had on health; the study determined that those cut from the program experienced a significant rise in blood pressure and deterioration of general health (Lurie et al.). The health of the poor undoubtedly suffers when they find themselves unable to pay for needed health care, and the costs in financial terms alone are likely to extend far beyond the money presently being saved.

Apart from the cost effectiveness of these cutbacks, to purchase cost containment at the price of unjustly restricting access to health care is a moral price too high to pay. A just and caring society would not respond to the financial crisis in medical care by leading us further down the path toward two societies—one rich and one poor, one with extremely good health care and the other without an adequate level of health care. Yet the United States seems headed in precisely this direction.

Christian stewardship will not deny scarcity and will look to the efficient use of resources, but it will also not deny sanctity and will look to the distribution of resources in ways that honor the image of God in all people. "We are stewards," Calvin said, "of everything God has conferred on us by which we are able to help our neighbor and are required to render account of our stewardship" (*Institutes* III.vii.5). Even if scarcity means we cannot provide everything that medicine could do for all patients, sanctity means that to cut costs by depriving the poor of needed health care is inadequate stewardship. Concerns about efficiency must be joined with concerns about equity if we are to nurture a just society and be faithful to God in our stewardship.

The major approaches to cost containment—regulation, reimbursement reform, and competition—have been controversial in part simply in terms of their impact upon equitable access to care.[4] Regulation has attempted to control costs by setting standard reimbursement rates, preventing duplication of services through certificate-of-need programs, and preventing unnecessary use of services through Professional Standards Review Organizations (PSROs). Critics claim that the rate-setting commissions have undermined the financial solvency of some hospitals, especially hospitals serving the poor, where "cost shifting" had enabled them to underwrite the care of the poor by charging the rich higher rates. Certificate-of-need programs are sometimes accused of giving certain hospitals a competitive advantage in attracting both staff and patients. And many have charged that PSROs encroach upon the professional independence of physicians and, moreover, that PSROs are not themselves cost effective.

Reimbursement reform is an attempt to create incentives for efficiency in the provision of health care. The criticism is that the conven-

4. For a sympathetic account of the major approaches to cost containment, see K. Davis's "Cost Containment and Health Care in the United States."

tional system of fee-for-service reimbursement encourages hospitals and health-care professionals to spend more, expand services, and increase use. Accordingly, various forms of prepayment plans have been recommended and implemented: health-maintenance organizations (HMOs), preferred-provider plans, independent physician associations, and prospective payment according to diagnosis-related groups (DRGs). Advocates of HMOs and similar plans that charge an annual fee for all medical care during the year argue that these reimbursement systems provide incentives for keeping the subscribers healthy, encouraging preventive measures, avoiding marginally beneficial treatments, and using the most economical methods of diagnosis and treatment. Supporters of the prospective-payment plan utilizing DRGs, begun under Medicare programs in 1983, argue that the fixed rates require hospitals to operate efficiently in order to avoid losing money on patients. Reimbursement reform has reduced costs, although the extent of cost containment remains a matter of debate (Davis et al.), and the savings have resulted from reductions in the length of hospital stays and in the number of services utilized rather than from reductions in the actual cost per day or cost per service. Critics charge that the savings are in part attributable to the decision of some hospitals not to admit patients whose care is likely to cost more than the DRG reimbursement (instead, these patients are "dumped" on community hospitals) and the decision to discharge patients at the earliest possible time, sometimes too early. Similarly, they charge that HMOs have saved money by targeting healthy populations for membership, leaving the sickest to community hospitals and fee-for-service insurance plans.

A third approach to cost containment is to introduce competition into medical care, creating more of a medical marketplace. As reimbursement reform is designed to change the financial incentives for physicians and hospitals, so the competitive strategy is aimed at changing the incentives for consumers of medical care. One proposal would limit the tax-exempt status of employer contributions to health insurance. The objective is not (or at least not only) to increase tax revenues but to encourage the purchase of less comprehensive insurance plans with fewer benefits (the exclusion of reimbursement for drugs, for example, or dental care, or transplant surgery) and/or higher deductibles and co-payments. The idea is that, as insurance plans compete for clients and hospitals compete for patients, less comprehensive coverage will lower utilization and, finally, costs. A second strategy, now enacted into law, simply requires employers to offer employees options in health-care coverage. Conventional health-insurance coverage will have to compete with health-maintenance organizations and other prepaid group plans and less comprehensive insurance plans; the savings will be passed along to the consumer in either cash or other fringe benefits.

Concern about cost containment is legitimate and important, but it must be joined to a concern about equity. The jury is still out on regulation, reimbursement reform, and competitive strategies. Let the instructions to the jury include the examination of equity as well as efficiency. Let the jury be reminded not only of the scarcity of resources and the need to cut costs but also of the sanctity of the lives of the working poor and their children and the need to secure for them access to an adequate level of health care.

Certain strategies offer opportunities to pursue efficiency and equity together. Preventive measures such as immunization, nutritional guidance, adequate prenatal care, and the like are both cost effective and required by justice. Competitive strategies could support "Chevy-model" HMOs—relatively inexpensive programs with clearly limited coverage—which would provide primary-care practitioners to serve as "gatekeepers" for further medical intervention (to monitor whether further care is needed and to provide information on how to get it). A voucher system might be financed by tax revenues gained by eliminating the tax-exempt status of employer contributions to health insurance; such a system would enable the poor to join an HMO and to receive the level of health care required by justice. The prepayment strategy of such an HMO would serve to restrain use of expensive and marginally beneficial treatments. Management, caregivers, and members would know in advance the resources available for care, and the level of care would be determined accordingly, as in the British system. If only the very poor joined such an HMO, however, it might indicate the delivery of an inadequate level of care.

To be concerned about cost containment is legitimate and important, but even successful cost containment will not eliminate scarcity or resolve tragedy. Cost-effectiveness strategies will ordinarily favor programs of preventive medicine over care for chronic illness, because preventive medicine is cheaper and results in better health for more people. But physicians and nurses are not committed to the health of some distant patient or some statistical patient or society or some other group (say, the HMO membership) as a patient; they are committed to the life and the flourishing of the patient in front of them even while they recognize scarcity and acknowledge the moral necessity of containing the cost of treating that patient. And members of society show their care for one another and express and nurture bonds of compassion in community by allocating resources to those in the midst of suffering, not to prospective sufferers. To provide the best care for all is impossible; there are limits to our resources. But not to provide a costly but effective treatment cannot be called good. It can only be called tragic.

Justice and Access to Health Care

In any context of scarce resources, the notion of distributive justice is applicable, and decisions which violate that principle are not only tragic but wrong. But precisely what justice requires in the allocation of resources is a much-debated and very debatable topic. There is universal agreement about some obvious things. Everyone agrees that justice requires that we give all persons their due. But deciding what is due each one is difficult. Everyone agrees that justice requires that like cases be treated alike. But deciding what makes cases like or unlike is also difficult. Here, too, there is agreement about some obvious things: for example, to provide services to white or blonde or right-handed people while denying them to black or redheaded or left-handed people may be to treat like cases alike, but such treatment is nevertheless unjust, because these criteria are irrelevant to the distribution of medical care. They are *arbitrary* determinations of what are to count as "like cases," and they are, therefore, wrong. But what are relevant criteria? What makes like cases like in the distribution of medical care? Is the ability to pay, for instance, a relevant criterion? Is it just to provide medical care to some because they can pay for it and to deny it to others because they can't?

It is appropriate to distribute many things, including items from cookies to cars, according to the ability to pay. Distribution according to that pattern frequently creates an incentive for productivity and creativity which can ultimately advance the interests of everyone in society. But even the most ardent capitalist acknowledges the injustice of distributing some things according to this standard. Nearly everyone agrees, for example, that to provide police protection only to those who could pay for it would be unjust, and that to provide basic education only to those who could purchase it would be unfair. It is our judgment that the provision of at least a basic level of medical care is more like providing police protection and education than like providing Oreos and Oldsmobiles.

Medicine is important to people for a number of reasons, and some of those reasons are the very reasons that society uses to justify the provision of things like police protection and basic education to rich and poor alike. One reason that medicine is important is that medical care, like police protection, responds to threats against our basic well-being. Not providing basic medical care when it is the difference between life and death or health and illness would be like not providing basic police protection when it is the difference between life and death or between safety and injury. Of course, basic medical care, like basic police protection, can be overwhelmed by what threatens life and health, and there is always room for debate about how much each citizen has a right to receive. But few would dispute that all citizens have a right to a basic minimum of "preventive" police protection as well as to a certain amount of resources for emergency intervention when adversity requires it. We believe there is an analogous right to medical care. In Chapter Three (p. 79) we noted that sometimes when a society can protect against such serious threats to its citizens' well-being and refrains from doing so, one can argue that the omission is not simply failing to help but is causing harm. We suggest that, when basic and cost-effective preventive and therapeutic medical care is not provided to the poor of an affluent society, the omission causes as much harm as would the refusal to provide them with police protection.

Another reason that medical care is important is that it, like education, can provide and protect a range of opportunities. Health, after all, makes it possible for us to pursue other goods; without health our options and opportunities are severely restricted. The normative importance of at least approximate equality of opportunity in capitalist societies justifies not only publicly funded education for all but also, in our view, some degree of publicly funded health care (Daniels, "Health-Care Needs"). The meaning of normal functioning or well-working will differ for the young and the elderly, for the patient who is terminally ill and the one who is not, for the person who is disabled and the one who is not; and the opportunities and options available to people will also vary according to age and condition. But a just society owes it to people — young people, elderly people, disabled people, and dying people — to preserve and protect a range of opportunities appropriate to their age and condition. In Chapter Three (pp. 81-82, 88-89) we noted several ways of arguing that there is a positive right of access to those services — such as basic education and medical care — that are the foundation of fair opportunity in our society. Henry Stob observes that Christians have considerations that reinforce these arguments: each person "bears in his very being the image of God and . . . has been mandated and commissioned by his Creator to perform an important task in this world" (p. 133). We agree with Stob that this belief gives Christians a powerful reason for seeking social arrangements that provide equal opportunity for stewardship, including arrangements for access to the basic educational and medical resources without which the opportunity for stewardship is crippled.

Finally, medical care is important as a gesture of what it means to be a member of the human community. The ordinary human events of giving birth, suffering, and dying are extraordinarily significant points at which people express their interdependence. In providing police protection, members of a society say to one another, "We will protect you and your goods against violence," and in providing education, members of a society say to one another, "We will nurture your children." Likewise, in providing medical care, members of a society can say to one another, "We will care for you." In Chapter Four (p. 110) we suggested with Stanley Hauerwas that providing medical care is the way society unites itself with the suffering and says to them, "We will not abandon you." Thus the public commitment to provide medical care to those giving birth, those suffering, and those dying is an important gesture that reflects and affects fundamental attitudes about what it means *to be in covenant* with one another.

For all of these reasons we believe that a just society will secure access to an adequate level of medical care for all of its members. The patient's inability to pay should not prevent access to an adequate level of care, and market mechanisms for allocating health care cannot be relied upon to provide or promote justice. But none of the reasons we have cited requires that society provide whatever a patient wants or even needs in medical care. We do not have the resources to do that; moreover, we do not do that in providing such services as police protection and education. But society should provide a basic level of health care to all, along with a basic level of police protection and education. Justice requires it, and citizens have a right to expect what justice requires. In this we affirm the conclusion reached by the President's Commission for the Study of Ethical Problems in Medicine and Biomedical and Behavioral Research: society has an obligation to ensure "that all citizens be able to secure an adequate level of care without excessive burden" (*Securing Access*, vol. 1, p. 4). The President's Commission did not recommend "everything for everyone" or "equal access–equal care." It recognized scarcity, that we simply do not have the resources to do all we could do and all we would like to do for all patients. Scarcity requires placing limits on what we provide, but justice requires that in allocating scarce resources we *first* secure access to an *adequate level of care for all.*

Just what an adequate level of health care is will be contingent upon the availability of resources and the proven effectiveness of various forms of care, and it will surely be defined and refined as part of the political process. Of course, there are some clues in the reasons that health care should be funded about what should be funded. Because medicine helps people express care for one another in community, it is our view that access to a primary care-giver should be guaranteed to all. This primary care-giver, whether a doctor or nurse practitioner, would be a "gatekeeper": he or she would provide preliminary diagnosis, primary care, and information about whether further care is needed and where to go to get it.

Because medicine contributes to the protection of life and health, an adequate level of health care will provide protection against unnecessary health risks. Regulations to ensure safe food, drugs, and water, regulations to guarantee a safe environment and workplace, programs to provide immunizations and preventive medical services, education in good health habits—all would belong to an adequate level of health care. Because medicine secures a range of opportunities, medical and rehabilitative services that effectively restore or maintain normal functioning should be available to all as appropriate to age and condition.

In determining what an adequate level of health care should include, it makes good sense to begin with those aspects of health care that are most basic and beneficial and least costly. Given a reasonable base of medical care, many patients will experience little effect upon their health by any increase in medical resources (V. Fuchs, 19); income and education may be more important to the health of individuals than medical care itself. It is clear, for example, that environmental factors play a bigger role in heart disease and cancer than the "remedies" of surgery and drugs do. Our priorities for establishing an adequate level of medical care are roughly those of Pellegrino and Thomasma (242): first, access to a primary health-care practitioner should be provided to all; next, those treatments that can effect a radical cure or prevent occurrence of a disease entirely (immunizations, antibiotics) should be funded; and only then and if resources permit, the treatment of established serious diseases for which no radical cure is available should be included, followed by the more expensive and complex procedures of yet unproven benefit and the treatment of disorders that are minimally debilitating but not incapacitating or that require only self-care and symptomatic treatment.

An adequate level of medical care (Buchanan) will not include everything that modern medicine is capable of doing. It represents a "decent minimum" (Fried), which ought to be provided by all just societies within the constraints of scarcity. If an adequate level of health care is guaranteed to all, it would not be unjust to use market mechanisms to allocate health care above and beyond that level. Therefore, the public policy we, in accord with the President's Commission, recommend may be described as "two-track care."

In the context of scarcity, a public policy that allows for two-track care may be considered just if it provides an adequate level of health care for all. The current situation in the United States falls short of this standard. Nearly 25 percent of the population is without either private or public insurance and therefore without assured access to an adequate level of medical care. The uninsured include three groups: the temporarily unemployed, who, having lost their jobs, also lost their employment-based health insurance; those uninsurable for medical reasons, who, having lost their health, lost the interest of insurance companies as well; and the working poor, who, although they have a job and their health, nevertheless have no access to public coverage or group coverage and cannot afford the premium for adequate individual coverage (Council on Medical Service, 790-93).[5] Children account for nearly one-third (11 million) of the uninsured (Oberg, "Pediatrics," 568). Forty percent of all women giving birth in the United States are uninsured (H. Brody, 40). Each year five million people report that they did not seek medical care because of their inability to pay for it. In a nation in which many benefit from joint replacements, transplant surgery, coronary-artery bypass surgery, and cosmetic surgery, millions lack the financial or insurance resources to gain entry into the health-care system for even primary care. Mary O. Mundinger summarizes the current situation in the United States with some revealing statistics: "The federal government pays more for the health care of the middle class and the wealthy than it spends for the poor; tax deductions for health insurance cost the government $29 billion in 1982—$8.7 billion more than the federal bill for Medicaid, at $20.3 billion" (p. 46). The United States does not meet the standard of justice. It is time for public policy to make vigorous efforts to secure access to an adequate level of health care for all.

Christians will insist on justice within their own countries, but they will also look beyond their borders to the global village. In that global village many are poor, and very often their poverty quite literally makes them sick. The data give clear and compelling proof of the health risk of poverty (see Appendix C). Whatever index one uses—education, diet, life expectancy, birth rates, infant mortality, the proportion of medical-care practitioners to population—the poor in the global village are less likely to be healthy than the rich. Compare, for example, those who live in countries where the per-capita gross national product is less than $400 per year with those who live in countries where the per-capita gross national product is more than $5,000 per year. People in the poor countries die sooner (15 percent sooner). They have more children (twice as many), and they watch more of them die (nine times as many). They have

5. The Council on Medical Service of the American Medical Association estimates that in 1983 six million people were without health insurance due to temporary unemployment, one million were uninsurable for medical reasons, and forty-four million working poor lacked adequate coverage (p. 790).

access to fewer physicians (one-tenth as many) and fewer nurses (one-twenty-fifth as many). Their average diet not only fails to meet nutritional standards but also fails to meet the minimum daily caloric requirements. The poor countries have fewer resources than the rich countries, and a smaller percentage of these resources is spent on health care—less than 3 percent compared with the more than 10 percent spent by rich countries (see Appendix C).

The link between economic status and health indicators is strong, but it is not absolute. The people of some poor countries enjoy good health. Cuba and Sri Lanka have a high life expectancy, an intermediate birthrate, a very low death rate, an intermediate infant-mortality rate, and adequate diets. Sri Lanka has very few physicians but a moderately high number of nurses; the good health in Sri Lanka is a tribute to social and political policies that have provided an equal distribution of minimal health care and have emphasized preventive public-health measures, particularly clean water supplies. Cuba has also successfully made health care a high priority and has secured equitable access to it (Eckholm, 23-24; Newland, 15-16). Conversely, the people of some wealthy countries have poor health. In many oil-exporting countries, which have become wealthy only recently and in which the wealth is in the hands of a few, the health of the masses is very poor. For example, although the per-capita wealth of Oman, Libya, and Saudi Arabia exceeds that of most industrial-economy nations, their health indicators more closely resemble those found in countries with low-income and lower-middle-income economies.

Another way of drawing the contrast between the health of people in rich nations and the health of people in poor nations is to compare the causes of mortality and morbidity in rich areas with those in the poor areas of the global village. In most poor nations the leading causes of mortality and morbidity are parasitic diseases and bacterial and viral infections. These diseases are largely the result of impure water, and they threaten life and health because of a lack of antibiotic drugs and a lack of modestly trained health-care practitioners to administer them. Most of the viral diseases could be prevented by simple vaccination programs. Thus the diseases that most threaten life and health in developing countries can either be prevented by education and vaccination or be treated and cured by relatively inexpensive medical care. By contrast, the principal threats to life and health in developed countries are the diseases associated with affluence and longevity — namely, cerebrovascular diseases (heart attacks, strokes, atherosclerosis) and cancer. The causes of these diseases are manifold, and prevention (while our best hope) requires major alterations in lifestyle. Treatment is expensive, seldom cures, and establishes a continuing and costly dependence on health-care practitioners.

In the global village we confront again the scarcity of health-care resources and the sanctity of each person whose life or health is threatened. Scarcity and sanctity contain the makings of tragedy—goods conflict and cannot all be chosen—but decisions and distributions that fail to meet the standards of justice remain not only tragic but wrong. If Christians recognize the image of God in all persons and the face of Jesus in the poor and hungry and sick, then they will surely care for them, at least insisting that justice be done for them. Christians must work—and insist that others work with them—toward protecting the life and health of the world's poor, toward securing opportunities for the world's poor, and toward expressing in a global village our membership in one community with the world's poor. That requires of Christians—and others—a global concern for health care.

The quest for elusive justice in health care would be well served by acknowledging the legitimacy of "two-track care" globally as well as nationally. Justice does not require that everyone in the world have access to the same medical care; it requires that everyone have access to some "decent minimum," an adequate level of health care. And as we have said, just what an adequate level of health care means will be contingent upon the availability of resources and the proven effectiveness of various forms of care; moreover, what it means will be defined and refined as part of a political process. Just what an adequate level of health care means, therefore, may differ among nations and may differ notably between rich nations and poor nations.

Although the notion of an adequate level of health care is relative, it is not altogether without direction. Every government of every nation owes it to its citizens to work to provide the basic necessities to maintain and restore health; that is, every government owes it to its citizens to work to provide a clean environment, sanitation facilities, access to decent housing and good nutrition, and primary medical care, including vaccinations and antibiotics, simple medical treatments, and preventive medicine. Most of this primary medical care could be delivered efficiently by nurses or specially trained public-health-care workers; and for the most part it could be brought to the recipients rather than requiring the recipients to come to special institutions.

Such medical care would be accessible and relatively inexpensive in comparison with importing the hospital-based and physician-dependent medicine of the West into poor nations. But "relatively inexpensive" does not mean "cheap"; such a program would require a substantial increase in the resources made available for health care—an increase that may require a reordering of a government's priorities and a reorienting of its sense of responsibility to and for the people. Effecting such changes in other nations' governments is beyond the power (and responsibility) of people (including Christians) in the West, but we are not totally without power (or responsibility) to make a difference in health care in poor nations. Christian medical missions should focus not on the miracle-working modern medicine of high technology but on the decent minimum. Rather than building acute-care hospitals for secondary and tertiary care and staffing them with physicians, missions should give priority to training and sustaining field workers such as nurses and primary-health-care workers, who could bring the decent minimum to villages and homes. Politically, efforts can be made through the governments of developed countries, the United Nations, and the World Health Organization to encourage and assist poor nations to secure access to such a decent minimum for all its citizens. A developed country, for example, might insist that a tenth of any grant in aid to a developing nation be spent on basic or "first-track" health care until the developing country is committed to spending 5 percent of its gross national product to secure an adequate level of health care for all its citizens.

The notion of an adequate level of health care gives direction and guidance to the allocation of resources for medical care even when resources are very limited. But the notion of the decent minimum must grow as a nation's economy grows. When resources are sufficient to fund additional medical care of proven effectiveness, then the decent minimum increases. In developed countries like the United States and Canada, the decent minimum of health care, the first track of the two-track system, should include most forms of secondary and even some forms of tertiary care. In the end, however, the duty to protect health and life is limited by the mortality of human beings; accordingly, while therapies of proven effectiveness should be included in an adequate level of health care, heroic and extraordinary forms of medicine should not be. The duty we have to gesture care for each another as members of one community would suggest the wisdom of including hospice care for the dying and at-home nursing care for the chronically ill as part of the decent minimum and eliminating funds for medical care that could be only marginally beneficial to such patients. The duty to secure a range of opportunities will vary with the age and the condition of the patient.

The precise contours of the first track may differ considerably from country to country, but the notion of an adequate level of health care is universally applicable. The means of financing the first track may also vary from country to country, but the commitment to secure access to it for all citizens must be constant.

The second track, of course, will also vary from country to country. Part of what belongs in the second track in developing countries will belong to the first track in developed countries. But no country will have the resources to fund all that medicine could do or might want to do for all patients. In many countries this second track will include artificial organ transplants, multi-organ transplants, heart bypasses, and kidney dialysis—at least for some patients.

Scarcity requires placing limits on what medical care governments provide and licenses a two-track medical-care delivery system, but justice requires that the first track be our first priority, that we *first* secure access to an adequate level of care for all. Only by so doing will we honor the vision of the physician Luke, who saw that to welcome Jesus and to watch for the kingdom he announced is to care for the poor. Only by making the first track paramount will we affirm the sanctity of all those who need medical care. But the recognition of the legitimacy of limits and the moral necessity of justice—and the policies they form and inform—do not eliminate tragedy. Physicians and nurses profess to offer their best efforts with their best tools to all patients, but to provide the best care for all is impossible because there are limits to our resources. To provide a decent minimum or an adequate level of health care for all is possible and, we have argued, required by justice. Nevertheless, not to provide the "best" care for a patient is not good. It remains tragic. The conflict between the intention of physicians and nurses to do their best for each patient and the restraints imposed by scarcity, which require that medical professionals do less than the best for some, make medicine a tragic profession.

The Future of Medicine

The constraints of justice and cost containment are just that for medicine —constraints, not virtues. Public policy based on considerations of justice and cost containment will set the limits within which medicine may act, but medicine must act with integrity within those limits. This is an important assertion, because medicine's financial crisis has created an identity crisis. Rival and alien stories are being used to understand medicine and to shape its response to the financial crisis. The rational and impartial principles of efficiency and justice are legitimate responses to scarcity, but the demand that medicine treat them as sufficient threatens to alienate medicine from itself, from its own moral interests and loyalties, from the projects and passion that give it moral character. Medicine's response to its current financial crisis may well determine the character of our children's medicine.

Medicine *will* respond to limits and make allocations in ways that express its sense of identity and its values. The questions "What is medicine?" and "What shall it become?" have become crucial in the financial crisis.

Many are suggesting that medicine should be understood in terms of the omnipresent American story of the marketplace, in which the seller gets rich by supplying what the buyer wants. According to this story, medicine simply is (or will become) a commodity that may be bought and sold to satisfy consumer desires, a collection of skills to be hired to do the bidding of the autonomous ones who pay. The marketplace story of medicine is told and lived by the for-profit hospitals that are multiplying across the country. The for-profit hospital chains, many of them now listed on the New York Stock Exchange, have discovered and demonstrated that there is still money to be made in medicine. Under pressure from stockholders to show a profit, many of these for-profit institutions limit their patient population to as few Medicaid and uninsured patients as possible, eliminate those services with a low profit margin, and "dump" inadequately insured and otherwise financially risky patients on other hospitals. The 1983 Annual Survey of Hospitals by the American Hospital Association estimated that public hospitals accounted for one-third of all care delivered without compensation, although they accounted for only 18 percent of all charges. Whereas public hospitals delivered uncompensated care that amounted to 11.5 percent of their total revenues, for-profit hospitals provided uncompensated care amounting to only 3 percent of their revenues (Inglehart, "Medical Care"). Perhaps even more telling are the decisions of for-profit hospitals to refuse emergency-room admission to those who have a "negative wallet biopsy" and to dump them instead on the nearest hospital that will accept them. Cook County Hospital in Chicago alone received 6,769 transfers in 1983, 87 percent of which were transferred for lack of adequate medical insurance. Twenty-four percent of those were transferred in medically unstable condition (Schiff). These refusals to care for the sick seem reprehensible to many professionals as well as to much of the public, but such refusals are quite coherent with the marketplace story of medicine.[6] It is little wonder that, as the stock of for-profit

6. Uwe E. Reinhardt, a health economist at Princeton, recently cited "dumping" as a symptom of a larger attitude of social Darwinism, which shows little concern for the poor and helpless. He describes the 1980s as the era of selfishness, in which the wealthiest nation in the world denied health care to its poor.

hospitals advances, many public hospitals are closing their doors—or else adopting the management style of the for-profit hospitals, ruefully appropriating the marketplace story of medicine.

The marketplace story of medicine will not sustain the dispositions of care and trust that have sometimes marked the covenant of physician and patient. Marketplace medicine will become a medicine in the service of the rich and the powerful while the poor and the weak watch and pray. Already, as George Annas puts it, "the new cry is to keep the uninsured and the poor out of the emergency room, based on Economic Law Number I of the House of Adam Smith: Poor people can't pay" ("Adam Smith").

Medicine must reassert its identity as a profession prompted by compassion and practiced to provide care for those who are sick, an identity born of and nurtured by its covenant to care—and to care intensively —for those in the midst of tragedy. It may not adopt the marketplace story as its story. Christians will point hopefully beyond tragedy and in the meanwhile nurture and sustain medicine as a watchful profession. The Christian profession and Christian professionals will acknowledge that they are enlisted on the side of life and health in a world where death and evil still apparently reign, and they will own a story elegantly told by the physician Luke, a story of good news to the poor, the sick, the despised, and all those who do not measure up to conventional standards or add up to marketplace profit.

In response to the financial crisis and in its rejection of a marketplace identity, a watchful medicine may honor and applaud efforts to assess cost effectiveness and guarantee everyone access to an adequate level of health care. But medicine may not identify with the impartial perspective that prompts these proposals. Medicine must remain a special covenant between a professional and a patient. It must not define itself as a purely political or economic relationship. Medicine must preserve its own identity, honor its own covenant with the sick, and sustain its own integrity, even when public policy—good public policy—imposes constraints which produce moral ambiguity for medical professionals.

It is not just the future integrity of medicine itself that is at stake; the success of public policy may well rely on the integrity of medicine. A lively sense of medicine's covenantal identity and an awe-filled sense of the sanctity of all persons needing medical care may keep a two-track medical-care delivery system from becoming a two-class system. At least such a watchful medicine would serve to remind the rest of us not only of scarcity but also of sanctity, of the tragedy and moral ambiguity of allocation decisions in which life and health are at stake.

A lively sense of medicine's professional identity may also preserve us from a society in which cost effectiveness *alone* determines the fate of those who presently suffer. It may preserve us from a society so focused on efficiency and prevention that it is prepared to turn a deaf ear to those who suffer now for the sake of avoiding more suffering in the future. At least such a medicine might force the rest of us to ask whether a society that can ignore a cry for help even as it "maximizes protection" against future suffering is the sort of society we want to be or become. Medicine must remain true to itself, to its covenant—for its sake and for ours. The financial crisis may be an opportunity for medicine to reassert its identity, not by denying the limits of resources, not by denying mortality, not by overcoming tragedy, but by signaling care for one another in the midst of tragedy.

A watchful profession will sustain and be sustained by the virtues we listed at the end of the last chapter: truthfulness, humility, gratitude, care, respect, and courage. We may now add another to that list in response to the financial crisis: cost conscientiousness, or stewardship of resources. The watchful physician and nurse can contribute to the careful and efficient use of resources. They can have—and ought to have—a "cost conscience," cultivating diagnostic and therapeutic elegance, rejecting the techno-logic that "if we can, we must," avoiding shotgun work-ups and roulette therapy (Pellegrino, "Medical Morality," 11). They can refuse to practice defensive medicine, which orders the additional test as a protection against liability even though it is of no reasonable benefit to the patient. A physician and nurse with a cost conscience will not give in to the patient's every whim as if they were little more than hired hands. Rather, they will stand firm in their refusal to make use of unnecessary testing or therapy even if the patient wishes it. They will, for example, avoid the temptation of over-prescribing drugs to those patients who have difficulty coping with the problems of everyday life. They can work to minimize institutional waste and overuse. They can work cooperatively to identify and educate physicians who overuse resources. They can put creative effort into cost-containment research and prevention programs. Finally, they can rigorously assess new and current technologies (Relman, "The Future"; Leaf). These stewardship efforts are in keeping with good patient care; they do not require tragic choices. Making these efforts avoids not only costly medicine but bad medicine, medicine that is indefensible both economically and clinically. However, despite the good they do, these efforts are not final solutions to the problem of scarce resources; they will not finally eliminate the necessity of tragic choices.

When scarcity and sanctity meet, we cannot eliminate tragedy, but we may not deny it, either. Doctors, nurses, and hospital administrators need the virtue of truthfulness to face the limits imposed by mortality and finite resources and to resist the temptation of denying those limits either to patients or to the public or to themselves.

The twin to truthfulness is humility, the readiness to acknowledge that human beings are not gods but finite and mortal creatures of God, in need of God's care and watching for God's future. When a dying patient needs a listening ear, and two monitors need constant watching, and Mr. Brown needs some reassurance and a backrub, and ten other patients need ten other things—all at the same time—then perhaps the Messiah can handle it all, but one nurse cannot. And the doctor—no matter how good her tools, no matter how competent her skills—cannot always give happy endings to the sad stories people tell with and about their bodies. It is the Messiah, not the doctor, who will usher in a new heaven and a new earth where "death shall be no more, neither shall there be mourning nor crying nor pain any more" (Rev. 21:4). Sometimes the doctor must watch and pray like the rest of us.

But there is a Messiah—Jesus—and the truth of his reign can sustain truthfulness about the limits imposed by finite resources and human mortality. There is a Messiah, and that truth can nurture and sustain the humility of following and serving him even as we wait for him.

Following and serving Jesus even as we wait for him have always demanded the disposition to care. Watchfulness supports the virtue of care in medicine, care even and especially for those who cannot care for themselves, effective and efficient care provided with the best tools and skills one can secure for patients. Watchfulness nurtures care in medicine, care for people who are numbered among the least, care for people in the pain of their labor, care for people in the anger of their premature dying. Watchfulness sustains care, care for people in the filth of their vomit and care for people in the stench of their incontinence. A watchful profession will profess to care, will publicly promise to care, even when it cannot or may not cure.

Finally, piety must be added to our catalog of virtues. What we mean to invoke is not any affected religiosity but what Calvin called "that reverence joined with love of God which knowledge of his benefits induces" (*Institutes* I.ii.1). There is nothing alien to medicine in such piety. After all, the story of medicine begins with God's care, and it will end with the new heaven and the new earth when death, disease, and pain will be no more. While we wait and watch for that day, piety can nurture and sustain not only truthfulness and humility but also gratitude for the opportunities to care within our limitations, respect for the sanctity of each person as an embodied self and as the image of God, and a sense of God's forgiveness in the midst of moral ambiguity.

A faithful medicine will allocate the resources provided and limited by public-policy decisions in a way demanded by its character, its identity, its virtues, and its profession. It will not leave allocation decisions to the marketplace or deny sanctity by using social-worth or social-benefit criteria in distributing resources. It will rely instead upon medical criteria and medical judgment. Medical techniques and procedures will be used only on persons who may significantly benefit from them. But these criteria may define only the group of candidates eligible for scarce medical resources. Ordinarily, random selection should be the method used to draw specific patients from within the target group. When scarcity dictates that not all can receive maximal treatment, sanctity ordinarily requires random selection, because it forbids godlike judgments that one person's life is "worth" more than another's (Ramsey, *Patient,* 256-59; Childress, "Who Shall Live"). Random selection— and perhaps only random selection—can sustain a relationship of truthfulness and trust between medical professional and patient. Random selection—and perhaps only random selection—will sustain a capacity to care even for those whom medicine cannot afford to cure. Random selection will encourage us to find less costly ways of responding to the threats to human life and flourishing that menace those about whom we care but whom we may not cure. At the very least, random selection will force us to acknowledge the tragedy of our limited resources.

When goods collide and evils gather, we may not deny either scarcity or sanctity. The best we can do is to act with integrity in tragedy, with faithfulness to our identity. But the very identity of medicine is what is at stake; the financial crisis in medicine is an identity crisis. Clearly, medicine must choose and own an identity. It faces two futures—one, as a marketplace commodity; the other, as a watchful profession.[7]

---

7. Parts of this chapter are revisions of A. Verhey's "Sanctity and Scarcity."

7. On Having Children and Caring for Them: Becoming and Being Parents

Now Adam knew Eve his wife, and she conceived and bore Cain, saying, "I have gotten a man with the help of the Lord."

(Gen. 4:1)

Everyone has heard of new versions of the Bible—the Revised Standard Version, the New International Version, the Jerusalem Bible, the Cottonpatch Version, to name only a few. Some time ago in *The Wittenberg Door* yet another version was announced—the Valley Bible, "a really tubular Bible, for sure" ("'Totally Awesome,'" 22).

Everyone has also heard about new versions of procreation. In 1978 a new version was announced that went something like this:

> Now Gilbert Brown took his specimen bottle and filled it with sperm, and the sperm were placed in a little glass dish along with an ovum which had been surgically removed from his wife, Leslie Brown, and, behold, after the egg was fertilized, it was implanted into the wall of Leslie's uterus and grew. And she bore Louise Brown, saying, "I have gotten a little girl with the help of Drs. Steptoe and Edwards and, oh yes, God—a really tubular non tubular little girl, for sure."

That, of course, was not the first new version of procreation—nor the last. Since Genesis, humans have developed a wide variety of new versions of procreation, new beginnings of life. Already in Exodus there are midwives, and over time people have increasingly subdued the natural processes of human begetting and brought them more and more under human control, until today it is possible to intervene at a number of different points of the reproductive process in a number of different ways and for a number of different reasons.

Human Control over Procreation

A comprehensive catalogue of these new versions of procreation and the possible reasons for them is beyond the scope of this chapter; some sampling must suffice. (See, further, Andrews; Lebacqz, 3-15; McCormick, *How Brave a New World?* 306-35; Schneider; P. Simmons, 159-63.)

People can intervene at the stage of birth by fetal monitoring and by various techniques of delivery, including, for example, Cesarean section. The new versions of procreation employed during pregnancy include hormonal therapy to sustain a pregnancy, amniocentesis and chorionic villi biopsy to diagnose abnormalities in the fetus, abortion to end a pregnancy, intra-uterine surgery to repair certain congenital defects, and embryo transfer to move the embryo from a petri dish to a womb, or from one womb to another, or from either a petri dish or a womb to the freezer to preserve it for later implantation. With regard to conception, people can intervene not only to prevent it by a variety of contraceptive measures but also to accomplish it—by hormone therapy, surgical repair of the fallopian tubes, artificial insemination, or in vitro fertilization.[1]

This is, it may be said again, only a sampling—and a sampling of present capabilities. In the future, genetic therapy, cloning, and artificial wombs may be added to the list. The list of human powers enabling us to intervene purposefully in procreative processes is sure to grow even more rapidly than the list of new versions of Scripture, but not perhaps any more rapidly than the list of reasons for developing and using these new powers.

Again, it is necessary to be satisfied with a mere sampling. The good sought and the purpose of these powers might be safeguarding the health and well-being of the child; enabling a childless couple to circumvent their infertility[2] and to have a child conceived with their own seed; enabling a childless couple to have a child conceived with donors' seed; enabling a couple to have a particular sort of child—say, a boy or a "normal" child or a gifted child; enabling a single person to have a child; or

1. Artificial insemination is a relatively simple procedure in which a syringe is used to deposit sperm in a woman's reproductive tract at her time of ovulation. The male providing the sperm may be either the husband of the prospective mother or another donor, and the woman receiving it may be either the wife of the sperm supplier or a surrogate mother. In vitro fertilization, the technology of Louise Brown's marvelous conception, uses an egg surgically removed from either the wife or a donor, fertilizes it with sperm provided by either the husband or another donor, and implants the fertilized egg in either the wife or a surrogate mother.

2. Estimates of the percentage of couples with infertility problems range from 7 to 15 percent (P. Simmons, 157).

enabling prospective parents to make an informed choice about whether to conceive when they may be at some genetic risk or to make an informed decision about therapy or abortion on the basis of a prenatal diagnosis. These could be called "personal" purposes (although they also have social dimensions simply because they involve the social roles of husband, wife, and parent), and they could be contrasted with an assortment of "societal" purposes. The good sought might also be predominantly social after all: to enable society to avoid the genetic disaster some have predicted if we continue to treat those who would otherwise die from certain genetic diseases; to enable society to avoid the costly care of persons who are retarded or disabled when there are many other demands on our resources; to enable society to reproduce geniuses or good soldiers or short and strong people to work the mines; to enable society—to quote Joseph Fletcher—"to offset an elitist or tyrannical power plot by other clonors" by "cloning top-grade soldiers and scientists" ("Ethical Aspects," 779). (It has been seriously suggested that there may one day be a "reproduction race" and a "cloning gap" as crucial to national security as the "missile gap" and the "arms race" putatively are today.)

This list of purposes for revising the old version of procreation is, as previously noted, only partial. It does not include, for example, some of Joseph Fletcher's most imaginative hypothetical cases or the situation of the couple who needed a son to secure a huge inheritance.

Of the new versions of the Bible, some are good and some are appalling. The same can be said about new versions of procreation: some of them are good, and some of them are appalling. But which ones, and why? Granted that people can do a number of things in begetting children that they never could do before, the question arises, *May* they do them? Should we use these new versions of procreation, and to what end?

Public Discussion of Human Procreation

It is not as though this chapter initiates public discussion about the new beginnings of life. On the contrary, the discussion of these powers has been vigorous and often rancorous. Indeed, although the vehement ill will that characterizes the rhetoric about legislative initiatives to license or limit these powers[3] is morally irresponsible and publicly unhelpful,

---

3. For a discussion of the legislative proposals concerning reproductive technologies, see P. Donovan. The need for some legal framework for regulation of these technologies is becoming increasingly clear, but there are a number of very difficult legal issues,

the rancor of such discussions signals that the issues have touched a nerve, that some deep and old questions about the kind of society we are and want to become have been reopened. The public discussion, however, seldom raises those questions candidly. It has focused instead on two issues, those of freedom and utility—that is, of protecting autonomy and of weighing risks against benefits.

It is not difficult to substantiate the importance of both freedom and utility. The issue of freedom comes up again and again: proponents of abortion based upon the results of amniocentesis defend abortion in terms of freedom of choice; couples desiring to use the new reproductive technologies defend them in terms of their freedom to do what they can to have a child (or the child of their choosing); single people have begun to insist on an equal freedom to have children. The issue of freedom has clearly been central to the public discussion.

The only issue that has perhaps come up more often is utility, the calculation of risks and benefits. In vitro procedures were discussed initially in terms of the risks to which the embryo was subjected. The question was often posed, "Are parents *free* to put their prospective child at *risk* for the sake of having one?" When the risks were shown to be within the range of the old versions of procreation, public opposition to in vitro fertilization diminished. The calculation of risks and benefits has also dominated public discussion of amniocentesis, experimentation on fetuses, contraceptive technologies, and so forth.

---

especially when the technologies involve donor seed or a surrogate mother. A sampling of the nettlesome legal questions to which there are currently no uniform legislative answers includes these: Should payment to donors and surrogates be illegal? Can a preconception agreement be enforced if a surrogate mother decides to keep the child she carries and bears? May donors later assert paternity or maternity rights? Are donors altogether free of responsibilities of paternity and maternity? May genetic screening be done on donors and their seed? Should it be required? Which genetic traits may be tested? Should the offspring from any one donor be limited? Should records be kept? Who should have access to such records? Does a person require the consent of a spouse to donate seed? May embryos be frozen for later use?

The bizarre case of Judy Stiver was one indication of the legal muddle. She entered into a $10,000 contract with Alexander Malahoff, agreeing to be artificially inseminated with Malahoff's sperm and to carry his child. When the baby was born with microcephaly and a serious infection, Malahoff refused to consent to treatment of the child. The hospital sought and won a court order to care for the baby. The Stivers wanted their money, but when genetic tests proved the baby was not a result of the artificial insemination but of Judy Stiver's intercourse with her husband, the Stivers took custody of the baby, and Malahoff kept his money—or most of it (the lawyer's fees were not refundable). Malahoff is reported to have said, "Instead of a baby, I ended up with a lawyer." One problem in this legal muddle is that babies and the yet unborn don't have lawyers, but everybody else does.

Society seems to have decided that these two issues—freedom and the calculation of risks and benefits—are the issues that need to be raised if society is to get its moral bearings, and perhaps this is not surprising. Since the Enlightenment the project of philosophical morality has been to identify and justify some impartial and rational principle that we can and must hold on the basis of reason alone, quite apart from our loyalties and identities, quite apart from our particular histories and communities with their putatively partial visions of human flourishing (MacIntyre, *After Virtue*, 36-79). Contemporary moral philosophy tends to present two such basic principles, autonomy and utility. The principle of autonomy, with its heritage in Kant, emphasizes the freedom of persons and the duty to respect the equal freedom of all others (Chapter Three, pp. 78-82). Utilitarianism, with its pedigree in Mill and Bentham, emphasizes doing that act (or following that practice) which will bring the greatest happiness and the least harm to the greatest number (Chapter Three, pp. 71-73). Judging from public discourse, the public has not decided whether Kant or Mill is right, whether freedom or utility is the right moral principle. But the public does seem to have decided that the Enlightenment was right, that public debate, including the discussion about new versions of procreation, should be limited and guided by impartial rational principles—specifically, the principles of freedom and utility.

We do not mean to overlook or underestimate the strengths of such a position—especially in a pluralist society. Indeed, we have contended that respect for freedom and concern about consequences are important—indeed, critical—moral principles. But we have also contended that at least sometimes an impartial perspective and the impartial principles such a perspective sponsors are insufficient. The insufficiency of such a perspective ought to be readily acknowledged by persons and communities with particular loyalties and identities, with particular visions of human flourishing, with specific moral convictions and passions. Such persons and communities want to live with integrity, not merely with impartial rationality.

The insufficiency of an impartial perspective becomes quite apparent when the new versions of becoming (and being) parents are discussed. For one thing, the ways the impartial principles are applied to the new powers of procreation depend on partial and particular perspectives on the future, on technology, and on nature and human nature. For example, the initial weighing of the costs and benefits of in vitro fertilization depends in part on whether a person looks at the future optimistically or pessimistically; it depends in part on whether a person sees nature or the mastery over nature as crucial to human flourishing; it depends in part on whether a person sees the normatively human as rational control over nature or as embodied participation in nature. The insufficiency of an impartial perspective and the principles it sponsors shows up as well in the failure to raise candidly in public discussion the sort of questions these new versions of procreation make fundamentally important. Publicly there is considerable discussion of utility and freedom, but there is precious little discussion of the appropriateness of certain dispositions toward the future, or of the fittingness of certain perspectives on nature and human mastery over nature, or of the wisdom of particular visions of what sort of persons and communities we should be and become. The insufficiency of the impartial perspective shows up, then, when it neither raises nor replies to such fundamental questions about new beginnings of life.

But the insufficiency of these principles shows up most tellingly when role relationships like those of parent and child or husband and wife or doctor and patient are treated simply as contractual relationships between free, independent, autonomous individuals or merely as instrumental relationships designed to achieve some extrinsic good. All persons with experience in a family know that they are not as autonomous and independent as they sometimes like to think they are, that their interdependence is to be nurtured as well as acknowledged, and that happiness is an inadequate goal. And if the principles of freedom and utility are insufficient to account for the good life in a family—let alone to nurture and sustain it (Hauerwas, *Community*, 155-74)—then they are probably also insufficient for public discussion of the new ways of becoming parents. We will not and may not disown a respect for freedom and a concern for consequences, but we must and we will own more profound convictions about what it means and what it takes for human beings to flourish. Then we may invite people to live in the faith and in families with integrity, not just with impartial rationality.

So much for observations about public discourse concerning new versions of procreation. Perhaps these observations have established an agenda for public discourse and communal discernment; at least they have established an agenda for the rest of this chapter. We must deal with freedom and utility, but beyond that we must deal with fundamental issues such as our disposition toward the future, our disposition toward nature and mastery over it, our disposition toward our children, and our disposition toward one another. Having done so, we may be more discerning about some of the new beginnings.

Toward a Christian Perspective

Freedom

We have already observed the importance of freedom in the public debate—and we have already suggested that the principle of freedom alone is insufficient for thinking about what is morally at stake in becoming and being parents.

It is important, first of all, simply to restate the moral significance of freedom in the Christian perspective. Faithfulness to God the provider, we have said (Chapter One, pp. 13-15), will nurture and sustain the disposition to honor the freedom God gives. Recognition of the image of God in human capacities for understanding and willing, we have said (Chapter Two, pp. 57-66), will nurture and sustain the disposition to respect the freedom of agents. Christian convictions and commitments will not permit people engaged in moral reflection to ignore the issue of freedom, nor will they permit people engaged in the moral life to be content when human freedom is violated. And respect for freedom also warns against unwarranted intrusions into the privacy of procreative decisions. The rub comes, of course, with the word *unwarranted.*

When respect for freedom is taken to be a sufficient principle and when freedom is understood as the capacity of neutral agents to will what they will, unconstrained and uncoerced, then the only warranted intrusion into the privacy of procreative decisions is the protection of the equal freedom of another person. Whatever one decides about the personhood of the fetus or embryo or fertilized egg (an issue we discussed in Chapter Two, pp. 34-48), one surely must agree that a child not yet conceived is not a person. Since many procreative decisions are made even before any child is conceived, they can presumably be made freely, without any regard for the equal freedom of another person. Therefore, it looks as though there is no warranted intrusion into the privacy of reproductive decisions about whether or when or how or why to have children other than the insistence that those who are making the decisions be "consenting adults."[4] Such a perspective runs the risk of enthroning subjectivism because it judges a decision to be right solely upon the fact that it was freely made.

However, we have not taken respect for freedom to be a suffi-

---

4. This conclusion, however, is invalid. Even if a prospective parent has no obligation to an embryo as a person or as a potential person, in deciding to have or attempt to have a child, a parent does have obligations to the future person who may be the consequence of a procreative decision.

cient moral principle, nor have we understood freedom to be the freedom of neutral agents to will what they will, unconstrained and uncoerced. Certainly persons must respect others, and that surely entails
that they must respect the capacities for agency in other persons. But persons are always more than their rational autonomy. Persons must also
regard others and respect others as *embodied* persons; people are not, for
example, to deprive others of bodily necessities. And persons must regard and respect others not only as free individuals but also as "members one of another," as members of communities at least some of which
are not of their own choosing. Indeed, when one acknowledges—as we
must—how the exercise of agency is dependent upon and restricted by
biological, cultural, and social conditions, it is clearly insufficient and
probably denigrating to construe respect for persons simply as respect
for their individual freedom.

Freedom itself, we have said (Chapter One, pp. 13-14), is better
understood in Augustinian fashion, not as the unconstrained choice of
a neutral agent to will what he will but as the capacity of an agent precisely to establish a self, to set that self upon some "good," to determine
an identity in one's choices, and then to will and to act in ways consistent
with the established self. Such an understanding of freedom illumines
reproductive choices in two ways.

First, it suggests that reproductive choices must be considered
and evaluated not simply as discrete and uncoerced choices but as
choices that establish ways of *being* parents as well as ways of *becoming*
parents. A decision about the reason to become a parent or about the way
to become a parent establishes a parental identity and helps determine
subsequent parental choices. The woman who chooses to have a child
using sperm donated by a Nobel-prize winner in chemistry, for example,
is probably more likely than other mothers to enroll her child in the
seven-day seminar entitled "How to Multiply Your Baby's Intelligence,"
sponsored by the Better Baby Institute (see Traub). The choice about how
and why to become a parent affects the sort of parent one subsequently
will be; it already establishes a parental identity. We will have to return
to the issue of whether there is any moral wisdom about being a parent
that could guide and limit choices about becoming a parent, that could
warrant "intrusions" into the privacy of procreative choice. For now it
is enough to observe that an Augustinian understanding of freedom will
not be content simply to raise the procedural question of whether the
person deciding is a "consenting adult"; it will demand consideration of
the very issues from which the procedural question withdraws, including the issue of the sort of parents people should be and become, and the
sort of parenting upon which people should set themselves.

The Augustinian understanding of freedom illumines reproductive choices in a second way: it alerts us to the danger of manipulatively establishing an identity for a child in particular decisions about how and why to have one. It is important that this point not be misunderstood. We do not see the goal of parenting as bringing a child to "mature" and "neutral" adulthood, when he will suddenly be capable of making and be expected to make "free" decisions, unconstrained and uncoerced. Such is the vision of parenting among those who take freedom to be a sufficient principle and who define freedom in terms of neutral agency; parents who share that vision want to bring their children up in an atmosphere of religious neutrality so that, when they are mature, they will be able to decide for themselves whether to be religious or not. But such is not our view. Freedom is important, but not sufficient, and freedom is always the freedom of established selves. So we are prepared to acknowledge and affirm that being born into a family establishes an identity for a child, provides a history and a community in terms of which the child must learn to understand himself or herself. And we affirm the baptismal vows of Christian parents to bring their children up in the faith, to instruct them in the faith, and to lead them by example into a life of Christian discipleship. A parent may and must initiate a child into communities and histories and so into an identity (Hauerwas, *Community*, 165-66, 173-74), but a parent also may and must nurture the capacities for agency which make it possible for the child to own that identity as his or her own—or to stand against it. Most parents know this, and the Christian faith insists upon it. A Christian identity that is not freely owned is not a Christian identity. A Christian parent properly concerned to lead her child into faith may not substitute behavior modification techniques for religious instruction and example, however effective such techniques may be, for a child is led into faith only if his understanding and will are engaged, not if they are circumvented and repressed. A Christian parent properly concerned to lead her child into faith may and must nurture and engage the child's capacities for agency—even if doing so enables the child to stand against a Christian identity—in the confidence that the Truth needs no other power (Hauerwas, *Community*, 174).

Some of the new reproductive technologies, however, make it possible for parents to establish an identity for a child without involving or inviting the development of capacities for agency in the child. To clone a human being, for example—whether a good soldier or a brilliant pianist—establishes an identity for the child that is not freely owned by the child and that does not invite anyone to nurture and engage the child's capacities for agency. The purpose, after all, is to produce a good soldier or a brilliant pianist, and the procedure fails if the one designed to be a good soldier becomes instead a brilliant pianist or a brilliant pacifist. Such a child's freedom will not be nurtured; it will be—and must be considered as—a threat to the success of the reproductive procedures. A genetically engineered child may properly feel used, a means to another's end. Any sort of genetic designing for the sake of specific limited goods—say, the breeding of short and strong people to work the mines—runs the same moral risk of manipulation, manipulation likely to be continued as parents circumvent and repress the child's capacities for understanding and will, manipulation properly to be abhorred and resisted, lest children become merely means to their parents' ends.

But the examples need not be as preposterous as cloning pianists or breeding people to work the mines; our new power of sex selection runs the same risks. It is questionable whether a sexist society is capable of using this power justly (let alone wisely). If, as studies show, firstborn children tend to be aggressive and competitive and next-born children tend to be docile and compliant, then the power to select the sex of children may be influenced by society's sexist preference for boys as first children and girls as second children. The procreative choice is, then, not simply the choice of a neutral agent but the choice of a self established (in part at least) by the sexism of society. Furthermore, the power of sex selection may even nurture society's sexism, because it may sustain the arbitrary expectations of and demands upon little boys bred for competitiveness and little girls bred for docility, which is to say that specified sexual identities and characters would be manipulatively established for children.

The risks, then, are that certain of the new versions of procreation can establish and manipulatively determine important aspects of a child's very self, and that certain new ways of becoming parents can establish and determine a way of being parents. If a fetus is "bred for" military duty or the concert hall or work in the mines or "male aggressiveness" or "female docility," then the child's life is likely to be continually molded toward that end. If in becoming a parent one breeds for such things, then in being a parent one is likely to demand and expect such things, to be disposed even to circumvent and suppress the child's developing understanding and will in order to achieve such things.

Freedom is an important but insufficient principle for making decisions about procreation. In public discussion of the new procreative powers, the burden of proof must not be borne only by those who would "limit freedom"; it must be shared by those who would ignore or deny the embodied character of human nature, reducing persons to their capacities for rational choice, and by those who would ignore or deny the natural—indeed, biological—communities by which persons are "members one of another," reducing persons to autonomous individuals and human communities to contracts.

Utility

We have already noted the importance of utility to public debate and observed that whenever a new version of procreation is introduced, it is likely to be assessed in terms of its "risks and benefits." But the weight of such arguments, frequently and conventionally taken to be compelling, should be reassessed; the limitations and ambiguities of such arguments should not be overlooked.

First, utility calculations, or assessments of risks and benefits, often ignore a basic moral question, the question of distributive justice. It is not enough to count up the risks and benefits; it is necessary also to ask "Who bears the risks?" and "Who stands to benefit?" and "Is this distribution just?" For example, when Joseph Fletcher writes that "if the greatest good of the greatest number were served by it," he would "vote" for genetically engineering people for specific tasks like "the testing of suspected pollution areas or the investigation of threatening volcanoes or snowslides" ("Ethical Aspects," 779), then it is important to ask whether it is just to assign one human being certain risks in order to benefit others. A good person may sacrifice his interests for the sake of another's good, but conscripting a person, even a good person, against his will or without his knowledge, to the service of others, even a great number of others; forcing upon one human being risks for the sake of a good, even an important good, in which that one does not share—that is unjust. The point is applicable to research utilizing embryos produced by in vitro fertilization. Some such research may lead to genuine benefits, but it is not fair to impose the "risks" of research on those who cannot voluntarily assume them for the sake of benefits in which they will not share.[5]

Second, utility calculations, by their very preoccupation with the values that people *achieve*, often ignore or deny another basic moral question, the question of the values people *express*. An action may make sense as an effective and efficient means to achieve an end but still be questionable in terms of the values it expresses or fails to express. The new versions of procreation may make it possible for a couple to have a

---

5. This point tells against the policy recommendation of both the Ethics Advisory Board for the U.S. Department of Health and Human Services and the British Warnock Report, which would permit fertilizing ova in vitro, using the embryos for experimentation, and then destroying them before fourteen days.

particular sort of child, but the questions to be asked include not only whether this would be a benefit and who would be benefited, but also what version of parenting such a decision expresses. In procreative decisions people not only attempt to achieve some goal; they also express some of their deepest convictions and values—convictions, for example, about nature and human nature, about children and about their relationship with children, and the like. These are issues to which we must return. For now it is sufficient to point out the insufficiency of utility calculations and to warn against the possibility of distorting what is morally at stake if that insufficiency is not recognized.

Third, the very language of *risks* and *benefits* is deceptively simple. A more adequate assessment would deal more honestly with the issue of the probability of consequences, both good and bad; it would consider harms as well as risks, and hopes as well as benefits.[6] The deceptively simple categories of risks and benefits force people to regard harms as though they were only possibilities and hopes as though they were already certainties (May, "Right to Know," 198). The language thus tips the scales in favor of the research or the innovative intervention into reproduction that is being assessed. Consider, for example, research on embryos produced by in vitro fertilization. If such research takes some *risks* with some embryos for the sake of the *benefits* of a cure for cancer or a remedy for genetic diseases, then the research sounds morally plausible. But the "risk" (being washed down the drain) is a certainty for these embryos, whereas the "benefits" (cures for cancer and genetic disease) are far from being probable. If we speak of the research as "harming" embryos in the "hope" of gaining some knowledge that may possibly contribute to a cure for cancer or genetic disease, then such research sounds much more dubious morally. If people were more careful with their language, they might also be more attentive to an old medical and moral (and biblical; Rom. 3:8) principle that says, Do no harm.

The uncertainty of certain risks and hopes ought also to be acknowledged. People may not know all the risks until they have taken them. The issue then is not only whether certain well-defined risks may be taken for the sake of some clearly known probability of benefit; in some cases the issue is exactly *what* the risks and legitimate hopes really are and whether we can get to know them morally. To be sure, any new procedure involves some uncertainty about risk, but with new

6. Some cost/benefit analyses deal in quite sophisticated ways with the issue, weighing the probability of harms and benefits as well as their magnitude, and some analyses categorize risks to unconsenting subjects as harms (in our view, properly). The point here has to do with ordinary discourse—in which the comparison of "risks" and "benefits" is often misleading.

beginnings in life, even if people learn that the risks are minimal, the stakes are very high. Or, to put it more elegantly, although the probability of harm may turn out to be small, the magnitude of the possible harm may be very great. After all, people are tinkering not just with biology but with their natures, with institutionalized habits of bearing and rearing children, with the very notion of what it means to be a parent.

Finally, it should be observed that the weighing of harms, risks, hopes, and benefits is indeed an important matter, but it is *not* a purely technical matter. The application of the "impartial" principle of utility depends on profound convictions about the future and about technology and about parenting. The people who weigh the risks and benefits differently do not have different information or different scientific methods: they have different perspectives, different dispositions, different convictions. To these issues we must now turn.

The Future

The assessment of risks and hopes is not a purely scientific matter; it depends in part upon a person's perspective on the future. Optimists are disposed to react to new versions of procreation with confidence and hope. Pessimists are disposed to react to the same new powers with anxiety and fear. Their perspectives on the future affect their assessments of the magnitude and the possibility of harms and benefits.

In 1978 those who celebrated the birth of Louise Brown, the world's first "test-tube" baby, pointed to a healthy baby girl and envisioned many other childless couples being helped by this procedure to have the baby for which they longed and prayed. And it did seem wrong somehow not to rejoice with the Browns, not to join them in celebrating human ingenuity and divine goodness and a beautiful little girl, not to join them in the hope and vision of other childless couples having their babies. On the other hand, those who reacted with horror and alarm shared a different vision, a vision of egg banks, surrogate mothers, classified ads announcing "eggs for sale" and "celebrity seed wanted" and "wombs for rent," sex choice, quality control, and the creation of a real London Hatchery and Conditioning Center to match the fictitious one in Aldous Huxley's *Brave New World*. And that vision has not lost its plausibility or its horror—especially for the pessimists.

We shall do best, however, to avoid the fateful script of either the optimists or the pessimists, as though either progress or catastrophe were inevitable. G. K. Chesterton once said "that the optimist thought everything good except the pessimist, and the pessimist thought everything bad, except himself" (p. 66). There is wisdom there, a wisdom borne out by many discussions of new versions of procreation; both optimistic proponents and pessimistic opponents have sometimes been guilty of moral and intellectual pride. There is also a marvelous—even if accidental—insight in the child's definition that an optimist is the person who looks after your eyes and a pessimist is the person who looks after your feet. That combination of vision and pedestrian realism, of hope and prudence, is the appropriate perspective on the future, especially for the Christian community, which knows both the common grace of God and the intransigence of human pride and sloth.

That said, it may be remarked that the American Christian community seems particularly tempted to a kind of optimism called "possibility thinking," which presumes the inevitability of success if people just put their minds to it instead of to negative thoughts. According to that perspective, people can "turn scars into stars," to quote one exponent. We think that view lacks realism, and we fear that it simply fuels our culture's confidence in technological progress and our society's notion of reproductive success. Thoughtless reproductive interventions may leave scars no one can turn into stars.

Technology and the Mastery of Nature

One's assessment of the new versions of procreation also depends in part upon one's disposition toward nature and human control over it by means of technology. Those who celebrate the new procreative powers often celebrate knowledge as control over nature for the sake of human welfare. Those who resist the new powers often celebrate nature itself and demean the new powers as violations of the natural order and natural processes.

The celebration of technology in Western culture most likely takes its pedigree from Francis Bacon (1561-1626), for it was Francis Bacon who first construed knowledge as power over nature and linked power over nature to human welfare (May, "Right to Know," 194). Since then the Baconian project has celebrated human mastery over nature (Ramsey, *Ethics*, 139, 256). From the perspective of the Baconian project, all dignity belongs to human persons, who are set over and against nature. The natural order and natural processes have no dignity of their own, and that which commands no respect may be mastered.

There can be no denying that the Baconian project has contributed to human well-being; we have already celebrated the new possibilities that medical technology provides for intervening in the sad stories people tell with and about their bodies and for giving these stories happy endings. But there can also be no denying that technology does not always bring well-being to human beings; the tremendous water and air pollution that has resulted from technology is hardly promising to human welfare; human beings, after all, are a part of creation, and its abasement is their abasement, its destruction is their destruction.

The close links between knowledge and control over nature and human welfare forged by the Baconian perspective make intelligible the foolishness of otherwise brilliant people. No thoughtful person, for example, would accept the techno-logic that "if we can, we may," for every reflective person knows there are many things we can do that we ought never to do. But some brilliant scientists seem to follow this techno-logic. The same Dr. Edwards who presided over the conception of Louise Brown had said in a 1966 article in *Scientific American*, "If rabbit and fly eggs can be fertilized after maturation in culture, presumably human eggs grown in culture could also be fertilized, although obviously it would not be permissible to implant them in a human recipient. We have therefore tried to fertilize cultured human eggs in vitro" (p. 80). He moved from *can* fertilize to *may* fertilize with apparent ease. Twelve years later, in spite of how obvious it had been in 1966 that it would not be permissible to implant the fertilized egg in a human recipient, he moved from *can* implant to *may* implant. The move from *can* to *may* is intelligible if, and perhaps only if, the Baconian project is accepted—that is, if knowledge is power over nature and power over nature entails human welfare. Knowing how to implant an egg fertilized in vitro was not the end of the story, of course. As Dr. Edwards said later, "The procedures . . . open the way to further work on human embryos in the laboratory" (Edwards and Sharpe, 87). Again he has some scruples about some of the "further work," especially about creating hybrids of human beings with other animals, but one wonders whether the scruples will dissolve again along with the technological obstacles as scientists expand what they *can* do. Edwards says at one point, "Scientists must maintain their right to exercise their professional activities to the limit that is tolerable by society" (p. 90). One might suppose that this sounds promising, that Edwards recognizes some limits besides what scientists can do, but the attitudes of society, according to Edwards, simply lag a little behind the technological achievements of its scientists and "struggle to catch up with what scientists can do" (p. 90). *Can* still implies *may*, and the public philosophy needs to catch up. The tail wags the dog—and let the dog beware.

Even among those who reject the techno-logic that if we can, we may (as all do, upon reflection), the Baconian project affects our culture's perspective on technology. It is popular to think of technology as society's "toolbox" (e.g., Mesthene, 26). In this view, any new technology is just a new tool introduced as an option for people and society to use as they see fit. How the tool is used will depend on the values of the individual or society. We will make what we want with it. Indeed, if we master enough tools, we may yet learn to master the world, to achieve human well-being, to build a new world, a new age. The assumption is that the development and use of technology are simply functions of our values, simply a way to get what we already want. But such a view of technology is naive and, when applied to new versions of procreation, dangerous.

Against such a view of technology it seems clear, first of all, that although technologies are introduced as increasing our options, they can quickly become socially enforced. The automobile, for example, was introduced as an option to the horse, but the horse is no longer an option; the automobile has become socially enforced. Genetic counseling was introduced as an option for prospective parents, but already some are insisting that parents have a *duty* to be informed and, given certain risks, a duty to avoid childbearing (D. Callahan, "Science," 6).

Second and more important, against the view of technology as society's "toolbox" it may be observed that although technologies are introduced to get things people want, they seldom satisfy wants—at least not for long. If people can travel faster by car than they can by horse, they want still faster cars. And if people can have a child when they could not have one before, they are tempted next to want a particular kind of child—say, a bright, blond boy, but surely no "mishap." Technology does not only attempt to satisfy wants; it also stimulates them (D. Callahan, "Science," 6). Technology is a shaper of life and values as much as it is a function of them. The new versions of procreation will shape and form a view of becoming and being parents as much as they are a function of a desire to be parents.

But it is not just scientists who have taken as their own the Baconian project. There are philosophers and theologians who lead the cheers for technology, for knowledge as power over nature, and for power over nature as implying human welfare. Joseph Fletcher, for example, has said, "Man is a maker and a selector and a designer, and the more rationally contrived and deliberate anything is, the more human it is" ("Ethical Aspects," 780). The implication is obvious, but no less remarkable for all that: "Laboratory reproduction is radically human compared to conception by ordinary heterosexual intercourse. It is willed, chosen, purposed and controlled, and surely these are the traits that distinguish *Homo sapiens*. . . . Coital reproduction is, therefore, less human than laboratory reproduction" (Fletcher, "Ethical Aspects," 781). Even the language used is significant. People used to beget children, or procreate; now, according to Fletcher (and, we fear, common usage), people reproduce children—like some furniture manufacturer.

But as image-bearing creatures of God, persons are children of nature as well as children of spirit. Persons are embodied, and for embodied persons to put hope in the Baconian project is presumptuous and foolish. It is presumptuous because embodied persons are plainly *part* of nature; persons transcend the natural order in certain important ways, but they can never live simply "over against" nature; they can only live in the embodied state that depends on nature. It is foolish because, ironically, it makes people even more dependent upon external objects, even if these objects are of their own making and choosing and owning, and it does not entirely release them from their dependencies upon the natural world. We also reject the Baconian project with respect to new beginnings of life.

On the other hand, it will hardly do to adopt a casual anti-technological spirit, to be content with slogans about "playing God" when people intervene in natural processes, to raise the cry "It's not nice to fool with Mother Nature"—unless along with that goes a willingness to call respirators, dialysis machines, insulin, and penicillin illicit. Embodied persons are children of spirit as well as children of nature, and it is slothful to suppress and refuse the dominion that has been given to humanity as a mandate and a blessing. The question should not be whether human beings will "play God" or not—God settled that issue by making us image bearers and stewards. The question should rather be whether or not persons are exercising their God-given dominion responsibly. It is moral sloth and folly to reject medical technologies, including reproductive technologies, simply because they interfere with natural processes.

Of course, one need not demand obsequious subservience to Mother Nature everywhere to call attention to the moral significance of the "natural end" of human sexual intercourse. The natural-law tradition of Roman Catholicism, for example, has insisted that sexual intercourse has by its very nature unitive and procreative ends. To separate the unitive and procreative ends of human sexual intercourse is "unnatural" and wrong. Thus contraception is wrong because it represses the procreative purpose of human sexual intercourse (Pope Paul VI), and technological reproduction is wrong because it takes procreation out of the context of human sexual intercourse with its unitive purpose (Pope Pius XII, "To Catholic Doctors"; "Apostolate," with reference to artificial insemination using the husband's seed).

It should be noted that not only Roman Catholics have been concerned about sharply distinguishing the sexual act as a gesture of covenant fellowship in marriage from the sexual act as the generation of human life, or distinguishing "love making" from "baby making." Paul Ramsey (*Fabricated Man*, 38-39) and Leon Kass ("New Beginnings," 53-56) claim that moving generation into the laboratory is dangerous precisely because it suppresses the biological, sexual, bodily meaning of marital love. The child conceived in the laboratory may be the result of a loving decision and welcomed into a family to be sustained and nurtured, and so it is quite proper to say such a child is a product of marital love. But the meaning of "marital love" in this context has subtly shifted. It no longer has both natural and spiritual components; it no longer has its bodily connotation and, therefore, its full human connotations. The case is just the reverse of the way our society trivializes sex—by suppressing its personal and spiritual components, making sex a technology of pleasure —and no less dangerous, according to Ramsey and Kass.

The position of Ramsey and Kass has much to recommend it. It is based not so much on the inviolability of natural processes as on the recognition that human beings in sexual intercourse are always both children of nature and children of spirit. That is the moral wisdom of Ramsey and Kass's position, but this wisdom seems to us to provide and sustain moral caution about reproductive interventions, not to insist upon a moral prohibition. Natural processes, after all, are not inviolable for Ramsey and Kass; neither would prohibit, say, delivery of a viable fetus by Cesarean section if it was medically indicated for the mother or the child, even though the procedure may suppress the biological and bodily meaning of "giving birth." And neither Ramsey nor Kass does in fact prohibit artificial insemination when the husband's sperm is used. So not even the procreative process is made sacrosanct by their—and our—appreciation of the fleshly and bodily character of marital love; only a caution, not a prohibition, is appropriate here. The course of wisdom is neither to make natural processes normative nor to dismiss them cavalierly as merely physical.

In lovemaking and in baby-making, we are children of nature and children of spirit. Neither may be reduced to mere physiology nor elevated to pure spirit. In our view they belong together not because they are essentially or "naturally" joined to each other but because they both belong to marriage. Marriage, with its vows and demands of covenant fidelity—"till death do us part" and "for better or worse"—is the appropriate context for both lovemaking and baby-making. When lovemaking takes place in a context other than marital fidelity, it is diminished and distorted, reduced to a biological urge, a natural necessity, a technology of pleasure governed only by the requirement that it take place between consenting adults, or, at best, to a romantic quest for intimacy without a commitment to continuity. But there remains in every act of coitus, and perhaps in the vulnerability of nakedness and any clumsy gesture toward lovemaking, a sign of God's intention for sex, for there remains an implicit exchange of trust and commitment. To ask during the intimacies of making love "But will you love me tomorrow?" is to impugn the *committal* of the act (Hauerwas and Verhey, 15).

Lovemaking belongs to marriage; and so does baby-making. When baby-making takes place in a context other than marital fidelity, it too is diminished and distorted, reduced to mere physiology or to contract, to a marketable reproductive capacity or to a technology of producing children without a commitment to care for them when they are not what we want. But there remains in every act of parenting, even in the "mere" donation of gametes, and perhaps in the very vulnerability of children and in their curiosity about their genetic parents, a sign of God's intention for sex, for there remain implicit responsibilities and commitments. Imagine a child asking a sperm donor or an ovum donor or a surrogate, "But will you care for me?" Acts of parenting may not be reduced to mere physiology or to mere contract. Children have a place in the fidelity of marriage, and they extend that fidelity to faithfulness in a family. Children have a secure place when there is a commitment to continuity in a marriage, and they extend that continuity to another generation. Lovemaking and baby-making are not necessarily joined to each other, but both must be joined to the covenant fidelity of marriage and family. Neither may be reduced to nature or set over or against nature as purely spiritual and "free." So we urge that the new powers be used only within marriage, and we caution against donor sperm, donor ova, and surrogacy.

In summary, then, part of what is at stake in the new versions of procreation is the image that people have of themselves in relation to nature and to their own powers of mastery over nature. One perspective, the Baconian project, sets people *over and against* nature, as controllers and possessors of it for the sake of human well-being. Another perspective puts people *under* nature — making them obsequiously subservient to Mother Nature — because it prohibits interference with the natural order and natural processes. But the Christian story puts human beings *in* nature, exercising stewardship over it, responsible to God in covenant faithfulness.

The sort of dominion that keeps faith with God the creator and provider will be more care-taking than conquering, more nurturing than controlling, more ready to suffer patiently with nature than to lord it over and against nature. A dominion that serves God will be prepared to acknowledge that human beings are only creatures themselves, as fallible as they are finite, ultimately dependent on God the creator and on the creation that God has put in their care. A dominion covenanted to God will not presume that the fault in the world is a part of creation to be remedied by human ingenuity. It will recognize that the fundamental problems of coping with human existence do not permit technological solution, that greed and pride and ennui are not technological problems awaiting a quick technological fix but human faults that can conscript technology into their service. Such a dominion will be able to recognize that the habit of the Baconian project of looking for the quick technological fix is folly—and reproductive interventions feed on that folly. It is God, not technology, that brings in the new age. Technology has brought real and significant benefits, but it is folly to be confident that it will always bring well-being in its train or that, if it doesn't, some new technology can correct the harm. For all its accomplishments and for all its promises, technology has yet to deliver people from their finitude or to the truly good—and it never will. Recognizing the limits of technology, people may be able to lower their expectations and demands of it and to respond in other ways to human problems.

Children and Parents

The new versions of procreation have confronted people not only with the question about their relationship to nature and technology but also with questions about their relationship to their own children. We have already asked, May people sharply distinguish between the sexual act as an expression of covenant fellowship and the sexual act as the inception of human life? Now we must also ask, May parenting as an act of begetting be distinguished from parenting as a vocation to nurture? May the biological relation be separated from the social relation? Surely in adoption procedures those relationships are sundered, and Christians celebrate the hospitality that adoptive parents show to children not biologically related to them. Indeed, the relationship of human beings to the heavenly Father is celebrated as an adoptive relationship. But it is important to observe that what is celebrated is not the sundering of genetic and social relationships but the gracious character of the covenant relationship of adoption, the fact that adoptive parents as imagers of God love their children, whom they are under no prior obligation to love, as though those children were theirs by birth. But biological parents are by virtue of being biological parents under the obligation to love and nurture their children as their children. Sometimes that duty can be impossible or very difficult to fulfill, as it is when parents die or when a parent is herself or himself still a child; sometimes it may even be that the obligation to love and nurture the child is best fulfilled by giving the child up for adoption. But such cases are tragic ones, where goods collide, duties conflict, or evils gather. Begetting is not merely biological and physical; it is essentially parental, entailing obligations for nurturing the child. However, the very desire of many couples to have a child biologically "their own" suggests that parenting is not altogether abiological. Indeed, in vitro fertilization and artificial insemination were first defended in terms of a crucial relationship between biology and parenting. The phenomenon of bonding during pregnancy and at birth also suggests the embodied character of the relationship of parent and child. Bonding is not just an abstract moral and spiritual commitment; it is borne and nurtured by carrying and caressing, by the surprise and delight of "quickening," and by the patient endurance of sickness and pain for the sake of another. The point is not that bonding is simply physical or that a physical relationship (e.g., a newborn laid across the mother's warm abdomen) works automatically and magically to achieve a spiritual relationship. The point is rather that the relationship is not purely spiritual and that the acts of begetting may not be treated (and dismissed) as merely physical.

The relationship of parent and child can begin adoptively, of course, in the voluntary consent of an adult or a couple to nurture and care for a child not biologically their own. Such consent to care for a child, to be parent to a child, cannot be demanded or expected. Ordinarily, however, the relationship of parent and child begins biologically in the "physical" relationship of parents to children. Such a relationship is not simply created by the voluntary consent of independent adults to care for the child born to them; the relationship antedates the consent. When parents assent to care for a child born to them, they do what may be demanded and expected of them: they promise fidelity to an identity and a relationship already and "naturally" established.

These remarks do not prohibit in vitro fertilization or artificial insemination, even adoptively, but they do provide a strong caution against using donor seed and surrogate mothers, and they make morally questionable the decision to donate seed or to lend a womb as though a biological relationship with a child carries no burden or obligation.

The question of the social relationship of parents and children is itself at stake in the new versions of procreation. Human beings are seizing control of procreation, gaining power to intervene purposefully in the begetting of children precisely when society is more confused about parenting than ever, and the new powers only add to our confusion. For example, after John Fletcher interviewed a number of parents who were undergoing amniocentesis and contemplating abortion, he declared that even a responsible decision to undergo amniocentesis and to contemplate abortion "permanently altered" the relation of the parents with their children, even though it "does not lessen the affection they bear for their children" (pp. 457-58). It's a stunning point, but quite obvious in a way. Imagine trying to explain to a young child that Mommy is not going to have a baby after all because a test showed the baby was sick or not normal or defective. Even if the mother doesn't say, "So the doctor killed it," even if she just says, "So the doctor took it away," the relationship of uncalculating nurturance and basic trust has been threatened. Imagine the child's insecure questions: "What if I get sick?—Do I measure up?" The point is not that all reproductive interventions (or even all abortions following amniocentesis) are immoral; indeed, we do not think they are. The point is rather that without greater communal wisdom about parenting we will not be able to limit or guide such powers properly, and we fear for our capacities to learn that wisdom in the midst of public enthusiasm about reproductive technologies. The technology now commended as a way of becoming parents, a way that not too long ago did not exist, may well shape our way of being parents. Biotechnical parenting may tempt us to view our children as a human achievement rather than as a gift of God and as the basis of hope rather than as a gesture of hope in God.

Few parents think anymore that children are parental property, to be disposed of as parents wish. Today the confusion stems —especially among the compassionate—from the view that parents have the awesome responsibility of making perfect children (through our reproducing) and making children perfect (through our parenting), of assuring them a happy and successful life, or at least the capacity to attain and to conform to the American ideal of "the good life." But this account of parenting as the awesome responsibility to make perfect children and to make children perfect turns our children into products, into human and technological achievements. Such an account may encourage—and finally require—the abortion of the unborn who do not meet our standards, the neglect of newborns with diminished capacities to achieve our ideal of "the good life," and the pursuit of technical possibilities of genetically improving our children. Such a view of parenting and of children may finally reduce our options to a perfect child or a dead child.

But children are begotten, not made (O'Donovan, *Begotten or Made?*). They are gifts, not achievements. To the old assumption that children are the property of parents, to be disposed of as they choose, the Christian church has always said no, for our children are first of all God's, not ours. Children have a heavenly Father who would nurture them and who entrusts them to us as gifts. Today the Christian church must tell that story to contradict the idea that parenting is an awesome responsibility to make perfect children and to make children perfect.

The language of "gift" is important but tricky. It is not used in Christian discourse to confer ownership, as though children were a birthday present we can exchange or return for cash. It is used to confer stewardship: we receive children in trust from God, and with the gift always comes the claim of God. So we receive children with delight and sobriety, delighting in the loving hand of God, which gives them, soberly responsible before the claims of God, who entrusts them to us. Of course, Christians call many things "gifts of God": food, friends, recreation, life, work—indeed, all the good things of life. It would seem we so stretch the language of "gift" that we make it trivial and powerless to speak of children as "gifts." But when we call anything "gift of God," we call ourselves to relate to it as it is related to God. To call so many things gifts does not diminish the power of the language; it acknowledges that we are indebted in many things and made stewards in many things, that we are to relate to many things—indeed, all things—as they are related to God. So the language of "gift" nurtures the disposition to relate to children as children related to God.

And no Christian can forget that Jesus, in whom God's future reign already made its power known, took little children in his arms and blessed them (Mark 10:13-16). There must have been babies there, and more than one with a dirty diaper, yet Jesus took them in his arms. There must have been toddlers, curious and energetic, crying occasionally and interrupting often. "Women are meant to deal with them," the disciples must have thought, but Jesus blessed them. And there must have been boys and girls, taking an infrequent break from playing tag and catch or standing on the sidelines because a limp or a disease or something else made them unwelcome in the game, and Jesus laid his hands on them. Other shocking behavior of this Galilean had hardly prepared people for this. Sure, he made the last first—but kids? Sure, he exalted the humble —but kids? Sure, those who didn't count for very much in other stories counted with him—but dirty-diapered, sweaty, silly, obnoxious kids? Yes, and he made it clear that to be his disciple, to welcome the kingdom, means to welcome, to serve, and to help little children.

No Christian can forget that when the Spirit works in our hearts, we cry "Abba! Father!" (Rom. 8:15; Gal. 4:6). And no Christian should forget (although some have) that God is like a mother, too: we are promised that as a mother comforts her child, so God will comfort us (Isa. 66:13). The images of God as mother can protect us from abusing the image of God the Father. We abuse that image when we think it means that God is literally male. In whatever ways God is like a father, God is not male like an earthly father. God transcends human gender—and the image of God as mother can remind us of that. More important to our present purpose, we abuse the image of God the Father when we interpret it in flawed and misleading terms. From Roman to Puritan times a father was an authoritarian, totalitarian head of a family. Since industrialization, a father has been mostly absent, working outside the home to earn a living for the family. The modern father is alternately indulgent, the one to ask when mother says no, and demanding, the one whose affection is contingent on success. But none of these images of father is what Jesus had in mind when he called God "Abba" and taught his disciples to do the same. *Abba* might best be translated "Papa" or "Dada." It's the first word for father that a little Hebrew child would learn to say. This image of father is the image of one who cares, one who carries, one who loves, one who can be trusted to provide uncalculating nurturance. It is, speaking culturally, a very motherly father whom Jesus taught us to trust and to love.

The language of "gift" calls upon us to relate to our children as little ones related to God, to the God invoked as "Abba" and known in Jesus, who blessed little children. It is no accident, then, that the language of "gift" involves acceptance of our children as given. We do not regard them as products, as achievements, and we may not beget them as though they were. Children are gifts, not products—they are not of our choosing, not under our control, not necessarily the children we want or expect or would choose if we could. Children are gifts, not products—and therefore they always have a measure of independence from us and from our rational choices. To regard children as gifts may be necessary if children are to be regarded as ends in themselves and not merely as instruments for achieving parental ends.

It is not because they always bring happiness that children are to be regarded as gifts. Sometimes children bring pain and suffering, but they are nevertheless always gifts from the loving hand of God. Indeed, even as parents endure the pain and suffering of having and caring for children as given, children are the most precious gift of all, for they teach us to love those who are not (and refuse to be) just as we wish. The language of being "entrusted" with children, then, points not toward the impossible responsibility of making perfect children and making children perfect but toward the duty and the surprising joy of nurturing those who are given. Parents are entrusted with children as gifts from the loving hand of the Father. And the Father's uncalculating nurturance is still the place to learn parenting, to learn to love the imperfect, the snotty-nosed, and the just plain snotty. Christians call God "Abba" and learn again and again in addressing God the sort of uncalculating nurturance and basic trust that should mark the relation of parents and children.

The tasks of nurturing children do not turn them into products, but they do involve support for the child as given. A parent covenanted to a child as given need not—and, indeed, may not—be altogether passive and "accepting." A parent may and should nurture the child so that the child as given can not only be but also flourish. And a parent may and should enlist the help of others to enable the child as given to be and to flourish within the limits of the world's finitude and the child's condition. A parent entrusted with the gift of a child must foster the excellence and well-being of the child as given, enlarging the capacities of the child as given and helping the child to fulfill the promise the child has as given.

But the "as given" prevents this parental activity from becoming demonic, from turning the child into a product and making acceptance and affection contingent upon the success of the interventions. Being entrusted with a child as a gift will require nurturing, but not nurturing undertaken as though all value rests on the success of making the child as given into something more or better, "as though the imperfect materials themselves had to be surpassed for anything good to come of the life" (May, "Parenting," 154).

A related but distinct confusion about parenting today is captured by the assertion "Our children are our hope for the future." Christians can only regard such a view of children as blasphemous and foolish. It is blasphemous because Jesus is our hope for the future. It is foolish because our children are destined for suffering and death like the rest of us. The view that our children are our hope for the future can only make more urgent the awesome responsibility to make perfect children and to make children perfect, for so much is at stake. And to deny that view takes a good deal of pressure off parents. Children are not the hope for the future—Jesus is. And because that is so, Christians are free to delight in children as gifts from God's gracious and nurturing hand. This world is not yet God's unchallenged realm, and we may not beget or rear our children in this world as though they can be spared suffering and death. There is wisdom about parenting in the Passover ritual that requires the children to eat bitter herbs with the rest of the family, reminding them of the suffering of the community of which they are a part. But God does reign—even over a world marked and marred by suffering—and he will reign. And Christians sign and seal their confidence in God's future by having and rearing and loving children. Children are not the basis for our hope; they are a gesture of our hope in God.

These remarks are not meant to imply a prohibition of technologically assisted procreation. Indeed, as long as Christians think of children as gifts of God and of having children as a gesture of our trust in God's future, Christians will welcome the ministry of physicians to infertile couples who long for a biological child of their own—will welcome the capacity to repair fallopian tubes, for example, or to regulate hormones, or to use a married couple's gametes in artificial insemination or in vitro fertilization to circumvent certain problems of infertility. And as long as Christians delight in the adoptive love of God, they will welcome the ministry of adoption agencies and celebrate and delight in the inclusion of an adopted child in a family and in the community.

Ministry to the childless, however, must involve more than technology and adoption. Christians may not be insensitive to the profound and sometimes desperate longing of some childless couples for a baby of their own, and ministry to them must start by attending to the ways in the common life of the church that people remind them of their childlessness and even subtly and unfairly rebuke them for it. Family gatherings and society meetings in which the topic of children dominates the conversation can be very painful to the childless. Well-intentioned advice that it is time to begin a family or that a couple is "trying too hard" may tear at their sexuality and self-esteem. Ministry to the childless demands sensitivity and care, a readiness to listen, to appreciate the pain and suffering, the grief over the child of promise they lost by never having (Van Regenmorter and Van Regenmorter). Ministry to the childless will not belittle their sense that their childlessness is a lack—children are, after all, a gift of God. But ministry to the childless will acknowledge and engage the gifts, including the gifts of nurturance and care, which the childless may have in abundance.

The Christian community may and must say clearly, both to those with children and to those who are childless, that children are not the basis for hope, that children are not the hope of the world and not the hope of a person's or a couple's flourishing. The child on whom the world's hope—and theirs—depends has been born "unto us" (Luke 2:11) —whether we have children of our own or not. And since then childbearing is no longer the necessity and the duty it was in the old covenant (Barth, 266). In the church it cannot be a fault to be infertile. Those with children, then, must work against aspects of a common life that force the childless to the margins. And both those with children and those without may and must set their hope on God, not on children. Then the whole

Christian community may avoid both excessive expectations of the children they have or still dream of and excessive anxiety about their flourishing if the children they have do not "measure up" or if the child of their dreams never comes.

Society and Children

If the family is a microcosm of society, then the new versions of procreation confront us also with the question of the sort of society we want to be and to become. Our dispositions toward each other will affect and be affected by the new reproductive powers. If amniocentesis with a view to abortion subtly affects the parent-child relationship, the same power subtly affects our relationships with all weak and handicapped people, with retarded and unlovely people, with outcast and unacceptable people, and perhaps with new categories of people—unwanted, unchosen, and "carrier" people. God knows we find it comfortable and convenient to ignore and avoid them now. Our new reproductive powers promise (or threaten) not only to ignore them but even to eliminate them, and the reservoirs of affection that help sustain the parental role are simply not present in society.

As reproductive technologies tempt us to think of our own children as products and to pin our hopes on them, society may tempt us to think about our children in terms of "quality control." The technologies introduced to increase the options of parents may easily lead to social expectations to exercise and social sanctions for not exercising the "option" of amniocentesis and abortion when a mother is at risk of having a child with, say, Down's syndrome. Perhaps it is unnecessarily melodramatic to envision a society that refuses to share the burden of care for "reproductive products" who do not meet standards, but our dispositions toward children in our present society hardly make it implausible (Hauerwas, *A Community of Character,* 187-94). And if society refuses to care for the genetically retarded or diseased, then it will be unfair to ask parents to heroically bear the burden alone. The issue is what kind of society we want to be and become: a society that cares for and nurtures children, including its so-called "defective children," or a society that "produces" children and cannot tolerate the "defective" or allow them to exist.

The issue bears on questions of funding quite immediately. We should not allocate public funds for reproductive technologies—say, for in vitro clinics and in vitro research—before we have provided a minimal standard of prenatal and postnatal care for the poor and decent support services for families with disabled children. The children of the poor are gifts of God as well, even if the world regards them as no great human accomplishments, yet the infant mortality rates among the poor are scandalous for a society with the resources to develop in vitro fertilization clinics. Children with disabilities are gifts of God as well, even if they bring more pain and suffering with them than the children their parents wanted. For society the most precious gift of all may be the lesson to care for those who are not as we wish them to be.

Commercial contracts for donor seed or for surrogacy also raise the question of the sort of society we want to be and to become, because such contracts make it attractive to the poor (especially poor women) to treat their reproductive capacities, their bodies—themselves—as marketable commodities to be purchased by the rich. If we would turn from being or becoming two societies—one affluent and free and the other poor and at the disposal of the rich—then we must turn against the commercialization of surrogacy.

Conclusions and Cautions

The new versions of reproduction have made some enduring moral questions urgent. The irony is that at the very time the issues are so urgent, we as a society are ill prepared to deal with them. We have magnificent tools, but we don't know what we're building or whether what we're building will be habitable. We're making great time, but we don't know where we're going.

If we lack the ultimate wisdom to be able to settle these enduring moral issues, then the best penultimate wisdom is caution. Nothing we have said requires installing a permanent red light against new versions of procreation. Almost everything we have said would argue against installing a green light. The signal here is amber. Caution is called for. It is a caution born of humility rather than fear, but it is caution nevertheless.

Along the way in this chapter we have suggested something of the shape of that caution, the shadows cast by that amber light. We have suggested that the burden of proof be shifted, that it be borne not only by those who would "restrict freedom" and "restrain progress" but also and equally by those who, in the name of freedom, establish a manipulative and calculating relationship with children and by those who presume that all technological innovation entails human well-being.

We have suggested respect for embodied selves, a reticence to separate either lovemaking or baby-making from marriage, and a reticence to sunder the "natural" or bodily relationship of parents and children from the social obligations and roles of parents and children. So we urge that the new powers be used within the context of a covenant of marriage, and we caution against donor sperm, donor ova, and surrogacy.

We have insisted that children be regarded as gifts of God, not as human achievements, and that they not be regarded as our hope for the future. To regard children as gifts will affect our motivation for having children and may free us from inordinate anxiety about *whether* we have children and *what* children we have. Such conviction may sustain in our culture an otherwise unsustainable courage to be cautious, to say no to technology and its promises, and an otherwise unsustainable courage to assent to a covenant with the children we are given, to promise the sort of uncalculating nurturance that can evoke and confirm the trust of children.

We have urged establishing social support for the children of the poor and for children with disabilities before public funding is allocated to research and development or clinical use in reproductive technologies.

We have flashed a few red lights along the way. We would prohibit the use of embryos procreated in vitro for experimental purposes. What we learn from them may be important and useful, but it is wrong to begin human life with the intention of discarding it once we have used it. We would also signal a stop to commercial contracts for surrogacy.

All these cautionary words must finally be joined with an exhortation to preserve and to cherish some ancient wisdom. The wisdom about the future is hopeful realism. The wisdom about nature is that we are creaturely stewards. The wisdom about parenting is nurturance and trust. The wisdom about one another is the care and respect we owe each other, especially the weak, "the little ones." Such wisdom and the corollary dispositions it suggests will not tell us exactly what to do and what to leave undone with our new powers, but they will provide some guidance for and some limits to our powers, including the awesome new powers of reproductive technology, even when we cannot solve a quandary with a rule. A reproductive revolution—if such it is—will require wise people, not just clever ones.[7]

7. Parts of this chapter are a revision of A. Verhey's "The Morality of Genetic Engineering."

8. *Abortion: A Covenantal View*

Induced abortion is one of the most common medical operations; up to 55 million abortions are performed in the world each year, including approximately 1.5 million in the United States and over 65,000 in Canada (Krafrissen, 130; Wadhera and Nair, 97). These figures do not include the (possibly higher) number of human zygotes that die as a result of intrauterine devices (IUDs) and other abortifacients. And, of course, these figures do not include spontaneous abortions, which, as we noted in Chapter Two, may be the fate of over 70 percent of fertilized human ova. Although, as we also noted in Chapter Two, some theories about the beginning of personhood may imply a responsibility to try to reduce the number of spontaneous abortions and may imply that the use of IUDs ought to be forbidden, this chapter will focus on the morality of induced abortions.

What is it about abortion that leads 20 percent of Americans to think it should be legal in all circumstances, another 20 percent to think it should be illegal in all circumstances, and most of them to hold a position (often tentatively) somewhere in between?[1] Some believe that "despite its capacity to attract major public interest and to sustain bitter public debate, abortion is not a serious moral issue" (Engelhardt, 242), whereas others believe that "the putrid decay in the open pits of Babi Yar and the sacrificial smoke that rose from Auschwitz were the effluvia of a spirit that now leaves like offerings in the pails of Pre-Term and the

---

1. From 1975 through 1988 these statistics did not change much, according to Gallup polls (see "Special Report: America's Abortion Dilemma," *Newsweek*, 14 Jan. 1985, pp. 20-29). A majority of Americans do favor a ban on abortions except in cases of rape, incest, or danger to the mother's life or health. Over one-third of those polled do have doubts about their own position, although over half do not. Approximately the same percentage that would permit abortion only in the previously mentioned circumstances are also opposed to reversing the Supreme Court's *Roe v. Wade* decision that allowed abortion choice ("58% Oppose Reversing Abortion Decision"). A scholarly and insightful summary and an analysis of much of American poll data on the abortion issue can be found in M. A. Lamanna's "Social Science and Ethical Issues."

incinerators of the Center for Reproductive and Sexual Health" (Burt-chaell, *Rachel Weeping*, 236).

Somewhere between these two viewpoints are the various middle positions held by those who believe abortion is a deep moral dilemma, who write books with such titles as *In Necessity and Sorrow* (Denes) and *The Ambivalence of Abortion* (Francke), and who are viewed by the extremes as trying ignominiously to be moderates on murder or mandatory motherhood. Emotions run deep in this dispute, and sometimes there is the temptation to dismiss opponents' views with ad hominem slurs: for example, pro-life activists are sometimes portrayed as Catholic housewives trying to legitimize their lifestyle by imposing it on everyone else, and pro-choice activists are sometimes portrayed as hedonistic yuppies wanting the pleasure of sex without its responsibilities, selfish enough to put their careers or BMWs ahead of their babies' lives.[2]

Recognizing that we are not immune to prejudice or emotionalism, we will try in the following pages to explain carefully our understanding of the main viewpoints on abortion. Where it is appropriate, we will explain our agreement or disagreement, and we will conclude with a summary of our position and its implications for social and legal policy. We believe that the three main areas of dispute in the abortion debate are (1) the nature and status of the fetus; (2) the nature of childbearing, of the family, and of social relationships; and (3) the predicted effects of various social and legal policies on abortion.

The Nature and Status of the Fetus

This section will be comparatively brief, because Chapter Two (pp. 34-48) discusses at greater length our view about the beginnings of persons as imagers of God.

Many — though not all — pro-choice proponents accept the "actualist" premise that, even if the fetus is an individual human being (in the genetic sense) from the time of its conception, it does not become an actual person until it either achieves the capacity to exhibit such person-making characteristics as self-consciousness and symbolic communication or has personhood conferred on it by its family or by society.

2. Neither the pro-life nor the pro-choice side accepts the possible implication that it opposes what the other side is labeled as favoring. We use the terms to denote the positions they are ordinarily understood to denote, without meaning to imply that either side is against life or against choice.

Until then it should be perceived as part of or, perhaps, the private property of the woman in whom it is growing or of the couple that produced it (Engelhardt, 219). The sorts of moral claims the fetus can make on others are like those of animals with similar levels of development and capacities for suffering (Engelhardt, 218). It has rights not to suffer and perhaps even not to be killed unjustly, but, as with pets, these rights can be overridden by the well-being or the nonarbitrary choices of its "owners." This position is compatible with society's conferring the protected status of personhood on infants and late-term fetuses, though such conferral is predicated not on the inherent claims of fetuses and infants but on empirical predictions about "slippery slope" dangers to society that would arise if killing fetuses and infants was allowed.

Many—though not all—pro-life proponents accept the "species" or "natural kind" premise that all individual members of the human species are actual persons from the time of their conception (or, at least, from the time of the fertilized egg's implantation).[3] Some pro-life proponents argue for conception as the beginning of personhood not on the basis of scientific facts or philosophical considerations but on the grounds that, whatever its *nature* may be, the human conceptus has the *status* of a unique relationship with God, who confers dignity and inviolability on it (Bajema, 39). Many of those who believe personhood begins at conception favor a "right-to-life" amendment which would explicitly make that belief part of the U.S. Constitution. Some pro-life thinkers see their position as compatible with allowing abortion when the pregnant woman's life is significantly endangered, and some would even allow abortion in cases of rape, incest, or profound neurological defects in the fetus. Other pro-life proponents argue that it is debatable whether such exceptions are consistent with the belief that the fetus is as much a person as any other human being is. To them it seems wrong to kill one innocent person in order to protect another's life. It even seems wrong to kill an innocent person a few weeks or months earlier than that person would otherwise die in order to spare

3. Some of the most prominent pro-life proponents take what we called the earliest of the "stage" positions in Chapter Two. B. Nathanson, for example, argues that at implantation the zygote establishes its "nexus with the human community" (p. 217). He raises some of the problems that we did about thinking of all human fertilized eggs as persons that must be protected and cherished: "Many do not implant and are simply washed away. How would we deal properly with these lost conceptions? . . . Mourn and bury them? . . . Should we undertake a crash program to make sure all these fertilized eggs, as 'human beings' are saved and implanted? The disarray of this whole approach to life boggles the mind" (p. 214). Of course, those who believe personhood begins at conception might find it mind-boggling to think that the possibility of being washed away does anything to negate one's nexus with the human community.

another's life. Thus some pro-life proponents argue that even in the "hard" cases we must let God decide or let nature take its course. In spite of—or perhaps because of—this intramural debate, it is clear that the belief that all embryos and fetuses are persons commits many people to an unambiguously antiabortion stance. (In the next section we will examine the argument that the personhood of the fetus can be consistent with a pro-choice position.)

In Chapter Two we stated our doubts about both of the preceding positions on the beginning of personhood and our doubts about the efforts to locate a stage or decisive moment during gestation at which the fetus moves from having (almost) no moral status to having (almost) the status of a person. We also noted our agreement with some aspects of the gradualist position, which calls for an incrementally stronger conferral of protected status on the fetus as it develops. But our main point concerning the status of unborn human beings was that they are *potential* (not merely *possible*) persons; they *will* (not *can*) become persons in the normal course of their development, and by virtue of that fact they deserve some of the awe and respect due imagers of God. Although this view does not equate abortion with murder, it does imply that killing unborn human beings is an extremely serious moral and religious matter. However, the question of whether or when we should tolerate or cooperate with an induced abortion cannot be answered until we have considered the argument that circumstances surrounding a pregnancy can sometimes make abortion an acceptable alternative.

Conflicts of Interest and the Nature of Childbearing

For most Christian couples the question of the nature and status of the fetus does not normally arise. Although how and when a human being is conceived may be a matter of the parents' stewardly choice, once a human being is in the process of developing, it is usually received and nurtured as a gift from God. This response is probably not derived from any sense of obligation to love God or one's neighbor; it is more probably derived from the perception of the fetus as one's child, from such deeply embedded feelings as gratitude, awe, and protectiveness, and from the belief that the family is the institution that God uses to continue the line of his covenant. Even if a pregnancy is a surprise or a very mixed blessing, the nurturing response normally overwhelms any worry or frustration over whatever sacrifice may be required by the pregnancy and the resulting child. Christian couples seldom feel compelled to consider abortion as a way out.

But unfortunate circumstances can raise the question of the nature and status of the fetus, especially for unmarried women, who have 80 percent of the abortions in the United States. What are Christians to say when the fetus is perceived not as "our developing child" or as a surprise that can be coped with, but as a stranger or even as a catastrophe in one's life? Very few people argue that the threat of catastrophe motivates a high percentage of abortions today, but many pro-choice advocates—some of the most ardent of whom are willing to agree that if social conditions were properly supportive of pregnant women, abortion could be legally proscribed (B. Harrison, 18)—are "pro choice" primarily out of sympathy for the relatively few catastrophic cases. In our view, a responsible position on abortion must not merely note that most abortions are sought to avoid inconvenience rather than catastrophe; it must also respond to those cases in which the developing fetus is understandably perceived as a stranger and a threat—and the pregnancy as a catastrophe.

But even when the fetus is a threatening stranger, it is also an innocent and extremely vulnerable stranger, and a central thrust of the Bible is that vulnerable strangers are to be treated hospitably—are to be treated, in fact, as neighbors. To some extent, this response brings us back to the question of the previous section: Does the fetus have the nature and status that call for its recognition as a neighbor? We believe that, as a potential person in the vulnerable process of becoming a person, it has such a status. But what are we to say to those people, including Christians, who not only fail to recognize the fetus as child but also fail to perceive it as neighbor? How do we answer the question "Who is my neighbor?"

Appeals to the Parable of the Good Samaritan

Jesus' answer to the preceding question should help us decide which human beings are within the scope of our covenantal responsibilities. When the lawyer asks this question of Jesus in Luke 10:25-37, Jesus responds by telling the parable of the good Samaritan. This parable broadens our concept of who our neighbor is, but it does not do so by directly asserting that vulnerable strangers are neighbors that deserve our help. Rather, it suggests a revolutionary way of deciding the question—namely, that by *being* a neighbor to "outsiders" we will sometimes perceive them as neighbors in need. The Samaritan's willingness to be a neighbor to a vulnerable stranger enables him to see that the man who has fallen among thieves is his neighbor. One thing the story teaches might be stated like this: When in doubt, do not consult your categories of which human beings have what status; rather, respond in a neighborly way to a human being in need of help and see whether, during that response, you clarify your perception of who that being is. When in doubt, do not first classify and categorize; be neighborly toward the stranger in question and then see how your classifications are affected. The parable seems to apply the principle we noted in Chapter Two when we discussed persons with frailties and disabilities: how we perceive others often depends on how we respond to them and not just the other way around. In philosophical terms, ethics sometimes precedes epistemology and metaphysics.[4]

The boundaries of the covenantal community are not discernible in the abstract. One must act in certain ways to discover what they are. This does not mean that the actual boundaries are relative to how we act, that we must simply decide who is included, or that personhood depends on a social decision to confer it. Rather, it means that how we *know* what the boundaries are depends on the correlation between what we do and what we see. There are some kinds of beings—pets, for example—that no amount of anthropomorphizing can transform into persons or imagers of God. But there are others—including fetuses in the process of becoming persons—who as a result of neighborliness will be perceived as fully human and will be welcomed into full membership in the human covenantal community. If we nurture those who are in the process of becoming persons—even when we cannot do it out of instinctive love or out of gratitude for a gift or out of awe at what they are or out of a sense of responsibility for their existence, but do it simply out of neighborliness to a vulnerable individual member of our own species—we will discover the appropriateness of welcoming them into the community of imagers of God. The point is not simply that, by definition, if we nurture potential persons until they become persons, we will then perceive them as such. The point is also that by nurturing vulnerable humans in the process of becoming

4. That is, the question "How should I act?" precedes the question "What do I know?" and "What is the nature of that which I am encountering?" A similar point is persuasively made by O. O'Donovan ("Again: Who Is a Person?"), who gives a similar interpretation of the parable of the good Samaritan. O'Donovan argues that the appearance of human form commands a committed humane response, and the ensuing interaction (or lack of it) will determine the appropriateness or inappropriateness of the response (p. 135). Even if a criterion other than human form is used, it will rely on something that we can sense about the other, so it may be more correct to say that ethics, epistemology, and metaphysics are in reciprocal relationships.

persons, we will perceive their humanity and the appropriateness of treating them as neighbors.

Does this point imply that refusing to so nurture human beings in the process of becoming persons is tantamount to murder? Before we can answer this question, we must consider the analogy with which some pro-choice thinkers interpret the parable of the good Samaritan. The fetus is like the man in the parable who fell among thieves: for survival, it needs the mother's nurturing womb, just as the man in the ditch needed help from outside himself. The mother, they say, can choose to be either like the Samaritan or like the Levite. (For convenience, "the Levite" will be understood as including the priest.) The Samaritan, it must be noted, is commended by the parable, but the Levite, it must also be noted, is not condemned, for any Jew hearing this parable would recognize that the Levite was not violating his own code when he passed by on the other side. The Levite was committed to a strict code of behavior that included regulations against coming into contact with a corpse (which the wounded man could have been or could have become, as far as the Levite knew). Because of his career—an honorable one, in Jewish tradition — the Levite had an acceptable motive to avoid the vulnerable stranger alongside the road. It is true that in certain cases "uncleanness" was reversible (whether or not "corpse contact" was reversible, we do not know), but it would be understandable for the Levite to think that the delay caused by the cleansing rites required if he touched a corpse would be so costly to his career that he did not have a strict duty to help the stranger. To be a good Levite, he must simply keep some very strict laws; to be a bad Levite, he would have to violate one of those legalistic obligations. He could be a good Levite even if he did not risk making career sacrifices to provide help beyond the call of strict duty. Analogously, pro-choice advocates could give the epithet "good Levite" to any pregnant woman who declined to nurture the vulnerable stranger growing within her if continuing to nurture its development involved risking her career or making sacrifices beyond the call of duty. And even the parable of the good Samaritan, they would say, does not condemn a "good Levite."

But a woman may also choose to be the Samaritan of Jesus' parable. She may choose to sacrifice significantly in order to give the gift of life, and, pro-choice advocates argue, *giving* birth is and should only be a matter of giving a gift. It should be a matter of obligation only if a woman has explicitly assumed pregnancy as an obligation, such as by signing a "surrogate mother" contract or by intentionally inviting a fetus to depend on her. If she has not assumed such an obligation, then if she decides not to make significant sacrifices in order to provide that gift, she fails to be a good Samaritan (Thompson, 184), but that, pro-choice advocates would say, is not to be a bad Levite—one who fails to honor her previous obligations and commitments.[5]

According to this pro-choice view, it is wrong to make the status of the fetus the primary issue in the abortion debate; the primary issue is whether any woman should be *coerced* into making significant sacrifices to give a gift to someone else (though perhaps she should be encouraged to do so). According to this position, the beginning point of the debate should be the woman's point of view, and to assume that, because the fetus is a person, it can appropriate a woman's body without her consent is intrinsically sexist (B. Harrison, 16). Nowhere else in law (or even in morality) does society coerce the continuation of such an impingement. (This point is illustrated by the McFall-Shimp case discussed in Chapter Three, pp. 73-83.) Unless society would be willing, for example, to coerce a father to donate a kidney to his daughter who would die without it, it certainly ought not to coerce continued pregnancy just because the woman is a uniquely qualified organ lender (Mattingly).

Pregnancy and Sacrifice

The preceding pro-choice position claims that the notion that pregnancy involves only minor inconvenience (less, say, than bone-marrow or kidney transplants) and not significant sacrifice ignores both common sense and the scientific discoveries that bear on the responsibilities of a woman giving the gift of life to another. Common sense recognizes that pregnancy is not just a matter of letting the fetus grow on its own; it reminds us that "labor" is just that—labor; moreover, labor can involve great pain and varying risks to life and health, often preceded by months of discomfort such as nausea, backaches, cramps, loss of sleep, and dramatic body changes that can be regarded as highly undesirable. All of this, of course, will be very visible to society, whose reaction, depending on circumstances, can range from solid support through amused tolerance to venge-

5. In accord with much of the literature on good Samaritanism, we interpret it as the willingness to make significant sacrifices to help others, including strangers, and we interpret Levitism as the restricted ethic of helping friends, family, or tribe and not harming strangers, including not causing harm to them in the act of refusing to help them when contractual relationships create legitimate expectations to be helped. (Chapter Three explains how not helping can sometimes be a form of harming, and later in this chapter we refer to an argument that much of what passes as good Samaritanism could be construed as good Levitism.) One could interpret Levitism not as a minimal ethic but as an alternative ethic that has strict requirements which forbid Samaritanism in certain circumstances. We do not discuss this interpretation because it is rarely relevant to the abortion debate.

ful punishment. Furthermore, recent scientific studies recognize the many ways the fetus can be affected by the pregnant woman's lifestyle and career. Of course, many restrictions on activities during pregnancy have long been regarded as reasonable and inevitable, and the list of such restrictions is growing. For example, we now know that smoking causes perhaps 50,000 miscarriages each year in the United States—and low birth weight when it does not kill (Ravenholt, "Addiction Mortality," 711), that drinking while pregnant can be as harmful as drinking while driving, and that both recreational and therapeutic drugs can cause fetal defects.

A patronizing response might be that it would be good for a woman to immediately cease such habits anyway, but we should appreciate the effort that such a change involves. Moreover, the occupational risks (to the fetus) can be even more difficult to avoid. Women constitute close to 45 percent of the civilian work force and heavily populate occupations that are hazardous to fetal health because of exposure to radiation and to substances such as benzene, lead, anesthetics, and hair spray.[6] So, in addition to the traditional requirement to leave her job for at least a few weeks (often with no benefits and no guarantee that she will get the job back), today's pregnant woman must struggle with her own conscience or with her employer over leaving or changing her job for the entire pregnancy. The economic implications could be severe for career women and those who need their jobs for survival or self-respect. In fact, surveys find that 94 percent of pro-choice women work outside the home, whereas only 37 percent of pro-life women do (Luker, *Abortion*, 195), which may be the reason why many women regard an unwanted pregnancy not as a surprise that can be coped with but as a tragedy that threatens to drastically undermine their well-being (O'Connor, 108).

Nowadays women are often asked to sacrifice even more extensively than in years past because perinatology has made the fetus into the "second patient," whose medical interests can call for therapeutic interventions that are costly to the woman. Already women have been legally coerced into having Cesarean sections to protect the baby being born, and the New Jersey Supreme Court has ruled that a Jehovah's Witness may be coerced into violating her religious beliefs by being forced to have a blood transfusion to protect her fetus's life (Annas, "Forced Cesareans"). The growing prospects for fetal surgery could force this "consent" issue much more often. Even if our society avoids legally enforceable "prenatal contracts" that spell out maternity conditions, a

---

6. For a perceptive analysis of how recent knowledge regarding the fetus is affecting the abortion debate, see D. Callahan's "How Technology Is Reframing the Abortion Debate."

caring woman who is bringing a fetus to term will increasingly feel a responsibility not just to change her lifestyle to avoid harming the fetus but also to submit to surgical and other therapeutic interventions to help it[7]—truly significant sacrifices.

Given the preceding considerations, the conclusion of many pro-choice advocates is that society may and perhaps should encourage pregnant women to be good Samaritans and sacrifice in order to give the gift of life to someone else, but that, at least until the sacrifice is more equally distributed, the decision should be the woman's. Otherwise, her autonomy is violated in a way that male autonomy is not violated in such analogous situations as the McFall-Shimp case.

Responsibility and Sexuality

One difficulty with the preceding pro-choice argument is that in most cases of pregnancy the couple willingly took the chance to create a

---

7. In 1986 a legal precedent was set when Pamela Rae Steward was charged with being criminally liable for the death of her son Thomas, who was born brain-dead and was found to have amphetamines in his body. (In 1980 a Michigan court ruled that parents can be cited for neglect if a baby is born addicted to drugs, but the Steward case is probably the first criminal prosecution for fetal abuse.) Steward was charged not only with fetal abuse via drug abuse but also with disobeying doctors' advice about how to avoid complications that might be caused by her diagnosed condition of placenta previa, which required her to stay off her feet, avoid sexual intercourse and street drugs, and get immediate medical attention for hemorrhaging. Prosecutors charge that she took amphetamines, had sex with her husband, and waited twelve hours after bleeding began to call paramedics. A conviction would have given her up to a year in jail and a $2,000 fine. Although a judge dismissed the charges, Steward spent six days in jail before her bond was reduced. (This information was culled from "Mother Charged after Baby Born Brain-dead with Drugs in System," "Judge Dismisses Pregnancy Abuse Case," and the articles by Begley and Chambers et al.)

The logic of both the pro-life and the pro-choice positions is certainly compatible with asserting a moral and legal obligation to protect developing human beings during their biologically most important and vulnerable growth stages. (The difference between the positions is not whether one may willfully harm—through omission or commission—a human being that one has decided to bring to term, but whether the latter is a matter of choice once a human being has been conceived.) Indeed, that one must protect a fetus to whom one has decided to give birth is a point that both sides have powerful reasons to accept. Some physicians have argued for the enforced hospitalization of a pregnant woman whose behavior threatens her fetus (Mackenzie and Nagel). Others worry about reducing "the woman to what current obstetrical language calls 'the maternal environment'" and about eventually requiring prenatal contracts in which a woman, her attorney, and the attorney appointed as fetal guardian are informed by a fetologist about the conditions to which she must adhere during the pregnancy (Rothman). Covenantal ethics would avoid legal contracts, but responsible women will probably continue to learn more about how they should change their behavior or lifestyle to enhance the welfare of fetuses they carry.

human being who would neither exist nor be vulnerable if they had not taken that chance. Even if they took reasonable precautions against pregnancy (and there is plenty of room for debate about what is "reasonable" [Luker, *Taking Chances*, 110]), they seem to be responsible for the fetus's vulnerability in a way that Shimp was not responsible for McFall's need or a father for his daughter's bad kidneys. If we alter the transplant analogies so that the prospective donor is responsible for the prospective recipient's distinctive needs, we may well agree that the former should be required to sacrifice to help the other, whose specific vulnerability he or she caused. Of course, in the case of pregnancy, the male can escape responsibility in a way that the female cannot. This fact may imply that society should be willing to provide the support that some irresponsible males evade, but it does not seem to eliminate the woman's responsibility except in such cases as rape.

Some pro-choice writers raise questions about the lengths to which a woman must go to avoid such purported responsibility. Judith Thompson approaches the idea by analogy. She asks us to imagine that "people seeds" float in the air like pollen and that, in spite of our putting up fine-mesh screens, one gets in when someone voluntarily opens a window. Would we say that person is responsible for the seed's "rooting" just because she took the small but real chance that a seed would get through the protective devices if a window was opened for fresh air, which she does not absolutely need? Thompson's implication is that of course the window opener is not responsible for the seed's rooting; after all, she even cooperated in installing the protective screens. When someone else declares the window opener to be responsible for the seed's "rooting" because the protective screens were not adequate for the job, Thompson asks how far we have to go to ensure perfect protection. That is also her question about sexual responsibility: What measures does a woman have to take to be considered sexually responsible? Does responsibility require that she go so far as to "avoid pregnancy due to rape by having a hysterectomy, or anyway by never leaving home without a (reliable) army"? (p. 182).

Thompson's point raises fundamental questions about sexuality and its relation to childbearing and the family.[8] Most Christians agree

---

8. Thompson's point raises related questions about the concept of responsibility. In a sense, the victims of crime are (partly) *causally* responsible for being in the wrong place at the wrong time. But if they had the right to be there and if they took reasonable precautions against being victims, they in no way are *morally* or *legally* responsible for what happened. To think otherwise is to engage in the all-too-common practice of blaming the victim, a practice that confuses the above-mentioned senses of responsibility. The question of whether a couple is morally (and not just causally) responsible for the existence of a zy-

that procreation is not the sole or even the most important function of sexual intercourse. Indeed, most agree that Christian couples have the stewardly privilege and even responsibility to use contraceptives (or, at least, calculated timing) so that they can enjoy and strengthen their emotional bonds without overwhelming their or the earth's resources by having numerous children. The question is whether sexual intercourse should be *completely* separated from procreation and childbearing so that it may be enjoyed even when there is not or cannot be any commitment to giving birth to a human being that, despite reasonable precautions, may be created. Is there a natural and appropriate connection between sexual intercourse and possible procreation—say, like the connection between eating (even careful eating) and possible weight gain—or is it an accidental connection so bothersome that its severing can be accepted even when the means involves the death of the fetus? If a strictly erotic model of sexuality—emphasizing play, passion, self-expression, and romantic games—is combined with a voluntary contract model of ethics — emphasizing individualism, which limits commitments and obligations to those explicitly agreed to—everyone (who survives) may feel less threatened and more fulfilled. If such a model of sexuality is recommended, then abortion can be celebrated as the technological fix that finally allows human choice to dominate natural reproductive processes: it severs the inconvenient connection between eager orgasm and any undesired offspring.

Of course, one need not accept the preceding model in order to desire sexual activity without procreation. Loving couples can have good moral and theological reasons for wanting to postpone or avoid having children, and they may and should take all reasonable precaution to avoid conception. What "reasonable precaution" involves probably depends on how important it is to avoid conception, but personal control can be combined with contraceptives to all but eliminate the chance of conception. We admit that insisting on such discipline as an alternative to abortion requires a model of sexuality that takes seriously the connection between sexual intercourse and the possibility of procreation. And we favor a model that sees covenantal wisdom in connecting most sexual activity and passion with the sort of long-term commitment that is interested in or at least can cope with procreation. This wisdom does not view the threat of pregnancy as the "price one should pay for sexual pleasure." Rather, it expands the idea of sexuality to include the

gote when they took reasonable precautions to prevent conception cannot be answered without the discussion about sexuality and its relation to childbearing.

feminine experiences of childbearing and nursing, and it refuses to allow a cheap, violent technological fix to substitute for policies and institutions that can support women in their childbearing and nursing roles.

A number of feminists writing about the threefold sexuality of women—orgasm, birth, and nursing—have wondered why it is only orgasm—the dimension of female sexuality shared with males—that tends to be glorified, while the others tend to be denigrated as bondage to nature (S. Callahan, 237). One obvious response to this query is that, even if childbearing and nursing are uniquely feminine (and perhaps pleasurable) aspects of a broadened notion of sexuality, they do "bind" women in ways that orgasm does not. Pro-choice advocates, arguing that women should be no more bound by their sexuality than men are by theirs, contend that society should not force women to risk birth and nursing whenever they experience orgasm. Why should women, they ask, be forced to risk what men are not forced to risk for the same kind of experience?

Abortion on demand is a way of ensuring that women are not forced to accept the highly sacrificial, uniquely feminine dimensions of sexuality whenever they experience the dimension of it that men do. But it is also a way of ensuring that men and the rest of society are not forced to share the sacrifices. White, upper-middle-class males constitute the single group most consistent in favoring abortion on demand (and men as a group favor it more highly than do women as a group) (Elshtain, 59). Feminists need not be overly suspicious to wonder whether this statistic is due to these men's undying commitment to equal opportunity for women or to the fact that these men have much to gain and little to lose with abortion on demand.

Mary Meehan, a pro-life feminist, connects the Playboy philosophy and strong male support for abortion:

> Feminists often say that women should have a right to abortion on request because all of the burden of bearing children falls on women and because most of the burden of rearing them falls on women. The first point is undeniably true, the second often so (although it need not be). But many feminists overlook the point that abortion is a men's solution. This is especially the case when children are conceived outside marriage. So much stress is placed on the social and financial difficulties of women in this situation that we tend to overlook the problems of the men who are involved. Abortion is a much simpler solution for them because they do not have to undergo it. They merely have to encourage their female partners. Sometimes, they must pay for it, but $150-$200 for an abortion is far cheaper than paying child support for 18 years. As Juli Loesch said, "In the bad old days, if an unmarried

woman got pregnant, the father-of-the-child was expected to accept some degree of accountability." She added, "Now the responsible thing is to put up the cash for an abortion ('No hard feelings, OK?'); and if the man actually goes to the clinic with the woman—if he holds her hand—Why, he's a prince." This is the easy way out, the cheap way out. Prolife feminists believe it is no coincidence that the Playboy Foundation has put a great deal of money into groups supporting legalized abortion. The Playboy dream of carefree, no-fault sex has been realized at last. For men. (Meehan, 157-58)

We do not claim that the Playboy philosophy is the only or even the main motivation for the pro-choice position. But we agree with pro-life feminists that society should notice the coincidence and should also notice that abortion on demand is likely to impede rather than encourage the sort of laws, policies, and institutions that would share with women the burden of childbearing. When abortion is available as a cheap and easy (at least for men) technological fix, there is much less motivation for society to reorder its structures to provide such measures as pregnancy leaves, day-care centers, homes for unwed mothers, and legal means for requiring male progenitors to live up to their responsibilities. These measures are harder and more complicated than abortion—they seek to recognize that most sex is connected to possible procreation and seek to institutionalize the commitments required to cooperate with natural processes—but we agree that they operate more in the long-term interests of women than do policies that encourage women to kill the fetuses growing within them.

Abortion not only entails medical and psychological costs suffered mainly by women; it also encourages "short-term-commitment sexuality," which is probably not in women's long-term best interests. Men seem to be able or at least willing to play low-commitment sex games (often with younger women) much longer than women can, and easy abortion enables them to provide a "choice" that, if declined, can leave a woman to struggle on her own with the consequences of her own choice. Then the choice of abortion becomes a pressure, because the easy availability of abortion enables society to avoid the more difficult measures that recognize the link between sex and possible procreation.

We have argued for a view of sexuality that requires either a high degree of sexual discipline or some degree of mutual responsibility for the life of the potential person when pregnancy results. This conclusion is at odds with a pro-choice view that abortion is simply the refusal to give the gift of life. Usually abortion ends a life that, at least to some extent, a couple is responsible for having begun.

Failing to Help versus Harming

That abortion results in the death of a fetus creates another difficulty for the pro-choice view, one that is independent of the issue of responsibility. Certainly it is a difficulty for those who believe that their obligations extend beyond their voluntary contracts, that they may have a responsibility to make sacrifices when circumstances thrust vulnerable strangers upon them, and that God calls them and gives them the resources to live up to those wider covenantal responsibilities which the commercial contracts of possessive individualism cannot handle. In short, those who accept the covenantal ethics we outlined in Chapter Three would feel a responsibility to sacrifice in order to prevent the death of the fetus. Moreover, this wider notion of responsibility is sometimes translated by the Anglo-American legal tradition into obligations with legal force. Thus many states have what are called "good Samaritan laws." Given what we have said about good Samaritanism, it should be obvious that translating it into legal obligations is very controversial. Generally these laws apply to special situations, such as injury-causing accidents, and they require persons to provide the reasonable sort of help that would prevent significant harm to the victims. John Kleinig argues that the rationale for most of our laws—preventing harm—is also a rationale for some good Samaritan laws that require strangers to help the vulnerable even when there is no institutionalized relationship between victim and helper (p. 398). Likewise, Robert Goodin boldly but persuasively argues that the principle of "protecting the vulnerable," rather than the principles of voluntary contractualism and utilitarianism, is at the foundation of Western ethics and law. He sometimes calls this expanded notion of obligation "good Samaritanism," in order to argue in favor of the "good Samaritan laws" discussed by state legislatures. But he realizes that often the refusal to sacrifice in order to prevent harm to others is a violation of a duty more narrowly defined than what we call good Samaritanism. He believes that once people see the true foundation of their common moral sense, they will see that "what would ordinarily be described as merely ungenerous acts are actually far worse than that. They show us to be bad Levites rather than merely bad Samaritans" (p. 26).

So those who accept covenantal ethics, which includes the responsibility to be a good Samaritan, will avoid abortion even if it is thought of merely as the refusal to make significant sacrifices to help a vulnerable stranger. And those who accept Goodin's justification for good Samaritan laws, which might more accurately be called "good Levite laws," will avoid abortion insofar as it is thought of as the refusal to provide reasonable aid that prevents significant harm to the vulnerable.

But even those who believe that they have no responsibility to aid strangers should not assume that they may actively harm strangers in avoiding giving them aid. And most abortions involve actions that kill the fetus. Pictures of aborted fetuses and sonograms of abortions are sometimes used to show that the killing is violent and bloody, but, although that fact may be relevant to the bad psychological and social effects of abortion, it is not relevant to the main harm done to the fetus, which is death, no matter how painless and clean it may be. We will not here defend the claim that death harms the fetus; the pro-choice use of the good Samaritan analogy does not question whether death harms the fetus but whether one must sacrifice to avoid allowing harm to occur. Abortion, however, usually causes harm rather than merely allowing it to occur. Generally it does not merely foresee that harm but even intends it (the distinction between foreseeing and intending harm is an important one that we will use later in Chapter Ten); it intends harm to the fetus as a means of relieving someone from other harms or burdens.

Pro-choice advocates might object that the preceding point assumes that a positive action (a commission) that causes harm is somehow morally worse than a refraining (an omission) that merely allows harm to occur. They might go on to argue that, when all other morally relevant factors are the same, quite likely there is no big moral difference between harming through omission and harming through commission. Therefore, the objector might say, we should not attach any moral importance to the fact that abortion results in harm through commission rather than omission.

We are inclined to agree with this claim that omissions and commissions are morally equivalent when all other relevant factors are the same (which they seldom are). But this point is more troublesome than helpful to the pro-choice use of the good Samaritan analogy. Suppose the Levite could not continue his journey without stepping on the wounded man and thereby killing him. Even if people were convinced that stepping on (and thereby killing) the man and merely abandoning him were morally equivalent actions, they would be more likely to believe that it would be wrong to abandon him than to believe that it would be all right to kill him. (Indeed, both Goodin and Kleinig use this belief in their arguments that helping vulnerable strangers is a strict obligation.) Therefore, we are not convinced by the pro-choice argument that abortion is merely the refusal to be a good Samaritan and not the violation of a moral obligation that evn a Levite must obey.

At this point, pro-choice advocates might object that something has gone seriously wrong in our argument. They might fear that somehow our somewhat reasonable opposition to killing the fetus has resulted in the right of the fetus to appropriate someone else's body and "without the woman's consent, to suck her very life's blood; to use her digestive and cardiovascular systems; to dump wastes into her bloodstream, use her kidneys and respiratory and endocrine systems; to sap her strength, drain her energies, interfere with her basic mobility, and eventually send her to the hospital" (Hilbert, p. 18). The author of this letter has a point, and the reasons the pro-choice side can elicit popular support that is as highly charged and as morally indignant as the pro-life support is that it, too, is protecting a fundamental value. Even those states or countries that have good Samaritan laws recognize definite limits to the sacrifices one person is obliged to make in helping another. The abortion issue arouses moral indignation on both sides because it is one of the few dilemmas (the only one confronted by many people) in which forbidding a person to cause harm to another simultaneously coerces her to nurture the other, sometimes at great risk or sacrifice and always at the cost of having her body significantly and intimately changed.

Pro-choice writers can use other analogous though hypothetical situations besides the parable of the good Samaritan to convey their intuition that, given the costs of pregnancy to women, abortion should be seen as a permissible refusal to sacrifice rather than a wrongful causing of harm. Suppose, for example, that medical practice involves the risk (despite reasonable precautions) that patients' survival sometimes requires that they or some organism they need be physically united with their physicians (a given physician being the unique person whose body is required by a given patient) in relationships that cause and require significant bodily changes in and restrictions on the physicians analogous to those experienced by pregnant women.[9] Suppose such a condition requires that physicians make appropriate changes in their work habits and that it requires their taking a leave for at least a few weeks. Suppose further that it sometimes is discovered that the condition threatens the physicians' physical or mental health and perhaps even their lives. Would physicians violate their duty and their patients' rights by in-

9. Imagine, for example, that some sort of organism has to be implanted in the physician's body, an organism that will do roughly what fetuses do to women's bodies and that will have to be surgically removed after nine months for transplantation into the patient's body. This example is an adaptation of J. Thompson's (p. 174) famous-violinist example, in which you are asked to imagine that you wake up some morning and discover that a talented violinist has been hooked up to you and that he needs your body for nine months in order to survive. Our adaptation seeks to capture some of the role responsibilities that Thompson's does not. Why try to gain insight into an already complex issue by using such far-out examples? Those who use them believe that the special demands of pregnancy require such analogies if we are willing to allow our intuitions about them to inform our perceptions of the abortion issue.

sisting on having the choice, at least in some circumstances, to eliminate such a condition even if it meant the death of the patients?

We are not at all sure how to answer this question, which may say something about the usefulness of such analogies but may also say something about the dilemma posed when forbidding a person to harm someone else (for whom the former has some role responsibilities) simultaneously coerces that person to nurture the other even if doing so requires great sacrifices or risks. We suspect that if the physician situation just outlined arose frequently—even in a society with an individualistic voluntary-contract model of ethics—there would be a major social effort (involving paid leaves, career protections, etc.) to share the burdens of physicians. Certainly a society with a communal model of relationships and a covenantal model of ethics would help physicians bear the burden, not just with inspiring stories but also with adequate concrete help. Such encouragement and help would likely make physicians feel obligated to bear their part of the burden. But even in a covenantal society, it is doubtful that physicians would get charged with murder if they refused the burden, at least in the hard cases. Indeed, there would most likely be a great deal of debate over the extent to which the sword power of the state should get involved in coercing physicians to live up to their covenantal responsibilities. This debate would be especially vigorous if—to stretch the analogy—the patients were in a deep coma during the time they needed the physicians' bodies, a coma they would survive only if the physicians accepted the risks and sacrifices (analogous to those of pregnancy) that would give the patients the gift of life. And there would be legalistic questions about whether these human beings were still truly persons, since they would not have the capacities for personhood and never would regain them unless the physicians accepted the sacrifices involved in "resurrecting" them.

A Christian covenantal approach, as we argued earlier, would not insist on settling the issue by asking legalistic questions about the moral status of such human beings or by asking what are the relevant, enforceable rights and duties. The primary question would be not whether *they* are imagers of God with certain rights but whether *we* are imagers of a God, who has a bias toward welcoming vulnerable human beings into covenantal fellowship and who sacrificed himself even unto death to give life to those who did not deserve it or have a right to it. But such an attitude assumes distinctive moral and theological beliefs. In a pluralist society, the legalistic questions about enforceable rights and duties do get raised, and we believe that the pro-choice position is correct in asserting that nowhere else in law or morality do we mandate that people accept the kinds of risks and sacrifices that are sometimes coerced when abortion is forbidden. For that reason we believe that abortion is not the moral or legal equivalent of premeditated murder.

Summary

We began this lengthy section by observing that Christians will normally perceive unborn human beings as precious gifts in the process of being welcomed into the covenantal community. The question of whether the fetus's status as a potential person grants it rights that cannot be overridden by those of the pregnant woman normally does not even arise. But we noted that circumstances can cause that question to be raised. Next we used the parable of the good Samaritan to suggest that, even when the fetus is perceived as a threatening stranger, treating it in a neighborly way will usually enable a person to perceive it as a vulnerable neighbor deserving of life and respect. We then asked about the morality of not treating the fetus in a neighborly way, explaining a pro-choice interpretation of the same parable. This interpretation suggested that, given the costs of pregnancy for many women, abortion often amounts to the refusal to make significant sacrifices to give a gift to someone else; having an abortion under these conditions is the failure to be a good Samaritan, but it is not a violation of strict moral obligation. Our first objection against this pro-choice view raised the issue of responsibility for pregnancy. In countering a pro-choice argument that people are not responsible for pregnancy when they take reasonable precautions to prevent it, we endorsed a pro-life feminist view of sexuality, a view implying that it is unwise to completely sever sexual intercourse from responsibility for possible procreation. Our second objection to the pro-choice use of the parable raised the point that abortion causes fatal harm to the fetus and that therefore it seems to violate not only covenantal ethics or the rationale for "good Samaritan" (or even "good Levite") laws but also the obligation not to inflict harm on others. In response to a pro-choice argument that forbidding abortion simultaneously coerces a woman to accept an amount and type of sacrifice that is mandated nowhere else in law or morality, we agreed that this consideration implies that abortion is not the moral equivalent of murder. This point holds independently of our argument in the previous section about the status of the fetus, which also implies that abortion is not the equivalent of murder. But that section and this one both imply that at least some abortions are gravely immoral; the policy implications of this view still need to be considered.

Policy Implications

According to the sense of "respect" we discussed in Chapter Three, it should be clear that we respect particular ways of developing both the pro-life and the pro-choice positions. Sometimes, perhaps, ignorance, selfishness, thoughtlessness, or the refusal to understand the opponent's position is what determines an activist's view on the abortion issue. But extreme positions on both sides can be held by intelligent and knowledgeable persons of goodwill who are defending basic values and insights. We think that recognizing this fact could raise the quality of the abortion debate and help avoid reducing it to slurs or shrill rhetoric. As we noticed in Chapter Three, however, one sometimes has to be uncooperative with or intolerant of a position one respects because one believes that position to be, in fact, dangerous, even though it can be rationally defended. So we must ask not only whether we respect a position but also whether we can cooperate with it or tolerate its being acted upon.

We begin on the positive note: all sides can agree on a number of measures and policies that could reduce the tendency to think of abortion as a necessary, even if tragic, alternative.

First, it is time for unions, insurance companies, employers, and the government to recognize that women are close to one-half of the work force, that nostalgia or even good arguments for the single-worker (male) nuclear family are not going to change that fact, and that provision ought to be made to help women workers in their childbearing and nursing roles. It is easy to pretend that the latter are private matters, and one can give respectable arguments against paid pregnancy leaves, nurseries on the job, and public funding of policies that increase population in an overpopulated world. But we believe these arguments are overridden by the facts that 85 percent of working women become pregnant (Taylor) and that until they can combine job or career with having children (as males can), there will be substantial pressure for abortions, whether legal or illegal. Moreover, one can find good covenantal reasons as well as frankly prudential ones for society's being willing to share the joys and burdens of childbearing and child rearing, especially when so much of the child rearing is done in single-parent families. So we think all sides should support such measures as pregnancy leaves, nurseries on the job, flex-time and part-time job arrangements, and day-care centers.

A second area for cooperation is the discouraging of sexual activity among young teenagers. Children having children and children having abortions are both scandals. Rather than arguing about which one is worse, we should work against the causes. Sex education is nec-

essary but not sufficient. It will prevent pregnancies due to sheer ignorance (and ignorance about sex is surpassed in young teens only by
pseudo-sophistication about it), but by itself it will not necessarily discourage sexual activity. Among other things required is sexuality training that nurtures in girls the self-esteem that makes them abhor being
treated as sexual toys and in boys the consciousness of what a perver-
sion of manhood it is to associate self-esteem with scoring sexual points.
The task is huge and complicated, of course, especially given the high-
hormonal character of so much of the popular music, movies, and cultural values affecting teenagers. But there is some evidence that enough
people are deeply enough disturbed that the epidemic of teenage pregnancy could get the sort of attention the drug epidemic does. Both epi-
demics require alternative sources of fulfillment, which implies an educational and nurturing task that begins with early childhood. The size
and complexity of the task, while daunting, should also underscore its
importance and the need for cooperation.

Perhaps we are naive, but we hope that another area of cooperation is the discouraging of hedonistic egoism and possessive individualism, which reduce one's responsibilities to the rights and duties for
which self-interested parties voluntarily contract. We fear that this mentality not only makes choosing abortion much easier than it should be
but also undermines the sense of communal support and responsibility
that creates conditions in which most abortions become as undesired as
they are unnecessary.

Other areas for cooperation include supporting adoption as an
alternative to abortion (this requires providing psychological and institutional support for unmarried pregnant women); supporting basic research into genetic diseases, which are often the reason for abortion;
supporting many types of genetic counseling; and providing insurance
or institutional support for families of children born with disabilities or
serious medical needs.

Although there is much room for cooperation and although the
energy spent on this cooperation may well do more to prevent abortions
and provide choices than alternative expenditures of pro-life and pro-
choice energies, when it comes to abortion itself, there obviously is less
room for cooperation or even tolerance. We cannot agree with those who
are either intolerant of any abortions or tolerant of all abortions. Our
views on the status of the fetus and on covenantal responsibilities imply
that abortion is not murder but that it often is the sort of serious wrong
that ought to be both morally and legally restrained. So we cannot support either the right-to-life amendments or abortion on demand, but we
admit that these positions do have a clarity and precision that our posi-

tion, like all middle positions, lacks. The policy implications of our view, we admit, are very general, and they become more debatable as they become more specific. But we agree with a statement in an excellent study that independently reaches a position similar to our own: "General advice is better than bad advice" (Wennberg, *Life*, 122). So we will state what we believe can be reasonably inferred from our views about the fetus and about covenantal responsibility.

Suggested grounds for abortion generally fall into four classifications: (1) traumatic (cases in which rape or incest results in pregnancy); (2) therapeutic (the woman's life or health is at risk); (3) genetic (the fetus is deformed); and (4) socio-economic (giving birth would impose too great a burden on others). In certain tragic circumstances involving the first three categories we would regretfully recommend an abortion; in the sense defined in Chapter Three, we would sometimes cooperate with an abortion we would not recommend; and we would sometimes tolerate and even (rarely) cooperate with an abortion while recommending against it. In all four categories there are examples of abortion that we would both tolerate and cooperate with, but we would not necessarily be willing to cooperate with every abortion we would tolerate. The abortions we would cooperate with or even recommend are what are often called the "hard cases," which probably amount to only a small percentage of abortions actually performed. Unless otherwise stated, we are referring to first-trimester abortions or (rarely) those performed at least several weeks before viability. (The relevance of gestational stage will be discussed later.)

In cases of rape, we would cooperate with abortions and, at least in the cases of some young teenagers, recommend them. If the woman had the maturity, strength, and willingness to continue the pregnancy, she would be a heroine in our view. But generally in cases of rape, the responsibility to welcome developing human life into covenantal fellowship is overwhelmed by the violence of the act of rape and the scars that can result from a woman's being forced to continue to sacrifice her bodily integrity when it was so brutally violated.

We would sadly but strongly recommend abortion when a woman's carrying a fetus is a serious and undeniable threat to her life, because we do not believe God desires the probable sacrifice of a covenant member (especially one with many relationships and responsibilities) as the means of welcoming another being into the covenant, and we do not think that society should recommend such a trade-off. But such a risk is extremely rare. More often, therapeutic abortions are performed when there is slight or debatable risk to life or health. We would cooperate with abortions when there is significant threat to life or health on the grounds that the decision should be between a woman and her God whether she must take such risks in living up to the normal covenantal responsibility to nurture rather than harm a developing human life. Our idea of health as the well-functioning of the organism as a whole prevents us from specifying risk to physical rather than mental health; we see no sharp separation. However, not all mental stress should be thought of as a significant risk to health; it would have to threaten to cause some long-term or irreversible impingement on the well-functioning of the woman if we were to cooperate with an abortion on this ground. We admit that the impossibility of drawing clear lines here makes our position difficult. We rely more on the covenantal dispositions of the decision-makers than on unambiguous criteria for precise line-drawing.

We would recommend abortion on genetic grounds in those cases in which the fetus is not a potential person because deformities prevent it from coming even close to having God-imaging capacities. Therefore, we would recommend abortion for anencephaly, a condition that causes the lack of a brain, which occurs 4,000 times per year in the United States (President's Commission, *Deciding*, 1811). We would also recommend abortion in those rare cases in which life would inevitably be short and subjectively indistinguishable from torture (for example, in cases of Tay-Sachs, trisomy 13, and trisomy 18[10] [Jones, "Abortion," 181; VanDeVeer, 214-23]). It is an empirical question whether a given biological abnormality would preclude the possibility of the developing human being's ever being welcomed into covenantal fellowship or would make its experience for its entire brief life subjectively indistinguishable from torture. In the former case — when the fetus is not a potential person —the pregnancy would lead to what is appropriately called "meaningless life." In the latter case—when the infant would experience nothing but suffering—pregnancy would lead to what is appropriately called "wrongful life." (Of course, the latter's suffering can

---

10. See pp. 248-49 for a description and further discussion of Tay-Sachs disease. Trisomy 13 is also known as Patau's syndrome; it results when the fetus receives an extra copy of chromosome 13. Infants suffering from this syndrome have very abnormal brains and usually defects of the eyes, heart, kidneys, gastrointestinal tract, and urogenital system. Affected infants nearly always die within the first few days to first few months of life. (See p. 237 for further discussion.) Trisomy 18 is also known as Edward's syndrome; it results when the fetus receives an extra copy of chromosome 18, which occurs in approximately 1 in 3,500 births. The condition is characterized by congenital heart disease, difficult breathing, retardation, and so on. It involves both painful physical problems and an early death; it may be an example of a condition that involves both the lack of potential personhood and a life subjectively indistinguishable from torture. Most afflicted fetuses die before birth. Of those born live, 50 percent die in the first two months; 90 percent die in the first year. (See p. 237 for further discussion.)

sometimes serve social goods, such as giving a family or society a focus for loving concern. But it can also cause social evil, and, in any case, a fetus ought not to be brought to term simply because its suffering would serve others.) One should not argue for aborting Down's syndrome fetuses on the preceding grounds: they almost always can be welcomed into covenantal fellowship as persons and also generally have special ability for such God-imaging capacities as honesty and appreciating what one has. We are not here claiming that Down's syndrome fetuses should never be aborted on socio-economic grounds (see what follows); we are simply saying that such grounds should not be confused with abortion "on behalf of the fetus," which would apply only to those rare cases of wrongful life. It is doubtful that aborting in cases of spina bifida or hemophilia can be justified as preventing wrongful or even meaningless life. Even in clear-cut cases of wrongful life we would not *require* abortion (to prevent useless torture), simply because some people think every abortion is murder and because abortion is usually a technologically invasive procedure that requires informed consent. Chapter Nine gives a further discussion of genetic conditions and genetic abortions.

Can abortions ever by justified on the grounds that the fetus's future life would be too burdensome, not to itself (wrongful life) but to the woman, the family, or society (socio-economic grounds)? We cannot recommend abortions on socio-economic grounds as long as society will help women bear the burdens. However, it is the pregnant woman who bears and will bear most of the burden even when others do everything they can, so we would cooperate with abortion in those cases in which the pregnancy genuinely threatens to overwhelm the woman's or the couple's ability to meet the covenantal responsibilities already assumed. Before deciding that such a situation can never arise, one should talk with parents of a burdensomely disabled child who are asking about the impact of a second such child.

But hard cases like these probably represent only a small percent of current abortions. Abortion today is often being used as a means of birth control and as a matter of convenience, not as a necessity. This is wrong because it devalues human beings who are in the process of becoming persons and it violates or at least fails to live up to the responsibilities of covenantal fellowship. We believe Christians should argue and counsel against abortions of convenience and should simultaneously support those measures previously mentioned that would reduce the perceived need for them. But we do not believe abortions should be made illegal, at least not during the first trimester. Our primary consideration is that they do not constitute murder, for the two reasons already mentioned several times: a human being in the process of becoming a person is not yet a person, and to forbid harming that human being is to coerce a woman to nurture it with the amount and type of sacrifice that not even the strongest "good Samaritan" laws require.

But a wrong does not have to be murder in order to be criminal, so why not criminalize abortions of convenience, serious wrongs that they are? There are three reasons. First, the reasons we give for reverencing potential persons and for the covenantal model of the moral life require distinctive premises not widely shared in societies oriented toward individual achievement and voluntary contracts. In Chapter Three we argued against using moral or theological beliefs that are not widely shared as grounds for criminalizing behavior. Second, as Andrew Kuyvenhoven argues, there is a limit to using the law to regulate behavior even if the majority think a particular behavior is immoral: "The laws of our temporary society are not intended to . . . convert the lives of the citizens. That work is done by the Word and the Spirit of God. Laws are intended to protect the life of society" (p. 7). In a moment we will use this point to argue for regulating late-term abortion, but we do not believe that first-trimester abortions threaten the very foundation or life of society. We understand, however, that those who believe all abortion is murder would disagree with us; if we agreed with their view of abortion, we would probably agree with their efforts to outlaw it. Further, we understand that, in spite of the observation that actions must usually be "out loved" before they are outlawed, sometimes the law can be used as an educational and not just a protective device. But not if doing so would create chaos, which brings us to our third reason against criminalizing early abortions.

Some pro-life advocates believe that, since the majority of Americans are repulsed by the abuse of easy abortion and oppose abortion on demand, it may be possible to get a right-to-life amendment into the U.S. Constitution (Andrusko, 9). Other analysts believe that, if Americans have to choose between pro-choice and the criminalization of (almost) all abortions, the majority will choose the former (Lamanna, 13). We believe the latter prediction is correct. But suppose that, through the judicious use of one-issue voting (and surely a perceived massacre of the infants warrants one-issue voting), abortion was criminalized. The prohibition of early induced abortions would no doubt result in massive civil disobedience and, we think, insurmountable difficulties in enforcing the law and applying appropriate penalties. We believe that the law could not be enforced without serious invasion of privacy. We believe this prediction to be correct even if the law managed to avoid treating the use of IUDs as assault with a concealed weapon. And, depending on how severe or lenient the penalties would be, one activist group or another would find them totally unacceptable. Both of these results would seriously undermine respect for law. So we believe that early induced abortions should not be criminalized.[11]

At the same time, we believe that no health professional or private health institution should be required to cooperate with induced abortions. If one's opposition to abortion is such that one cannot in good conscience even refer those seeking abortions to cooperative professionals, one is obliged, we believe, to make that very clear at the beginning of a relationship with a pregnant patient (or one able to become pregnant). Patients should also be informed about one's possible refusal to cooperate with prenatal testing. (Since the issue of informing patients about prenatal testing is legally disputed, professionals would be prudent to consult with knowledgeable lawyers about how to state their stance to patients.)

Some have argued that, if early abortions are not made illegal, it is inconsistent to make late abortions illegal, because from day to day there are not enough changes in the fetus that would justify making illegal at a particular point what was merely a therapeutic procedure the previous week. One must be careful with such arguments; they can be used fallaciously—for example, to conclude that, if children do not have the right to vote as soon as they are able, then there is no point at which they could justifiably be given the right to vote because there are no dramatic shifts in development that would prevent arbitrary line-drawing. Although there is some arbitrariness in deciding precisely at which birthday society should grant the right to vote, there is no arbitrariness in agreeing that the appropriate age span is the late teens rather than the early teens or the middle twenties. Likewise, we are convinced that the "stage" and "conferral" considerations we discussed in Chapter Two, combined with the potentiality principle and the appropriate restrictions on causing suffering when avoiding the burden of nurturing, yield the conclusion that society should grant personhood to the fetus by the end of the second trimester of gestation. After that point the natural revulsion to killing what amounts to tiny babies could be overcome only by a callous disrespect for developing human life that would quite likely endanger the sanctity of young persons. The bloody history of the human race shows how fragile the respect for personal life is and how

---

11. Although in Chapter Two we expressed some doubts about the arguments that implantation marks the beginning of personhood, we believe those arguments are strong enough to leave the use of IUDs up to the informed conscience.

difficult it is to regain that respect in a society that loses it. Thus it is not arbitrary to insist that the line be drawn early enough to protect reverence (especially in medical personnel) for personal life, even if one can argue that the capacities for personhood are not achieved until after birth. We admit that, even if we could fully develop our argument here, it would involve using the empirical slippery-slope argument (see pp. 75-76), which means it would involve predictions about the social effects of practices. These predictions do not have the decisiveness that alternative positions on abortion have. But decisiveness is not the only or even the main virtue for a position on a very complex issue.

We agree that some of the "stage" and "conferral" considerations that imply the wisdom of granting personhood by the end of the second trimester can also be used to argue for an earlier time. Although fetuses neither have reached "quickening" nor are capable of being biologically independent by the end of the first trimester, they have developed the shape, organ differentiation, brain activity, and other characteristics that some have argued are relevant to their inherent or conferred status. Although we do not believe that such facts imply that abortions soon after the first trimester threaten the life or foundations of society (as we believe they could in the third trimester), we do believe that they could be used to argue for laws which express society's concern for developing human life. Insistence upon an "indications" policy (allowing abortion only for the sort of "hard cases" we discussed previously) after the first trimester would avoid many of the legal and social problems we claimed would result from granting personhood at conception, and at the same time it would express respect for human life that has developed the organ differentiation and biological capacities that are the physical foundation of personhood.

However, there are some reasons for wondering whether, in the United States and Canada (whose indications policy has been legally overturned), the political fight for an indications policy after the first trimester would be worth the energy it would require, energy that might be taken away from other efforts to reduce abortions. It would take much political work because it would be vigorously opposed by both the 20 percent who support abortion on demand and the 20 percent who support the right-to-life amendment (see p. 205). The former tend to compromise only to the extent of allowing an indications policy after the second trimester (the Supreme Court's 1972 *Roe v. Wade* decision), whereas the latter tend to compromise to the extent of allowing an indications policy only up to the end of the first trimester (Burtchaell, "Response," 66). Moreover, more than 90 percent of the abortions in the United States already are induced during the first trimester. The introduction of a policy for second-trimester indications would probably cause almost all women to seek first-trimester abortions and thereby to avoid the need to meet the requirements of the policy. The relatively few women seeking later abortions would likely meet whatever indications the policy required, which would no doubt be quite inclusive, or the policy would not have the political strength to be passed. It is doubtful, for example, whether a politically feasible indications policy could exclude abortions for cases of Down's syndrome or spina bifida discovered through amniocentesis. Moreover, an indications policy might increase illegal abortions among women who feel it is demeaning to have to argue their cases before screening panels, panels that inevitably would vary in how they applied the law. So we doubt that it is wise to work for an indications policy applicable during the second trimester, and the reasons we have given against criminalizing all or almost all abortions prevent us from arguing for an indications policy that would be applicable significantly earlier in gestational development. We think that most of what we say here also applies to the issue of whether Christians should strive to have the *Roe v. Wade* decision overturned and then fight for an indications policy on the state level.

In summary, our views on the status of the fetus and on covenantal ethics imply to us that people should choose abortion only in certain hard cases. Those same views imply to us that abortion cannot be equated with murder and that sometimes we should tolerate and even cooperate with abortions we would not recommend. Those views, combined with our views on the role of law and the effects we predict if (almost) all abortions were made illegal, imply to us that we should not support a right-to-life amendment that would grant personhood to fetuses from conception or implantation. All of the preceding views and a number of conferral considerations imply to us that personhood should be morally and legally granted to the fetus at the end of the second trimester, a position that seems to us to allow third-trimester abortions only when the fetus poses an undeniable and significant threat to a woman's life or when it is certain that the fetus is either not a potential person or would have a brief life subjectively indistinguishable from torture.[12] We question the wisdom of an indications policy for abortions during the second trimester.

---

12. We believe that these latter, rare conditions would also call for only ordinary medical care after birth, care that would seek to relieve pain but would not seek to prolong life with what are often called heroic or extraordinary measures (see pp. 275-76). Among the important morally relevant differences between a late abortion and infanticide is that forbidding the latter doesn't simultaneously coerce a woman to continue nurturing a fetus within her own body. What we said about profoundly retarded human beings (pp. 56-57) implies that ordinary care should always be provided them by a covenantal community.

We conclude this chapter by recalling the areas of cooperation that would reduce the demand for abortion. We support measures that enable women to combine childbearing and child rearing with jobs and careers. We support educational measures that help children and teenagers understand the implications of sexual activity, the short-sightedness of associating it with popularity and self-esteem, and the immorality of being irresponsible about it. We encourage personal and institutional commitment to covenantal ways of thinking that expose the poverty of reducing one's responsibilities to those rights and duties for which self-interested parties voluntarily contract. And we support measures that enable women to see adoption as a viable alternative to abortion, as well as other measures that help families cope with long-term burdens of rearing children with disabilities. A covenantal community can do more than all of this, but given the dispositions that characterize covenantal ethics, we believe it should seek to do no less.

9. Genetic Control and Counseling

Since antiquity people have observed that many characteristics of parents are inherited, for better or for worse, by their offspring. They have also frequently noted certain other curious regularities of inheritance, such as fatal bleeding following circumcision in the sons of sisters, as was recorded by a second-century rabbi (Rosner, 833-34). And people have often tried to assume some control over the characteristics of offspring, as did the patriarch Jacob, who by ingenious husbandry attempted to produce sheep that were "striped, speckled, and spotted" (Gen. 30:37-42). Only recently, however, have people really begun to understand genetic inheritance and to be able to exercise some control over it.

It was just over a hundred years ago that the Austrian monk Gregor Mendel formulated several hypotheses about inheritance based upon careful observations of the pea plants in his abbey garden. His hypotheses were the beginning of modern genetics. Today people take those hypotheses for granted as commonplace laws of inheritance and put them to work in many contexts—when they create hybrid corn or new strains of cattle, or when expectant parents talk eagerly about the likelihood that their child will have blue eyes or worriedly about the likelihood that the same child will have cystic fibrosis or sickle-cell anemia. It was just over three decades ago that James Watson and Francis Crick discovered the structure of deoxyribonucleic acid, or DNA, but in the last thirty years that discovery has triggered a veritable explosion in the scientific understanding of the molecules and the mechanisms of inheritance. With the rapidly developing new knowledge have come rapidly developing new powers. With the new powers have come new possibilities and new problems. In this chapter we will first briefly survey some of the new knowledge of genetics and then attend to the new powers such knowledge provides, attempting to think in a clear and Christian manner about some of the possibilities and some of the problems in human genetics and medicine. We will celebrate the possibilities these powers provide to nurture and sustain well-functioning, but we will also acknowledge the problems and the possibilities for harm in these powers.

Some Background in Genetics

In all living things, including human beings, physical traits are passed from parent to offspring through information encoded in molecules called DNA, deoxyribonucleic acid. The human body normally has forty-six molecules of DNA in each of its cells. Each molecule of DNA is "packaged" with protein into a *chromosome*. (These chromosomes are visible with the aid of a good light microscope.) Normally, then, human body cells *(somatic cells)* have forty-six chromosomes. The forty-six chromosomes are actually twenty-three pairs of chromosomes, one set of twenty-three chromosomes from an individual's father and the other set of twenty-three from an individual's mother. (The reproductive cells— the sperm and the egg, or *germ cells*—have only twenty-three chromosomes, unpaired.) Twenty-two of the pairs are called *autosomes;* the twenty-third pair is the *sex chromosomes* pair, containing a matched pair of "X" chromosomes in females (XX) but an unmatched pair of one "X" chromosome and one "Y" chromosome in males (XY).

Each chromosome, as we have said, contains one molecule of DNA. Each molecule of DNA consists of segments of encoded information called *alleles*. As the chromosomes are paired, so are the alleles. Each pair of alleles, one allele from the father and one from the mother, constitutes a *gene*. It is estimated that there are between 50,000 and 200,000 genes on the twenty-three pairs of chromosomes (McKusick, xvii-xviii). The genes determine traits of inheritance, from the number of fingers to height and intelligence. In each gene one allele is dominant and the other is recessive. Under certain known conditions (e.g., exposure to radiation or carcinogens) and often for no known reason at all, the encoded information may change. Such an alteration is known as a *mutation*.

Inherited traits are the result of the expression of the information in a pair of alleles, or a gene. A pair of identical alleles is an arrangement called *homozygous*; a pair of different alleles is an arrangement called *heterozygous*. The information encoded on an allele will always express itself in a physical trait if paired with an identical allele (in a homozygous arrangement). If two different alleles are paired (in a heterozygous arrangement), the information encoded on the *dominant* allele will express itself in a physical trait, but the information encoded on the *recessive* allele generally will be masked. The traits determined by homozygous genes and dominant alleles are sometimes normal traits and sometimes not. Sometimes, sadly, the traits can be a threat to human life or human well-functioning; sometimes information encoded in the genes can be expressed in impairments and disabilities and handicaps that are not inconsistent with human life or well-functioning but that are nonetheless burdensome to the individual affected and to those who care for that individual. (See the section entitled "Health and Persons with Disabilities" in Chapter Two.)

Estimates are that each person carries from five to twenty alleles for abnormal traits. Most of these, however, are not expressed, because they are recessive and combined with other alleles in a heterozygous arrangement. Alleles for abnormal traits may be passed from parent to offspring through the germ cells for many generations, and they may arise spontaneously through new mutations during the formation of germ cells. Since the recessive alleles for abnormal traits are expressed in an individual only when they are inherited from both parents, and since such recessive alleles are relatively rare, the probability of the expression of such alleles is quite low. The probability of the expression of rare recessive alleles increases markedly, of course, in incestuous relationships, a fact that has been observed from antiquity and that probably led to the ancient prohibition of incest.

There are three basic categories of genetic problems. The first category is made up of *cytogenetic conditions,* those conditions caused by an abnormal number of chromosomes. The second category is made up of *single-gene conditions,* those conditions controlled by a single gene. The third category encompasses *multifactorial conditions,* those conditions caused by the complex interaction of more than one gene and nongenetic (environmental) factors as well.

Cytogenetic Conditions

Abnormal cytogenetic conditions occur at conception whenever an individual receives too few or too many chromosomes. Most abnormal cytogenetic conditions are usually lethal in utero, resulting in spontaneous abortion (miscarriage). But some babies are born with such conditions, and these individuals will always carry their variation from the normal number of chromosomes and will express the overdose or underdose of genetic information in abnormal physical and/or mental traits. The severity of the abnormal traits will vary, depending on the particular chromosomes involved.

These conditions can be identified by a diagnostic test called a *karyotype,* in which the chromosomes of dividing cells are photographed, then arranged in pairs in an orderly fashion. A cytogenetic symbol system has been developed for recording karyotype findings. The first number indicates the total number of chromosomes in a somatic cell; combinations of X and Y indicate the particular sex chromosomes present; + and - designate an extra chromosome and a missing chromosome, respectively; and the last number identifies the particular number of the extra or missing chromosome. In cytogenetic shorthand, a normal male would be 46,XY; a normal female would be 46,XX.

Abnormal cytogenetic conditions in human individuals are frequently the result of one extra chromosome in every body cell, usually an extra one of the relatively small chromosomes such as chromosomes 13, 18, and 21. The single most common cytogenetic condition (approximately one in seven hundred births) is Down's syndrome, which is caused by an extra chromosome 21. A baby boy with this condition would be karyotyped 47,XY,+21. He most likely would be mildly to profoundly retarded, have a contented or happy disposition, and also might have congenital heart disease or an improperly formed digestive system. Edward's syndrome (an extra chromosome 18) is much rarer (one in eight thousand births) and much more of a threat to human life and well-functioning. A baby girl with this condition would be karyotyped 47,XX,+18; she most likely would be profoundly retarded both physically and mentally and would probably die in infancy. Patau's syndrome (an extra chromosome 13) is rarer still (one in twenty thousand births) and even more threatening. A baby boy with a karyotype of 47,XY,+13 most likely would have a particularly small head and would survive only briefly. All other trisomy conditions (an extra chromosome of any of the other autosomal chromosomes) usually lead to spontaneous abortions (miscarriages) of the affected embryo or fetus, though there are rare exceptions.

Abnormal cytogenetic conditions also frequently involve an extra chromosome or a missing chromosome in the sex chromosomes. For example, a person with Klinefelter's syndrome is a male with an extra female chromosome, karyotyped 47,XXY. The condition occurs approximately once in every one thousand births and usually leaves the man who has it mildly retarded and sterile. A person with Turner's syndrome is a female with a missing sex chromosome, karyotyped 45,XO. This condition occurs about once in every ten thousand births, and the female who has it is likely to be short of stature, sterile, and perhaps mildly retarded.

Sometimes more than one chromosome is involved in abnormal cytogenetic conditions. In fact, sometimes—although very rarely—there can be an extra set or extra sets of chromosomes, making a total of sixty-nine or ninety-two chromosomes in each body cell.[1] Fewer than one hundred such cases have been documented in medical literature; none of the children with such conditions survived beyond one year of life even when given intensive medical care (Blackburn et al., 252; Faix et al., 296).

Single-Gene Conditions

The category of single-gene conditions includes many diverse conditions ranging from very mild effects to very severe effects. The most recent systematic cataloging of single-gene conditions lists over 3,350 disorders.[2] Of these, approximately 1800 are inherited as autosomal dominants; 1300, as autosomal recessives; and 250, as sex-linked traits (McKusick, xi). Overall, approximately one of every one hundred births expresses some single-gene disorder (Wyngaarden, 118).

Obviously we cannot catalog all of these disorders here; some sampling must suffice. Among those inherited as autosomal dominant conditions are familial hypercholesterolemia (1 in 500 births), polycystic kidney disease (1 in 1,250 births), Huntington's disease (1 in 20,000 births), and Marfan syndrome (1 in 20,000 births).[3] Because autosomal dominant

---

1. It is called *aneuploidy* when the number of chromosomes deviates from the norm by just a few chromosomes, resulting in each somatic cell of the individual having 45, 47, or 48 chromosomes. It is called *polyploidy* when there is an increase in the entire set of chromosomes; *triploidy* is a polyploidy condition in which there are triplets of all 23 chromosomes, or 69 chromosomes total; *tetraploidy* is the polyploidy condition in which there are quadruplets of all 23 chromosomes, or 92 chromosomes total. Aneuploidy alone has been shown to account for some 50 to 60 percent of all spontaneous abortions, or miscarriages (Boue et al., 10).

2. Sometimes the affected gene may be a *regulatory gene*—that is, one which controls another gene, causing the controlled gene to be expressed at the wrong time or in the wrong amount, thereby producing abnormal effects. At other times the affected gene may be a *structural gene*—that is, one which produces a substance needed within the body, causing a defective gene product, which will have abnormal effects.

3. In *familial hypercholesterolemia*, an individual's body is unable to adequately regulate cholesterol levels and therefore has elevated serum cholesterol levels, frequently five to ten times greater than normal. This contributes to clogged arteries, which usually cause heart attacks, sometimes as early as childhood. *Polycystic kidney disease* is a group of conditions in which the kidneys develop many cellular masses known as cysts. Depending on the type of condition, the onset of symptoms may occur early or late, cysts may occur in other organs as well, and complications may include aortic, renal, or cerebral aneurysms. *Huntington's disease* (or Huntington's chorea) is a disease in which nerve cells degenerate, resulting in sporadic involuntary movements, gradual yet dramatic personality changes, and a slow deterioration of mental abilities, leading inevitably to a premature death; the average age of the onset of symptoms is the early forties—clearly after individuals have made most if not all of their reproductive choices. The "late" onset means carriers can pass the disease on to their children without realizing it. *Marfan syndrome* is a condition in which there is a disorder in fibrous connective tissue that results in dispropor-

conditions are caused by a dominant allele on a gene, people with these conditions have a 50 percent chance of passing on the dominant allele to their offspring; each of the children has a fifty-fifty chance of inheriting the dominant allele and, therefore, of having the same disease.

Among those diseases inherited through autosomal recessive alleles are sickle-cell anemia (1 in 625 births to American blacks), cystic fibrosis (1 in 2,000 births to Caucasians), Tay-Sachs disease (1 in 3,000 births to American Jews), cystinuria (1 in 7,000 births), phenylketonuria (PKU: 1 in 12,000 births), all types of mucopolysaccharidoses (1 in 25,000 births), all types of glycogen storage disease (1 in 50,000 births), galactosemia (1 in 57,000 births), and homocystinuria (1 in 200,000 births).[4] A

---

tionately long limbs, eye problems, and a weak cardiovascular system susceptible to heart-valve problems and artery aneurysms.

4. *Sickle-cell anemia* is a disease in which the beta-chain protein of the oxygencarrying component of red blood cells —hemoglobin—has a variation in just one of the 146 amino acids of which it consists. This seemingly minor variation in protein structure alters the oxygen-carrying capacity of the hemoglobin and decreases its solubility, causing the hemoglobin to precipitate, which distorts the red blood cells into sickle shape—hence the name. While sickling is a chronic problem for individuals with this disease, each person experiences acute episodes in which sickling is severe and life-threatening. *Cystic fibrosis* is the most prevalent genetic disease in Caucasians. The basic molecular problem of the disease has not yet been identified; it affects all exocrine glands and most other tissues and organs. Persons with cystic fibrosis have elevated salt concentrations in most secretions and a particularly thick mucous that lines the respiratory and digestive tracts. They usually experience severe pulmonary and digestive problems as a consequence, and their life expectancy is significantly reduced. *Tay-Sachs disease* is a disorder in which one enzyme is either defective or absent; this results in an accumulation of lipid, which becomes neurologically toxic. Several months after birth, a child with this disease ceases to develop mentally and gradually deteriorates to a premature death by age five. *Cystinuria* is a disorder in which the kidneys and intestines are unable to transport one or several amino acids appropriately. As a result, multiple cysts of these amino acids form, and these in turn may contribute to kidney impairment or even kidney failure. *Phenylketonuria* (PKU) is a condition in which one enzyme is either defective or absent, which results in an elevation of the amino acid phenylalanine in the blood. This, in turn, affects mental development. If untreated, infants with PKU will be persons who are moderately to severely retarded; if the condition is treated, mental development proceeds normally. Treatment consists of a diet low in phenylalanine from time of diagnosis shortly after birth until age seven, after which mental development seems unaffected by higher phenylalanine levels. A pregnant woman with PKU must resume a diet low in phenylalanine during gestation so the development of her child will be unaffected. *Mucopolysaccharidoses* are a group of disorders in which the concentration of specific biochemicals (mucopolysaccharides) builds up to toxic levels because of the absence of a functioning enzyme. Some disorders result in childhood death; others are less severe. All, however, are progressive in their severity. *Glycogen storage diseases* include a group of eight or more disorders in which the polysaccharide glycogen accumulates, usually affecting the skeleton, liver, heart, and/or muscles. Some of these disorders are severe enough to result in death in infancy; others are compatible with a long life. *Galactosemia* is a combination of several disorders in which the failure of an enzyme to function normally results in an inability to handle the milk sugar galactose. Untreated, galactosemia leads to cataracts, mental retardation, liver problems, and premature death; however, if the disease is

person must have two abnormal alleles to be affected by autosomal recessive conditions; thus, for offspring to be affected by a disease produced by these conditions, each parent must be at least a carrier. If both parents are carriers, there is a one-in-four chance that each child will be affected by the autosomal recessive condition (and a two-in-four chance each child will be a carrier).

Sex-linked conditions are determined by alleles on the X chromosome. Females have two X chromosomes and so are usually unaffected. Males, however, have only one X chromosome; every allele on the X chromosome, whether dominant or recessive, will be expressed in a male, since the allele has no matched allele on the Y chromosome. Accordingly, males are affected much more often by sex-linked conditions than females; for a male to be affected, it requires only that his mother be a carrier of one abnormal allele on her sex chromosomes. Examples of sex-linked conditions include two forms of red-green color blindness, glucose-6-phosphate dehydrogenase deficiency (1 in 20 births to U.S. blacks), Duchenne muscular dystrophy (1 in 7,000 births), two forms of hemophilia (1 in 10,000 births), and Lesch-Nyhan syndrome.[5]

---

treated with a galactose-free diet, all manifestations of it can be avoided. *Homocystinuria* is a disorder in which an enzyme facilitating amino-acid metabolism is absent or defective. This condition produces cloudy lenses of the eye and progressive mental retardation; some individuals respond to various treatments, whereas others do not.

5. The forms of *red-green color blindness* are highly variable in severity. Affected individuals experience difficulty distinguishing between the colors red and green. Some individuals perceive green as red (deuteranomaly); others perceive red as green (protanomaly). *Glucose-6-phosphate dehydrogenase deficiency* (G-6-PD) is a condition in which an enzyme is defective or absent. Persons with this condition usually have no symptoms unless they consume fava beans or are treated with the antimalarial drug primaquinone, in which case these persons suffer from mild to severe hemolytic anemia because of their inability to break down a toxic component found in the beans and the drug. *Duchenne muscular dystrophy* is a condition of as yet unknown molecular basis in which the person's muscles, including the heart muscle, gradually degenerate. This is a particularly severe form of muscular dystrophy that has been reported exclusively in males and inevitably leads to death by the late teens. *Hemophilia* includes two conditions in which a blood clotting enzyme is either defective or absent. Classical hemophilia, or hemophilia A, which affected the royal families of Europe, involves a specific clotting factor, Factor VIII; Christmas disease, or hemophilia B, is symptomatically similar to classical hemophilia but involves a different clotting factor, Factor IX. Both conditions involve an impairment of the blood's ability to clot internally as is normally required in bone joints and the intestines; treatment is expensive and involves infusions of the missing factor, which, until blood began to be screened for HIV antibodies in 1985, carried the risk of being contaminated with AIDS (4 percent of AIDS patients in the United States are persons with hemophilia). *Lesch-Nyhan syndrome* is a condition in which a deficient enzyme leads to an excessive accumulation of compounds that cause individuals so affected to manifest many neurological problems, including compulsive self-mutilation and mental retardation. Death inevitably occurs by the late twenties.

Multifactorial Conditions

Multifactorial conditions are caused by the complex interaction of more than one gene and of nongenetic (environmental) factors as well. Atherosclerosis and diabetes, for example, are multifactorial conditions. Spina bifida and cleft lip and cleft palate[6] are also suspected to be multifactorial conditions, although their genetic and environmental factors are less clearly understood than those of atherosclerosis and diabetes. Indeed, this whole category of conditions is not yet well understood. The complexity of several genes working together in response to environmental factors has so far largely frustrated attempts to understand these conditions.

Genetic Knowledge and Human Response

This summary of human genetics permits some general observations about human genetic conditions. The first general observation is that, although individual genetic conditions may be quite rare, taken together genetic conditions are quite common. We have seen, for example, that one of every hundred births expresses some single-gene disorder. Cytogenetic conditions are also quite common at birth, not to mention the fact that many (perhaps 50 percent) of all fertilized eggs have an abnormal number of chromosomes and therefore die, washed away in the menstrual flow before a woman ever knows she is pregnant (Boue et al., 1). When the frequency of multifactorial conditions is also taken into account, it is estimated that of the three million infants born in the United States each year, more than two hundred thousand have some faulty genetic condition (a ratio of one in fifteen). Some of those genetic conditions are not serious, but many are. It has also been estimated that genetic

6. *Atherosclerosis* is a disease more commonly known as "hardening of the arteries" and is recognized in the United States and Canada as a leading cause of death. In this disease, fatty deposits occur throughout arteries, threatening to block them off and rendering them brittle and susceptible to rupture (aneurysm). An occluded or ruptured brain artery will produce a stroke; an occluded heart artery will produce a heart attack. *Diabetes* usually refers to *diabetes mellitus*, in which the body is unable to regulate levels of the blood sugar glucose with the pancreatic hormone insulin. *Spina bifida* is a developmental neurological condition in which the base of the spinal cord fails to seal itself during fetal development. It can vary dramatically in its severity, from severely life-threatening to manageable with physical implications. *Cleft lip and cleft palate* are developmental conditions in which the septum between the lips and nose or mouth and nasal cavities fail to seal during fetal development. The two conditions can occur together or independently and are considered surgically correctable.

conditions account for 30 percent of the hospital admissions of children and 10 percent of the hospital admissions of adults (Clark and Gosnell, 120). Those who are seemingly unaffected by genetic conditions are still carriers of them; as we have observed, every person carries five to twenty deleterious recessive alleles, which may put their offspring at risk even if they themselves are unaffected; no one is genetically "pure."

Although the genetic conditions range widely in severity—from conditions that express themselves in extra fingers and toes (polydactyly) or color blindness, to conditions that are inconsistent with human well-functioning—the second observation is that many of the genetic conditions (and especially the cytogenetic conditions) result in significant morbidity and premature mortality. Except for Down's syndrome, most autosomal cytogenetic conditions are usually lethal in infancy or childhood (if the fetus survives gestation). Many single-gene conditions have relatively fixed and dismal prognoses. Children with Tay-Sachs disease, for example, have the prognosis of neurological and physical degeneration until they suffer their way to death, usually by age five. The stories told of children with many of these genetic conditions are very sad stories indeed.

Compassion and care have often been the response to the sad stories told of children with genetic conditions, and such compassion and care have often enlisted the aid of medical care, which has been successful in treating or managing some of these conditions. An infant with phenylketonuria (PKU), for example, can be placed on a special diet low in phenylalanine, and the serious mental retardation that would otherwise result can be avoided. A person with diabetes can be given insulin. A person with hereditary spherocytosis can have a splenectomy. Sometimes the only hope for managing a genetic condition requires medical care that borders on the extraordinary, as is the case when persons with familial hypercholesterolemia receive heart and liver transplants, or when persons with Wiskott-Aldrich syndrome or hereditary severe immune deficiencies receive bone-marrow transplants.[7] But — and this is the third general observation—medical care has not yet pro-

---

7. *Hereditary spherocytosis* is a condition in which a person's red blood cells are deformed, occurring as spheres rather than biconcave disks. The abnormal shape of these cells causes the spleen to attempt to remove them from the circulation, with the result that the spleen becomes engorged, tender, and susceptible to rupture. *Wiskott-Aldrich syndrome* is a condition in which there are inadequate levels of platelets (which are essential for proper blood coagulation) in the blood. Persons with this condition experience bleeding tendencies and are very susceptible to infections; the condition is almost invariably fatal within a few years. *Hereditary severe immune deficiencies* are a group of inherited conditions in which the immune system is impaired. David the "bubble boy" (see Box 9.2) is a specific, though very extreme, example of one of these disorders.

vided any cure for the genetic conditions themselves. Indeed, often there is not yet any way to manage or to treat the conditions, and the care that can be provided is palliative at best.

Given the frequency and the severity of these genetic conditions, it is little wonder that the new knowledge of genetics has been enlisted against these conditions and has provided new powers. It is those new powers that we now consider.

New Powers, Possibilities, and Problems in Human Genetics

Advances in genetic science have provided remarkable new powers: powers to diagnose certain genetic conditions in newborns, children, and adults; powers to diagnose certain genetic conditions even pre-natally; powers to diagnose the carriers of certain genetic diseases; powers to treat and even powers to intervene in the genetic endowment of our children, perhaps to cure certain genetic conditions and perhaps to "improve" on the genetic endowment, to design our children to our specifications. We will examine each of these powers in turn, ready to celebrate the new possibilities they provide to serve human well-func-tioning and human flourishing but ready as well to attend soberly to the problems they present.

Diagnosis of Newborns, Children, and Adults

The new knowledge of genetics has made possible the diagnosis of cer-tain genetic conditions in newborns, children, and adults—in many in-stances before the condition is manifested in its gross and health-threatening symptoms. An early diagnosis permits early therapy (if there is a therapy), and the earlier the therapy, the greater the possibility of alleviating or minimizing the effects of the genetic condition. The fa-miliar heel prick to test for phenylketonuria (PKU) in infants is a cele-brated example of such a genetic diagnosis. And it is properly cele-brated, because early diagnosis permits early therapy; the genetically based metabolic problem can be controlled by a special diet, and the brain damage that would otherwise surely result can be forestalled and thus prevented. Having a child with PKU is no longer a horror story, though it surely is a burden to prepare the special diet and make the child stick to it. Yet the burden can be borne in the confidence and hope that the child will flourish like any other bright youngster. The genetic test for PKU is now, of course, not simply an option that parents have in consultation with physicians; it is routinely done in the PKU screening programs mandated by law. We celebrate both the diagnostic test and the public policy for detecting PKU in newborns and for providing the possibility of their well-functioning.

Certainly there are features of the PKU genetic test that make it worthy of celebration. But the celebration of PKU screening has sometimes led to extravagant expectations of this power and to "a screening mentality."

Where PKU is concerned, the diagnostic test itself is inexpensive, safe, and accurate. The test distinguishes with great accuracy between those persons who will manifest the condition unless treated and those who will remain unaffected. But at present such diagnostic tests for other genetic conditions are rare; rather, there are sometimes false positives (people who erroneously test positive) and false negatives (people who erroneously test negative). One notorious example is the test for sickle-cell anemia that was used in the early 1970s in screening programs for blacks. The initial tests did not distinguish those who were carriers of the trait from those who were affected by it. As a result, there were many false positives, many who thought they were—and who were thought to be—diseased when they were simply carriers of a recessive allele for a serious genetic condition (and everyone carries some health-threatening recessive alleles).

Another point to consider is that the diagnostic test for PKU is directly related to an available effective therapy. In the absence of such effective therapy, the power to diagnose becomes considerably less advantageous. Diagnosis may indeed make for better genetic counseling, but genetic diagnosis without the possibility of managing or treating the disease risks stigmatizing the affected individuals rather than helping them and of increasing anxieties rather than alleviating them. Again, the rush to screen for sickle cell provides an example of how the dangers of stigmatization may be exacerbated by the presence of such a genetic test in a racist society. For a time in the 1970s, many blacks who were carriers had their insurance premiums raised and additional obstacles put in the way of employment (Childs, 104). About the same time, another clear example of stigmatization occurred when persons with the karyotype 47,XYY were presumed to be violent and antisocial because at one time a disproportionate number of people with this karyotype were found in penal institutions.

Indeed, a look at our language about people with genetic conditions suggests how facilely we stigmatize them. We too easily reduce such persons to their conditions, referring to the child with Down's syndrome as a "Down's child" or as a "mongoloid," or to a person with hemophilia as a "hemophiliac." It is too convenient to lump newborns with disabilities or handicaps into a single category and to call them all "defective neonates." But we must not forget that it is our children of whom we speak. We must not reduce individuals to their diseases. We must recognize not just a disease, a condition, a disability; we must recognize an individual, a person who has an identity and a name and not just a condition. To do so is a small gesture of care even if and when we are unable to cure. If we refuse to stigmatize people with genetic conditions, we may be better able to accept them; indeed, to recognize these persons as well as their conditions will make us reluctant to be content with acceptance only and ready to be advocates on their behalf, insisting that their birthright, too, is to grow and to flourish to the limits of their conditions.

Where there is a safe and accurate test for a condition and where that test is related to available and effective treatment, we celebrate this new power to diagnose newborns, children, and adults. Where such conditions are not met, we are more cautious than celebratory, and we are particularly concerned about the sort of mentality that would routinely screen for conditions for which there are neither accurate tests nor effective therapy. We are especially worried about the possibility that people who will eventually suffer from the onset and effects of a genetic disease will suffer the stigma of that disease even before the symptoms become apparent because others know that they are diseased and have a "genetic defect."

Prenatal Diagnosis

The power to diagnose certain genetic conditions has extended even into the womb. It is now possible to diagnose certain genetic diseases prenatally by means of amniocentesis and chorionic villi sampling. (See Box 9.1, p. 246, for an account of these and of ultrasound and fetoscopy, two other in utero diagnostic techniques.) All of the cytogenetic conditions and many of the single-gene conditions can be detected by these procedures. Some sex-linked diseases like Menkes' syndrome (approximately 1 in 40,000 births), a metabolic disorder that affects the absorption of copper and that is usually fatal before three years, cannot yet be diagnosed, but in utero testing can determine whether the fetus is a male (with a fifty-fifty chance of being affected) or a female (and, therefore, although perhaps a carrier, unaffected by the syndrome).

When power to diagnose in utero is celebrated, it is celebrated

Box 9.1   In Utero Diagnostic Techniques: Amniocentesis, Chorionic Villi Sampling, Ultrasound, and Fetoscopy

During pregnancy, the original fertilized egg grows and divides into the trillions of cells composing the newborn baby. Normally, all the somatic cells derived from the fertilized egg have the same genetic makeup. Approximately one week after conception, the growing mass of cells, called an embryo, implants in the uterine wall. Most of these cells will become the fetus and eventually the baby, but some will become protective membranes vital for the further development of the embryo into a fetus. Two such protective membranes are the *amnion* and the *chorion*.

The amnion is immediately adjacent to the developing human, encasing the fetus in the amniotic fluid. The amniotic fluid is mostly fluid, but it also contains some cells termed *fibroblasts*, which have been sloughed off from the developing human. In amniocentesis, a specially trained physician inserts a needle guided by ultrasound through the expectant mother's abdomen into the amniotic cavity and removes a small quantity of fluid with minimal risk to the mother and fetus. (There is approximately 1 percent risk of fetal mortality.) Amniocentesis is usually performed at fourteen to sixteen weeks of pregnancy, when the fetus is relatively small and the amount of amniotic fluid is relatively large. Because in any drawn sample there are too few fibroblasts present for immediate analysis, the fibroblasts must be further grown under laboratory conditions for several weeks before they can undergo DNA analysis or be analyzed for such things as chromosome number, sex of the fetus, and the presence of certain biochemical abnormalities. By this time the pregnancy is in the middle of the second trimester (F. Fuchs, 47; Chervenak et al., 305).

The chorion is a membrane just outside the amnion. Early in pregnancy, the chorion is intimately and prominently involved in forming a series of finger-like projections called villi, which form the placenta. At nine to eleven weeks of pregnancy, it is possible to insert a needle — either noninvasively through the vagina or invasively through the abdominal wall, the needle guided by ultrasound — to the site of these chorionic villi to remove a small sample. The cells so removed by this chorionic villi sampling technique are sufficiently plentiful to allow immediate analysis of chromosome number and fetal sex as well as biochemical analysis and DNA analysis. This technique, which is still undergoing clinical trials, appears to be only slightly more risky to the fetus than amniocentesis. It offers the distinct advantage of providing a diagnosis during the first trimester (Jackson, 39; Chervenak et al., 305), thereby providing more time for parents to adjust their expectations and consider their options, and permitting earlier intervention— possibly an abortion with considerably less risk for the mother.

Both of these techniques allow the prenatal diagnosis of all cytogenetic conditions and, at present, approximately forty single-gene conditions. Because of the expense and complexity of testing, a fetus is usually tested for only one or two conditions for which it has been judged to be at risk. A test which reveals that the fetus does not have a particular condition in no way guarantees that the child will be perfect.

While these two techniques provide for genetic observations of the embryo and fetus during development, ultrasound and fetoscopy actually provide a visual picture. Ultrasound is a noninvasive procedure whereby high-frequency sound waves are beamed through the expectant mother's abdomen. Through computer technology, the reflected sound waves are gathered, and a two-dimensional image of the fetus is constructed, based on the deflection pattern of the sound waves. Ultrasound is most frequently used to determine whether more than one fetus is present or what the gestational age of the fetus is. It is considered to entail no risk. A fetoscope is a slender steel tube with a glass lens; this instrument can be inserted through the abdominal wall to observe the fetus, take a skin biopsy, or sample blood. Both of these techniques can be used to look for major malformations, including hydrocephaly, spina bifida, and other neural-tube defects; ultrasound may also detect renal blockages, herniated diaphragms, and lung infections (Petres and Redwine, 768-69). Under rare circumstances, fetoscopy has been used surgically to correct some serious fetal defects. Fetoscopy carries the rather high risk of 11 to 16 percent fetal mortality (Filkins, 344).

Each of these techniques provides a means of "seeing" the developing fetus. Since amniocentesis, chorionic villi sampling, and fetoscopy involve some risk, these techniques are not recommended in standard medical practice unless a couple are known to be at risk for some undesired condition and are willing to consider abortion or are so emotionally concerned about the condition of the fetus that its further development would be jeopardized if the procedure was not performed. After such tests are performed, most parents receive the good news that their developing child is not affected, and the pregnancy is continued to term.

for the possibility it gives parents to make an informed decision about whether to carry a fetus to term, whether to seek special medical intervention, particularly at birth, or whether to abort. It is sometimes celebrated as the power to prevent birth defects. However, we are not ready to join the latter celebration.

We reiterate our concern about the accuracy of diagnostic tests and particularly about the difficulty of an accurate prognosis even for conditions where the diagnosis is certain. Down's syndrome, for example, can be diagnosed with certainty prenatally, but the prognosis ranges from mild to profound mental retardation. Our concern about the accuracy of prognosis, however, is not so strong as our intense concern about the relationship of diagnosis to therapy. When prenatal diagnosis is related to therapy, we are prepared to celebrate it, but we do not consider abortion to be therapy. When prenatal diagnosis helps to prepare parents for the demands of parenting a special child, we are prepared to celebrate it, but what we frequently see is a readiness not to be parents to a particular fetus with a particular diagnosis, and what we fear is a change in the disposition of parents—from the uncalculating nurturance which can evoke and sustain trust in children to a calculating nurturance which would abandon or abort the offspring that does not meet specifications (see Chapter Seven, pp. 184-91). If prenatal diagnosis were simply related to the prevention of birth defects, we would celebrate it with little reservation; but when this prevention of birth defects involves the prevention of the birth of the so-called defective and when it risks stigmatizing potential persons in terms of the birth defect they have, reducing them to their genetic condition, we cannot celebrate it without significant reservations.

We are not ready, then, simply to celebrate this new power, but neither are we prepared simply to condemn it. We are not prepared to celebrate abortion, with which prenatal diagnosis is so closely linked, but we are prepared to acknowledge some decisions to abort as tragic choices, choices where evils gather and cannot all be avoided and where goods conflict and cannot all be chosen. Indeed, it may be recalled from the previous chapter that, despite our general disposition to welcome nascent life, we would recommend abortions for some genetic conditions (Chapter Eight, pp. 226-28). If the fetus has a condition such as anencephaly or trisomy 18 that is seemingly inconsistent with the fetus's ever becoming a person or ever coming close to having God-imaging capacities, we would recommend an abortion. And if the fetus has a condition such as Tay-Sachs that can promise only an inevitably short life that is subjectively indistinguishable from torture, we would recommend an abortion. Such recommendations are, we think, morally legitimate even if they are not free from the moral ambiguity of tragedy, but they rely, of course, on accurate diagnosis. Thus, even if we are unprepared to celebrate without reservation this new power of prenatal diagnosis, we are prepared to acknowledge that it has a legitimate place in medicine and that it can be responsibly used.

One example of its responsible use may be seen in the voluntary screening programs for Tay-Sachs disease. Tay-Sachs, which occurs almost exclusively in Ashkenazi Jews, is inherited as an autosomal recessive condition; it is a terribly debilitating disease that strikes infants during the first year of life with progressive degeneration both neurologically and physically; it usually kills by age five. Diagnosis of affected fetuses can be made in utero by chorionic villi sampling at eight to ten weeks' gestation or by amniocentesis at fourteen to sixteen weeks' gestation. (Diagnosis at birth can be made by physical examinations and biochemical analysis; carrier parents can be identified by biochemical analysis of small blood samples.)

Before 1970 between fifty and one hundred children were born in the United States each year with Tay-Sachs disease. As a result of the widespread use of a voluntary genetic screening program in the ethnic community, in 1980 only thirteen children were born in the United States with Tay-Sachs disease. Such voluntary screening programs for Tay-Sachs are not limited to the United States. In 1981 voluntary screening programs in 102 centers around the world monitored 912 at-risk pregnancies, identified 202 fetuses with Tay-Sachs disease, and screened over 350,000 individuals, identifying 337 couples in which both husband and wife were carriers (President's Commission, *Screening,* 18-21). We are not prepared to call the abortions of fetuses with Tay-Sachs "good," but neither are we prepared to call a life subjectively comparable to torture "good." We recognize the tragedy of a choice among gathering evils, and we can recommend abortion only reluctantly and regretfully, but we do recommend abortion as a course of Christian faithfulness and fidelity in those rare and exceptional cases in which a genetic condition consigns an abbreviated life to such intense pain that life is subjectively comparable to torture, or consigns a brief life to such profound disability that the fetus will never develop God-imaging capacities, even minimally (further, see Bube, 160; Jones, "Abortion," 15; Jones, *Brave New People,* 176-81; Santurri, 129; D. Smith, "Abortion," 140).

It is an empirical question whether a particular genetic condition has such effects and whether there is indication for abortion. Some cases are fairly clear: Tay-Sachs disease does indicate abortion; Down's syndrome does not. Patau's syndrome does; cystic fibrosis does not. Some cases, however, are less clear and more morally ambiguous in our view. Take thalassemias, for example, and the voluntary screening program to diagnose these conditions. Thalassemias are genetic disorders in which the production of one of the polypeptide chains of hemoglobin, the blood protein that carries oxygen, is impaired. Thalassemias cause no mental retardation, but they do cause pain, disabilities, and death. Death frequently occurs prenatally or neonatally, but sometimes the afflicted live to the age of thirty. The pain is sometimes excruciating, but not always. These diseases always diminish physical capacities, but they are not necessarily profoundly disabling. No known therapy is any more than palliative. Even though these diseases can be profoundly disabling, the uncertainty of prognosis keeps us from recommending abortion. There are several kinds of thalassemias, and the empirical question needs to be asked about each type; perhaps the prognosis for some types is both so fixed and so dismal that abortion would be indicated.

Nevertheless, we cannot support or recommend the voluntary genetic screening programs for thalassemias like those introduced in Sardinia and Greece, where the frequency of thalassemias is quite high. Popular, intensive educational programs have been used in Sardinia to promote prenatal diagnostic testing and abortion to the point where 95 percent of the fetuses diagnosed as victims of thalassemias are aborted; the result has been that the incidence of thalassemias in live births has been reduced threefold, from 1 in 250 to 1 in 800. Claims are made that prior to the possibility of prenatal intervention, couples who were at risk had stopped reproducing (Williamson, 405). Now, as a result of the availability of prenatal intervention, such couples are again reproducing, and thus a large increase in the birth of normal children is reported. We are prepared to celebrate the birth of normal children, and we find plausible the suggestion that the power of prenatal diagnosis has led to the birth of many normal children to parents who would otherwise have chosen not to take the risk of having children, but children (fetuses) are not products to be exchanged for a better model or recalled when they do not meet specifications. We are prepared to recommend an abortion only in response to certain genetic indications such that loyalty to the child (fetus) itself sadly calls for it, and/or when the potentiality for personhood is absent.

But there are conditions in which loyalty to a child already born can tragically conflict with loyalty to an unborn child, conditions in which pregnancy itself—let alone the burden of caring for a child with a serious genetic condition—seriously compromises the capacity of a woman to fulfill covenantal obligations already assumed. A woman or a couple with a child with thalassemia, for example, or cystic fibrosis or Down's syndrome may find their capacity to carry the burden of caring for such a child genuinely threatened by another pregnancy and overwhelmed by the prospect of nurturing a second such child as well. Yet we are not ready to recommend an abortion in such a case. We recommend instead that the community share the burden of carrying and nurturing such children. The Christian community particularly — at least if it would be faithful to Jesus, who cared for the weak and helpless and those who did not count for very much according to conventional assessments—should share the burden of caring for persons with genetic conditions. If communities shared the burden, women and couples would have less reason to see their other covenanted loyalties compromised by pregnancy with and the birth of a genetically affected child. But when a community refuses or fails to share the burdens of care for such a child, then it strikes us as moral posturing for that community to condemn a decision to abort. Our point is not to recommend abortion in the absence of communal support; nevertheless, we would not condemn—and could cooperate with—a woman's tragic choice between conflicting loyalties when her resources of time and energy and compassion are limited and are neither sustained nor refreshed by the community in which she lives.

Of course, not every decision is a tragic decision. Some decisions to abort a fetus with a genetic condition are simply wrong. Even in tragic circumstances a careful weighing of the conflicting goods and gathering evils is required and may point the way toward a decision. A decision not to abort in tragic circumstances may be not only legitimate but heroic, involving a commitment to care that surpasses in selflessness and courage the more ordinary commitments of most of us; such a decision should be not only affirmed but celebrated. Such heroism may be society's best protection against the easy slide from "can" to "should"— that is, because we *can* diagnose prenatally and *can* abort, we *should* routinely do so. But in tragic circumstances a decision not to abort, though it may be legitimate, may also be rash, involving hopes and promises that surpass any human resources. Parents are not messiahs. Such rashness may be as dangerous to caring for the afflicted for whom there *is* hope as are the tools that make it possible to suppose we can eliminate "defects" by eliminating "the defective."

We celebrate without reservations not prenatal diagnosis but the coming reign of God. Faithfulness to God will not delight either in death or in suffering. Watchfulness will sustain care for the weak and helpless, including the little ones who do not measure up; but it will also nurture humility, the acknowledgment that we are not the Messiah, that we—and our children—are mortal and that our resources—even for our children—are limited. We do not celebrate the power of prenatal diagnosis, but it is our conviction that it can be used responsibly and watchfully.

Diagnosis of Carriers and Genetic Counseling

The new knowledge of genetics has provided the power to detect the presence of many genetic conditions in adults, children, newborns, and even fetuses; it has also provided the power to detect the carriers of many genetic conditions. Carriers are unaffected by the genetic condition they "carry," but they are at risk of passing on an allele for that genetic condition to their offspring. If two carriers of an autosomal recessive condition marry, for example, each of their children would have a one-in-four chance of being affected by that condition. The power to detect carriers is a remarkable one, and it is properly celebrated for the new possibilities it provides to prevent some serious genetic conditions and to avoid suffering.

The power is joined, of course, with other powers in genetic diagnosis and reproduction, providing an at-risk couple with some alternatives. The couple informed of the risks they must take with the health of their child if they choose to conceive one may instead choose to adopt, but they may also choose to conceive and then to utilize prenatal diagnosis of the fetus and perhaps to abort, and they may also now choose to circumvent their genetic risk by using donated germ cells (eggs and/or sperm). We have dealt with prenatal diagnosis already in this chapter and with technological reproduction in Chapter Seven, and we need not repeat our assessments of those new powers. The power to diagnose carriers, however, is not necessarily joined to abortion and to its moral onus; indeed, responsible decisions by carriers not to conceive could reduce the frequency of tragic decisions to abort on genetic grounds. Accordingly, the power to diagnose carriers may properly be celebrated.

Along with this new power has come a new specialist, the genetic counselor, although the new specialty is still in search of a professional identity. Currently, genetic counselors vary widely in training and qualifications and in the ways in which they understand their role. It is a remarkable new specialty, and it may properly be celebrated for the help it can give to couples in the anxiety of decisions about becoming parents. But this new power is not without its problems, and the new profession and the prospective parents who would use this power face some moral decisions that may be as important to the next generation as the new power itself.

One fundamental decision surely has to do with the professional formation of this new specialty, genetic counseling. Is it a value-free skill learned by special training and available for contract? Or is it part of the medical practice, profession, and calling we sketched in Chapter Four? It is our conviction that genetic counseling should be understood according to the model of medical covenant (p. 120; Weir, 90-95). The genetic counselor's loyalty, then, is not fundamentally to the human gene pool or to society but fundamentally to the vulnerable couple that seeks genetic counseling. And the relationship to that vulnerable couple is not simply contractual: the genetic counselor is not simply contracted to render technical services and to provide accurate scientific information and mathematically correct figures about risk. The relationship is professional and covenantal: the genetic counselor professes to care even when there is no cure and teaches not only genetics but also the good to which medicine is properly committed, the well-functioning of the sick and of those with impairments, disabilities, and handicaps. The medical professional is not relieved from covenantal duties of care and advocacy for the sick simply because he or she is a genetic counselor.

We think this view of the genetic counselor sheds light on some of the particular questions being faced by this new specialist. One of the debates among genetic counselors is whether counseling should be nondirective or directive, whether it should simply provide information and remain studiously neutral about questions of value or whether it should also give advice. A poll of genetic counselors revealed that a clear majority of them attempt to counsel in a nondirective manner. We doubt that genetic counseling *can be* value free; the tone of voice and body language of the counselor who is telling couples about a genetic condition subtly reveal evaluations. But the covenantal model also leads us to question the notion that genetics counseling *should be* value free. A contractual model may suppose that the clients have contracted only for accurate information and arithmetical assessment of risks, but a covenantal model would worry about the minimalism of such a supposition. We are not suggesting that genetic counselors have the right to impose their personal values on vulnerable couples, but we do think that the good which medicine professes can and should govern counselors' advice and that loyalty to vulnerable couples requires not just the thoughtfulness of scientific objectivity but also honesty and openness in the dialogue concerning the couples' value-laden decisions (Weir, 95, 109-11). A conversation in which there is candor about values—the values important to the genetic counselor as a medical professional, the values important to the couple who have been diagnosed as being at some genetic risk, and the values at stake in decisions about procreation—can serve autonomy and integrity rather than threaten them.

Another question being faced by this new specialty involves the limits of confidentiality. The requirement that genetic information about a couple or an individual be kept confidential is widely and properly acknowledged, but the limits of that confidentiality are a matter of considerable dispute. Confidentiality is an important moral rule because it protects the privacy and autonomy of individuals, because it nurtures and sustains trust in relationships, and because it is implicitly promised when a person gives or receives privileged access to the vulnerability of others. In general, it is properly the decision of the person whose truth it is, not the decision of the genetic counselor, whether or not to make that truth known to others. Of course, the genetic counselor may counsel the individual to tell others, and sometimes should — and quite "directively." Suppose, however, that an individual diagnosed to be a carrier of a serious genetic defect refuses to tell a future husband or wife or a brother or sister or a child about the condition. In cases where the risk of harm and the magnitude of the possible harm are great to others, we believe that the genetic counselor may and must break the confidence. (Indeed, the genetic counselor may break the confidence only if he or she must do so in order to protect someone from a high risk of serious harm.)

The new power to diagnose genetically poses questions of identity and duty not only for the new specialty it has created but also for the people who would utilize such power. Perhaps the first question is whether people should think it their *duty* to engage the service of a genetic counselor. The answer to that question is no. The "no" is loud and clear if the "duty" really masks a desire to be "procreatively risk free." No one is; there is no "genetically pure stock." The "no" is prophetic and adamant if the "duty" expresses a disposition to welcome only "perfect" children into covenant. When people acknowledge that God is the hope of the future and do not blasphemously claim that our children are, parents can be and will be less anxious about the genetic risks they take in having children and more ready to welcome a child "as given." Although we do not think people have a duty to seek genetic counseling, it is sometimes wise. Given finite resources of time and money and energy and compassion, when a family history gives good reason to suspect a serious risk of a serious disorder, it is wise to seek genetic counseling even if it is not, strictly speaking, a duty.

But when the decision has been made to see a genetic counselor, other problems of duty and identity quickly surface, as a single example demonstrates. A woman wisely went to a genetic counselor because her sister had given birth to a baby boy with hemophilia. She was told that hemophilia is a sex-linked genetic condition. She was also told that, since her sister was evidently a carrier, there was a fifty-fifty chance that she was also a carrier. If she was a carrier, any male child she bore would have a fifty-fifty chance of having the disease, and any female child she bore would have a fifty-fifty chance of being a carrier. She was then told that there is a test to determine if one is a carrier but that the test is not absolutely accurate. She also learned that there is no prenatal test for hemophilia. If she should become pregnant, however, a prenatal test could determine whether the fetus she was carrying was a boy—who would have a fifty-fifty chance of being affected. Finally, she learned that there is a range of severity in hemophilia, that many people with hemophilia do not have the most severe problems possible, and that even those who do can now be helped by quite effective (although very expensive) treatments. The woman then had to decide whether or not to be tested and whether or not to have children. We do not think this woman had a duty to be tested, but we would recommend testing in her case. And what if the (admittedly imperfect) test revealed that she was a carrier of the sex-linked condition for hemophilia? Then, although we do not think she had a duty, strictly speaking, to forego childbearing, we would have recommended that she do so unless she was prepared for the very worst and had the resources to deal with it, for we could not recommend abortion in her case (Childs, 113-14).

Christians may celebrate and use this new power to diagnose carriers whenever it can result in the avoidance of suffering without doing any harm. To be sure, a decision to forego childbearing is never an easy one. Moreover, sometimes the decision to forego childbearing is a cowardly refusal to take the risk of becoming parents without a guarantee of "the perfect child." But sometimes—when the probability of a genetic condition is high and where the magnitude of the harm caused by the genetic condition is great—the decision not to bear children is a heroic and selfless decision. There is no precise mathematical computation for such decisions and no neat formula to distinguish the cowardly from the heroic ones. In some cases the judgment is clear, but in more cases it is not. In the midst of such uncertainty, we may have to rely on character rather than on rules. It is good if the character on which we must rely has learned to celebrate something more and something other than the new powers of genetic diagnosis. It is good if the character on which we must rely has learned to celebrate the coming reign of God even though evil and suffering still assert their doomed power.

The Power to Treat (or Not)

In this chapter we have called attention more than once to our concern about the new powers of diagnosis when there is no meaningful relationship between diagnosis and therapy. Now it is time to call attention to the fact that the new genetic knowledge has provided some therapeutic powers as well as diagnostic ones and that it may yet provide the therapy to cure other genetic conditions.

So far, of course, none of the treatments cure or change the genetic condition itself. Some treatments do exist for single-gene and multifactorial conditions; these are quite remarkable and quite properly celebrated. The special diet for children with PKU enables those children not only to avoid profound mental retardation but even to flourish. Some other genetic metabolic disorders can be controlled by diet and the effects of the condition forestalled and limited. The success of insulin in the treatment of diabetes is well-known and properly celebrated. Surgical interventions can repair certain effects of genetic conditions, from removing extra fingers and toes to repairing the open back of a child with spina bifida. The power to intervene in the sad stories of many genetic conditions and sometimes to give them happy endings is remarkable, and we celebrate it.

Again, with treatment as with diagnosis, there are problems as well as wonderful new opportunities. The possibility of treatment means, in neonatal intensive care no less than in adult intensive care, the possibility of overtreatment. Some treatments can promise no genuine benefit to a child with a serious genetic condition and seem motivated by the mere presence of technological power, research interests, educational needs, and/or parental desperation. If treatment can promise no benefit to the child, it should not be offered. If therapy will do a child no good, it is pointless and cruel to risk adding to a child's suffering.

There are genetic conditions (for example, Patau's syndrome, Edward's syndrome, and Tay-Sachs disease) which can be accurately diagnosed and for which the prognosis of early death and profound suffering is quite fixed and certain. When a child's condition is terminal and treatment only adds to a child's suffering, then it should be withheld. There are cases in which to treat is to mistreat. Of course, parents and medical professionals always owe these little ones their care and their company, even if and especially if no treatment can cure them, even as and especially as parents and professionals "let them go." Sadly, some genetic conditions seem to put a child beyond the reach not only of our cures but also of our care. Even so, it is not neglect but care, not abandonment but company that must provide the context for decisions to withhold or withdraw treatment. The very preciousness and vulnerability of these children compel the decision to cease any intervention that has become only cruel. Of course, such decisions are tragic; the death of a child is never a "good," but it may sometimes be permitted to avoid the evils of a lingering dying and of a child's life being overwhelmed by the pain and suffering of a genetic condition and of treatment for that condition. Perhaps the saddest epitaph for a child is written as a result of overtreatment: "He died too late for grief" (Stinson and Stinson, 3).

But if overtreatment of individuals with genetic conditions is a possibility and a problem, so is undertreatment. A decision not to treat is not warranted simply because a child has a genetic condition that cannot be cured. Children with Down's syndrome, for example, do not have a terminal condition, and if such children suffer more than "normal" children, it is not because surgery pains them more but because "normal" people can be cruel and spiteful. Not to repair a heart defect or a digestive-tract defect of a newborn with Down's syndrome is wrong, not tragic. In general, treatment is indicated when the life that is prolonged will not be engaged merely in lingering dying, will not be overwhelmed by unalleviated pain, and will not be incapable of ever developing even minimal capacities for human relationships. Accordingly, treatment is initially indicated for a child with sickle-cell anemia or Duchenne's muscular dystrophy or cystic fibrosis. Of course, these diseases, too, may advance to a point at which treatment, though once clearly indicated, is clearly no longer indicated. Between those points there will be other points at which the indications to treat or not to treat are quite unclear.

The new possibilities of treatment, therefore, present not only problems of overtreatment and undertreatment but also the problem of irremediable ambiguities in treatment. Some new treatments, for example, are frankly experimental, promising benefit to some future child with a genetic condition but meanwhile having very doubtful or limited salutary effects for the child currently being treated. One thinks of cranial shunts for fetuses with hydrocephaly, of bone-marrow transplants for infants with Wiskott-Aldrich syndrome, of heart-liver transplants for children with familial hypercholesterolemia, of David "the bubble boy" (for his story, see Box 9.2, p. 258). Newborns cannot give informed consent to experimental procedures, and parents and physicians should not make medical heroes or heroines of children. Nevertheless, great risks may be taken where there is some little hope for a child's well-functioning. Still, those great risks may not be taken lightly, nor may the limits imposed by finite resources and the mortality even of children be ignored or denied. Sometimes the ambiguity of the situation is due to the uncertainty of prognosis. A child with Lesch-Nyhan syndrome, for example, is likely to be physically and mentally retarded and to engage in compulsive self-mutilating behavior. But while the syndrome always has some effect and cannot be cured, the severity of the effects can vary, and some children with milder forms of the syndrome are clearly not beyond the reach of human care or beyond the power of human control. To treat a newborn with Lesch-Nyhan syndrome may be to condemn a child to a life of self-inflicted torture; not to treat may be to condemn a child with a controllable condition to death. Such decisions, where prognosis is crucial but (so far) uncertain, are irremediably ambiguous.

Watchfulness in all these cases would nurture the disposition to care for little ones who are sick or weak or disabled. Such care would not deny the not-yet character of our existence or the simple fact that in this age our children cannot be spared death and suffering any more than the rest of us. Such watchfulness and care would prepare parents to let go instead of hanging on in desperation, but they would also be prepared to insist that doctors and others do what can be done to enable a child

---

Box 9.2   David the "Bubble Boy"[8]

On September 21, 1971, a baby boy was delivered by Cesarean section in a sterile operating room at St. Luke's Hospital in Houston, Texas. Named David, he was whisked away within minutes to a sterile plastic isolation bubble. David had an older sister and had had a brother, but his brother had died at five months from SCID, severe combined immune deficiency syndrome, an extremely rare condition (affecting 60 to 100 American newborns a year) that left his body incapable of defending him against viruses and bacteria. His brother had died a few days after a bone-marrow transplant had been attempted, using as donor his sister, who was histocompatible (their body tissues were sufficiently similar that it was reasonable to believe that an attempted transplant would not be rejected), but the transplant had come too late to protect him from previously acquired infections. Despite their experiences with their first son, the parents wanted another baby. Genetic counselors had informed them of their risks: a 25 percent chance of having an immunologically normal son, a 25 percent chance of having an immunologically normal daughter, a 25 percent chance of having an immunologically normal but carrier daughter (who would experience the same risks as her parents when she had children), and a 25 percent chance of having an affected son. They decided to take the chance, reasoning in part that, if they had another affected child, he might be histocompatible with his sister (a 25 percent chance) and be able to receive a bone-marrow transplant.

From his plastic isolator, David was tested. He was neither immunologically competent nor histocompatible with his sister. To remove him from his sterile environment was to sentence him to certain death from infections. The chances of finding a histocompatible bone-marrow donor were slim—approximately 1 in 32,000—but the parents and doctors chose to keep him in his polyethylene isolation chamber, and David became internationally known as "the bubble boy." Perhaps, they thought, a research breakthrough would eventually enable David to be freed from his sterile plastic womb, or a prospective donor might be located through tissue registries.

As ensuing weeks became months and years, David remained in his sterile environment, touched only through the plastic or with rubber gloves protruding into his plastic world. Toys, clothes, food, books — everything that entered his chamber—first had to be meticulously sterilized. When David became older, a plastic isolation chamber was constructed at his parents' home; later, NASA constructed a special space-suit that functioned as a mobile isolator, which enabled

---

8. The story of David's life and death, while highly publicized, has not been well documented. This account is based on the following references: "Baby David: Alive, Well and Waiting," "David's Debut into the World," "Monoclonal Antibodies Correct Severe Immune Deficiency," "Emerging from the Bubble," "Oldest SCID Survivor Dies," and "The Bubble Boy's Lost Battle."

David, for brief periods and with great restriction, to venture outside. Reports suggested that, despite his profoundly limited human contact, David was experiencing normal psychological development.

In 1981 the first bone-marrow transplant from a nonhistocompatible donor was made in a young girl with SCID after the donor cells had been treated with monoclonal antibodies developed through high technology (Reinherz et al., 6047). When this and several subsequent transplants were judged to be successful, David's parents and physicians decided to take the risk for David.

Bone-marrow cells were taken from David's sister, treated with monoclonal antibodies, then infused into David's bloodstream. When David became sick several months later, too soon for the transplanted cells to protect him or the success of the transplant to be determined, it became necessary to remove him from his sterile environment to adequately treat him. In a kind of second birth, he was delivered from his plastic womb to the real world. For the first time since his birth, he actually felt directly the hands and kisses of his parents. But a few days later infections overwhelmed his still-defenseless body, and on February 22, 1984, at twelve years of age, having spent all except the last fifteen days of his life in a plastic isolation world, David died.

David's case raises a host of ethical issues. Was the approximately $1 million spent on David well spent? Were David's parents given too much cause for optimism in their decision to have David in the first place? to raise him in isolation? to try the transplant? Did David's life have its own value and meaning, or was he a humanely treated "guinea pig" for the benefit of others (Lawrence, 74; Hamilton, 15)? Under what conditions should parents give informed consent for research or therapy treatments such as sibling bone-marrow transplants for their children?

to function and, within the limits of a child's condition and the world's fallenness, to flourish. Such watchfulness will not tell us exactly what to do in ambiguous situations, but the disposition of watchfulness is never more crucial than in situations where no rule can be formulated.

Such watchfulness will not be easy in a culture disposed to use technology simply because it is available, a culture ready to assess people in terms of their social worth, prepared to construe parenting as making perfect children and making children perfect, eager to construe medicine as skills for hire (to be contracted to do the bidding of the one who pays), a culture tending to identify "the good life" with unburdened individual self-fulfillment. A watchful people will resist these tendencies in our culture. Perhaps that resistance can be expressed in the words of a book or the phrases of a sermon, but it will be powerful only if watchful people nurture communities of care, communities in which the burdens of caring for children with genetic conditions are shared, communities in which the sometimes surprising joy of caring for those one cannot cure is celebrated, communities in which people are together advocates for the sick and weak before God in prayer and before the broader community in programs, policies, and practice.

The Power to Intervene: Power to Cure and to Design

All of the therapeutic powers mentioned so far leave the genetic condition of the child unchanged. The effects of the genetic condition are avoided or overcome in the best therapies, limited or controlled in the good ones, but the genetic condition itself remains. Now the explosive growth of genetic knowledge has provided an even more remarkable power, the power to manipulate the genetic material itself. This power may finally provide the possibility of a cure for some genetic conditions. It may provide as well the possibility to design the genetic characteristics of our offspring. It is a cause for great celebration—and a cause for great caution.

The attempt to control genetic inheritance is hardly new, as Jacob's attempts at animal husbandry in the Old Testament remind us. And the breeding of plants and animals has been quite remarkably successful. Farmers have selectively bred cows, pigs, and chickens based on their desirable traits (positive eugenics), and the new knowledge of genetics has enhanced this power. Researchers have produced new crop strains, some with special disease resistance, others more nutritious and more productive than the "natural" strains. They have also developed new strains of poultry that produce more eggs and new strains of cattle that produce more meat.

The possibility of selecting *for* desirable traits (positive eugenics) and selecting *against* undesirable traits (negative eugenics) also exists in the human species, of course. The attempts at positive eugenics made by Nazi Germany and American slave owners are well known and generally abhorred. The positive-eugenics proposal made by Nobel prize-winning geneticist H. L. Muller in 1961 was that the sperm of distinguished men should be frozen, placed in a special sperm bank, and donated to conscientious women who wanted to improve the genetic characteristics of the human race, but that proposal has not gotten a warm welcome from scientists, moralists (see Ramsey's lively critique, *Fabricated Man*, 22-59), or conscientious women. The negative-eugenics policy of requiring the sterilization of persons who are mentally retarded was once the law in some states, but such laws have generally been ignored or repealed. At present there seems to be no great public enthusiasm for eugenic programs applied to human beings.

Developments over the past few decades, however, especially recombinant DNA technology,[9] have opened up possibilities of greater and more specific genetic control in the foreseeable future. The greatest advances have been made with bacteria, yeast, and mammalian cell lines via the insertion of segments of genetic material from one species into another. In 1980 the U.S. Supreme Court judged that such life forms could be patented; among the patented bacteria are some that can ingest oil and others that produce bovine growth hormone (Sun, 150). The genetically engineered life forms have medical applications as well: among the patented life forms, for example, are a bacteria to produce human insulin and one to produce an analog of human growth hormone, yeast to produce human alpha interferon,[10] and a mammalian cell line to produce a hepatitis B protein. There are concerns about recombinant DNA technology, of course, but there is not space here to discuss the safety of the technology, the effect of releasing new life forms into the ecological system, or the wisdom of commercializing life forms. We recognize and celebrate the great benefit that bacteria-produced human insulin offers to diabetics who are allergic to bovine or porcine insulin. We are even prepared to celebrate the benefit that the bacteria-produced analog of human growth hormone offers to children whose genetic condition renders them hormone-deficient: previously they had to resign themselves to their size or seek the costly and risky human growth hormone isolated from cadavers.[11] It is not difficult to imagine, however, that parents of children of normal stature might seek this hormone in the hope of giving their children the advantages associated with height in our culture (Benjamin), perhaps even for a chance at a basketball scholarship. The celebration of possibilities for therapy needs to be joined with caution about the possibilities of designing our children.

Of course, it is not only on bacteria and yeast and isolated mam-

---

9. Recombinant DNA technology is the technical ability to isolate genes, synthesize genes, and move genes from one organism to another.

10. Interferon is a protein produced by human and animal cells in response to a viral infection which confers on cells of the same species resistance to infection by a wider range of viruses.

11. Until recently, human growth hormone was prepared from the pituitary glands of human cadavers. Over the last twenty years, some 10,000 persons have been treated for short stature, the average treatment lasting four years. In 1985 it was reported that three growth-hormone patients had died from a rare, slow-acting virus, suggesting that the supply of natural human growth hormone might have been contaminated. Accordingly, the Food and Drug Administration removed it from the market, thereby making the engineered hormone the only available treatment (U.S. FDA, 17).

malian cell lines that the new powers to manipulate genetic material have been used. Even as some scientists were re-engineering bacteria with genes from higher species, other scientists were seeking to transfer genes from one animal species to another. It was quickly realized that such transfers could be made into somatic cells (body cells)—in which case they would be passed on to daughter cells during normal cell division but would have no effect on the offspring of the recipient organism —or into germ cells (egg and sperm cells)—in which case they would be inherited by the conceptuses resulting from any fertilization in which these engineered germ cells participated. Although the transfer of genes into germ cells is technologically very difficult, the same effect can be achieved by placing the genes into an already fertilized egg; if the genes are incorporated into chromosomes of the fertilized egg, they are replicated as the fertilized egg becomes an embryo and a fetus and ultimately an organism that incorporates the transferred genes in both its somatic and its germ cells. To experiment, scientists microinjected first rat growth-hormone genes and later human growth-hormone genes into fertilized mouse eggs; the result was a high proportion of cases (70 percent) of oversized "supermice," which indicated the successful transfer and expression of growth-hormone genes from one species to another (Palmiter et al., "Dramatic Growth," 611; Palmiter et al., "Metallothionein," 809). Furthermore, that some though not all of the supermice passed the giantism trait on to their offspring indicated the successful incorporation of the genetic information into the germ line. Of course, there are problems and concerns with such powers, but, again, given the limits of this book, we cannot enter into that general discussion. But such powers, combined with human in-vitro fertilization, suddenly make genetic cures—and genetic design—seem technically feasible.

Indeed, it is now conceivable—even imminent—that clinical researchers may transfer normal genes into the somatic cells of an individual with a genetic condition in an effort to rectify the condition. "Genetic therapy" is now on the horizon. How shall we think of this new power and the possibilities it provides?

Imagine this. A child is born. His mother counts his fingers and toes, names him Adam, and announces, predictably, that he is the most beautiful child ever born. Hidden in his genes, however, is a defect that the doctor calls ADA deficiency. The mother does not understand all the doctor says about an enzyme called adenosine deaminase (ADA) or about the reasons it is crucial to the body's ability to fight infections, but she understands well enough that something sinister threatens to rob her child of promise and to condemn him to death before his second birthday.

If Adam were born last year, his mother would probably be

watching anxiously for the infection that would kill her son—and, if she were a praying woman, she would be praying for a miracle. If a child like Adam is born next year, however, his mother will be watching anxiously for the outcome of an experimental genetic therapy that may save her son—and praying for the doctors and scientists conducting the procedure.

Adam is an imaginary child, but ADA deficiency is real enough, and experimental genetic therapy may be attempted this year on a child, an "Adam," suffering from the condition. A special virus will be prepared. Using recombinant DNA technology, normal ADA genes will be spliced into a viral particle. Doctors will remove some bone-marrow cells from the baby and "infect" them with the specially prepared virus. The virus is supposed to be the delivery van, bringing the necessary ADA genes to the genetic structure of the child's bone-marrow cells. Then doctors will transfer the bone-marrow cells back to the baby and watch him carefully to check the ADA enzyme level, hoping that the ADA deficiency is corrected.

Perhaps it will work. Experiments on mice and monkeys suggest it may. Of course, the scientists will call it successful if any measurable level of ADA can be detected after gene transfer, whereas the parents will probably say the procedure worked only if Adam's immune system begins to function adequately. It is probably more likely to be a scientific success than a therapeutic one, but the parents of a child like Adam will surely pray for a therapeutic outcome. And Christians may join them, for the God in whom Christians delight and trust is a healer. Christians may pray in thanksgiving and petition that God's healing hand may touch children like Adam through these procedures. Christians may and should celebrate God's power to heal and welcome the new opportunities for healing that God provides. But Christians also may and should worry about the new path that genetic therapy blazes and about where it will lead. Christians need to think hard about how to use this new power God gives in ways that honor God and serve God's cause.

Such worry will be especially difficult and especially important in the midst of the public enthusiasm that will almost certainly accompany success in such experimentation. The enthusiasm will no doubt foster and promote extravagant expectations of the new technology and excessive confidence in it. Our imaginary Adam may be celebrated as a new beginning for humanity. The brokenness of the world may be understood as a genetic fault, and the new techniques as a genetic salvation. But Christians know and believe a different story, and they must be prepared to tell it and to live it in the midst of new genetic powers and possibilities.

In the context of the predictable public enthusiasm over success-ful genetic therapy, it will be crucial for the church to say soberly that "all flesh is grass," that all human genes direct people to their death, that human beings cannot create or sustain themselves, that they are depen-dent—in their strength as well as in their weakness—upon God.

Without such a reminder of dependence upon God and of re-sponsibility before God, people might celebrate the new powers and possibilities simply as a matter of human control rather than as therapy. Therapy, of course, requires control, but proper therapy also directs con-trol to the goods of life and health, to the goal of healing genetic disease. If people simply celebrate genetic control itself, human mastery even of *human* nature, we fear that they will lose the capacity to direct and limit this new power to therapeutic uses.

The gene therapy in Adam's case will be quite unique. It will be a first in human gene therapy, made feasible in large measure by the rela-tive simplicity of the gene involved. Scientists anticipate that gene ther-apy for most genetic diseases will entail four steps: (1) isolating and pro-ducing the normal counterpart of the defective gene, (2) getting the gene to the correct cells and having it remain there, (3) getting the gene to pro-duce its normal product in a properly regulated fashion, and (4) making sure the gene does no harm. In Adam's case, the normal gene has been isolated and produced, the virus vehicle has been designed, and the tar-get cells are exceptionally accessible, but the gene does not seem to be regulated—it is always "turned on." Yet, given the alternative of certain death, it is hard to imagine that the gene therapy may pose a greater harm unless it results in a prolonged dying with suffering. Most gene therapy for genetic diseases is anticipated to be much more complex than that for ADA deficiency, and most genetic control for designing humans to parental specifications is anticipated to be infinitely more complex. Things like intelligence and strength are not inherited through single genes but through multifactorial conditions, combinations of inherited genes and numerous environmental factors. Our ability to control and to design is limited by the complexity of many traits, so there are seem-ingly insurmountable technological and economic barriers that weaken the empirical slippery-slope argument that we are sliding into the genetic engineering of our children.

Still, we share some of the concerns of those who are worried about genetic design. There may be technological and economic barriers, but we should not rely on them to prevent what we ought not do. It may make little sense to worry about what we cannot do, but there are many things we can (already) do that we ought not do. Some designing is al-ready being done—for example, sex selection. But what is wrong with genetic design? In an earlier chapter we have attended to the way in which the designing of offspring corrupts the identity of parents and manipulates the identity of the offspring (Chapter Seven, p. 185). Here it is useful to borrow an argument from Alasdair MacIntyre (found in "Seven Traits"). Suppose, he says, that all the technological barriers have been overcome; suppose that we really can design human excellence by genetic intervention — indeed, that we can design traits of character. Which traits, he asks, should we select for our offspring? MacIntyre answers that question with a plausible list of traits. We should want our children to have the ability to live with uncertainty, with the unpredictability of the future. We should want our children to be able to be comfortable with a particular identity, a particular history and community, not to be "universal liberals," whose only appeal can be to impartial and impersonal standards. We should want our children to have the capacity for nonmanipulative relationships—that is, to be disposed *not* to make another merely an instrument of one's own preferences and desires. We should want our children to be disposed *not* to assume that knowledge is or ought to be power over nature. We should want our children to have the capacity to recognize and appreciate human finitude and mortality. We should want our children to have a disposition to hope in the face of the evil that tempts to despair. (This is not the Enlightenment's confidence in progress, which believes that it is only ignorance and irrationality that bar the way to human flourishing; it is rather the hope—sometimes against all calculation—that one's life and death will not be wasted.) We should want our children to have the readiness to endure conflict and suffering for the sake of goods that transcend happiness.

Having set forth the desirable traits, MacIntyre then draws a stunning but accurate conclusion. He says that, if we did so design our descendants, we would have contrived for ourselves descendants "whose virtues would be such that they would be quite unwilling in turn to design *their* descendants. We should in fact have brought our own project of designing descendants to an end." From MacIntyre's argument it must be clear that even if we *could*, we *should* never embark on such a project, for we would risk descendants who would be "ungrateful and aghast at the people—ourselves—who brought them into existence" ("Seven Traits," 7).

There may be technological and economic barriers on the slippery slope toward the designing of offspring, but the moral barriers may finally be more reliable and more stable. The technological barriers have consumed massive efforts by large teams of researchers over many years in attempts to learn how to effectively transfer a single, nonregulated gene. If this becomes technically feasible, it will require further efforts of Herculean proportion to extend these abilities to a regulated gene and even more efforts of logarithmic proportion to extend these abilities to multifactorial traits. Attempts to overcome the technological barriers will be accompanied by enormous costs—economic barriers. But technological and economic barriers are not insurmountable, and thus we ought not to rely upon them to regulate and control genetic powers if we have moral objections to their unrestrained use. Rather, we must work to articulate our moral reservations, because it will be the moral barriers that will be stable and reliable.

It remains crucial, then, that we celebrate not just the power of genetic intervention itself, not just the raw possibilities of human genetic control, but the therapeutic powers, the specific powers to intervene against genetic disease. Yet even if people celebrate not genetic control itself but genetic therapy, there is still some cause to worry, because the meaning of genetic therapy is dangerously slippery precisely because the definition of genetic disease is dangerously slippery. ADA deficiency is a disease, but is nearsightedness? Tay-Sachs is a disease, but is shortness? Our cause for worry lies in the fact that people may be inclined to call any slight departure from "normalcy" a disease and then attempt to justify genetic intervention for its remediation. Because "disease" and "health" involve evaluation as well as description, it will be crucial for the church to hear again God's word to Paul: "My grace is sufficient for you, for my power is made perfect *in weakness*" (2 Cor. 12:9; italics added). The faithful recognition that God's power does not despise weakness may keep people from calling "diseased" any who do not meet their standards or match their preferences.

God's cause, signaled in the healing miracles of Jesus and in the Resurrection, includes life and its flourishing in health. So Christians may join Adam's parents in praying that God's healing power may touch him before his death. But as Christians wait for God's final triumph, God's power is also revealed—decisively—in one who was despised and rejected, "smitten by God, and afflicted" (Isa. 53:4). At the final triumph (and Last Judgment), Christ will tell people that they met him in the sick and the weak, in "the least," as the world counts greatness. Then Christians may see even the "diseased" not just as victims of genetic accidents but as Christ's presence in the world. Then people may be called not only to heal and to help but also to care for those they cannot cure and to love those who do not meet their standards, whom they are too much tempted to call "diseased" in an anxious struggle to be free of them. If the Christian community tells and lives its story, it will counter the temptation to let the slogan "eliminate birth defects" slip into "eliminate what doesn't meet our standards and preferences" or slide still deeper into "eliminate the defective."

The celebration of genetic therapy must not blind people to the facts that the fundamental human problems are not genetic and that the fundamental remedies are not genetic manipulation. Delight in God's cause will incite Christians to try to change social values and social prejudices and to discern whether it is God's cause or a socially approved prejudice calling them to want to change the genetic structure of a child. They will express their confidence in God's power in their attempts to alter the dominant values of the culture even as those values encourage attempts to alter the genes of children.

The celebration of genetic therapy must not divert attention from the moral necessities of caring for those already afflicted with genetic and nongenetic diseases; or of protecting human beings from harm, including avoidable damage to human genes (through environmental pollution, for example); or of delivering the poor and weak from oppression, including perhaps those stigmatized as diseased or as "carriers."

Finally, the celebration of genetic therapy must not be allowed to nurture a disposition to bear and treat children as though they can be spared suffering and death. If we do, then we will finally transform procreation into laboratory reproduction and children into products. Of course, we will not and may not choose suffering or death for our children, but we may and must still care for children as a way of expressing our confidence in God rather than in human technology.

So we may pray that Adam will be healed and that we may have the wisdom and faith to direct the powers God gives toward God's cause. Such prayers will be the more urgent if we have the compassion to be concerned about Adam and the sense to worry a little about whether human beings are wise enough to control their own cleverness. Such prayers are fitting from those people of God who are aware of both the positive and the negative effects of the new technological powers of medicine discussed in this chapter.[12]

12. Parts of the last section of this chapter are reprinted from A. Verhey and H. Bouma's "Genetic Control: On Celebration and Caution."

10. Death and Covenantal Caring

Since the turn of the century, life expectancy in the United States has increased from 47.3 to 74.8 years. That is good news. A good portion of this gain can be attributed to nonmedical measures such as improved public sanitation. But much of it is also due to the increase in medical knowledge and to new medical measures such as antibiotics and inoculations, which made possible the highly cost-effective attack against infectious diseases that occurred during the middle of this century, the "golden age" of medicine (Fried, 30).

However, the fact of human mortality has not changed; we all die, and the advances of medicine and public health ensure only that we are more likely to die later of a degenerative disease than earlier of an infectious one. While we celebrate the good news about controlling the old infectious diseases, we must realize that similar advances will not be made against degenerative diseases. And when the highly technological tools of scientific medicine are aimed at degenerative diseases such as kidney and heart disease, the increase they bring about in the number of our days will not always be accompanied by health. Prolonged dying, helpless dependency on machines and unfamiliar people, chronic pain, social isolation, and the depletion of psychological, medical, and financial resources often accompany today's way of death. While we are glad that medical technology often gives a happy ending to sad stories, we must recognize that too often it provides an even sadder ending to already sad stories because of its capacity to intervene in a person's dying.

Society's current attitudes about the use of medical technology for extending human life are influenced by historical precedents and by sociological trends. In Chapter Five we noted that the Hippocratic tradition in the medical profession recognized that terminally ill patients were simply "overmastered by their diseases" and that the caring professional could do little but mitigate their suffering while allowing them to die. That the Hippocratic oath (Appendix D) forbade the giving of "a deadly drug" to such patients suggests it was reacting against an even earlier practice of actively and intentionally hastening their deaths. We also pointed out that, with the development of medical knowledge and technology and through the influence of Francis Bacon, the medical profession began to regard Hippocratic passivity in the face of death as the equivalent of neglect and inattention, and it began to resist death more aggressively—sometimes at any cost. The results were twofold: physicians were spectacularly successful in extending the life and the health of patients, and this encouraged the development of a "crusader" mentality, which tempts physicians to regard the patient's body as a battlefield on which all the weapons of modern medicine should be used to fight disease and extend life as long as possible. Add to these factors the evidence that physicians as a group may have a higher than average abhorrence of death,[1] and we begin to see why physicians often seem overly aggressive in their use of medical technology, even at times when it seems merely to prolong dying; we can also understand why many physicians view a patient's death as a personal failure.

But it would be highly inaccurate and unfair to suggest that this aggressive use of medicine is something that physicians foist upon a reluctant public. Although our lifestyles show us to be a death-defying society, we are also a death-denying society. Too many people believe that technology can rescue them from the effects of unhealthy practices such as smoking, overeating, and failure to exercise; too often patients and loved ones buy into popular notions of medical science and technology as the great cure-all; too many people begin to question their attitudes toward technology's role in sickness and in dying only after they discover that death cannot be denied, only delayed, and that during the delay health is sometimes denied. A consideration of some developments in the social connotations of the sick role and of the dying role will help to show what kinds of expectations sick persons and dying persons have—often because society expects them to have these expectations.

Dying Contrasted with *Being Sick*

Philippe Aries's account of changing Western attitudes and practices toward death and dying over the past thousand years chronicles how

---

1. This theme has been a recurrent one in the literature since D. Oken's 1961 study of medical attitudes led him to conclude that "among the motivations for entering medicine, the wish to conquer suffering and death stands high on the list. Practicing physicians are not the kind of persons who can sit quietly by while nature pursues its course" (p. 22).

the "art of dying" has moved from the circle of family and friends to the isolation of the hospital ward, and simultaneously from active personal participation in decisions concerning one's own dying to passive acquiescence to the decisions of others at the hospital.

In the United States one need look back only one or two generations to witness a shift in the social response to dying. Then, unlike today, a person's dying was openly acknowledged. In fact, dying persons— surrounded by family and friends, in the security of their own homes— occupied a privileged position from which they could orchestrate or at least actively participate in the events of their final days. Although vestiges of this way of dying may still be found in rural communities and urban hospices, it has all but disappeared with time.

What can account for this change in our way of dying? If Elisabeth Kübler-Ross is correct, our reluctance both to assign and to assume the role of dying may be traceable to a deeply embedded denial of death that seems to pervade American culture. Health fads aimed at arresting the aging process, grounded in our romantic view of youth, express a mentality and a value system that keep the cognitive knowledge of our own mortality from penetrating our psychic core. Some people even employ cosmetic surgery to disguise the signs of aging and impending death. Whether or not we actually deny death, the fact that most dying now takes place in the relative isolation of a hospital or a nursing facility rather than in the intimacy of the home allows many of us to avoid having to confront the dying of loved ones in a directly personal way. Blind faith in medical science has allowed us to delude ourselves into at least half-believing that sickness—especially our own—will never end in death, that withering and dying can be conquered. The optimistic strains in our culture have come to regard technological advances as the answer to our problems of disease and malfunctioning and have allowed us to lose sight of the importance of the involvement of an individual in his or her own dying. The diminution of religious faith can also account for our fear of death and our unwillingness to participate with others in their dying. Finally, the recent and rapidly growing body of literature on biomedical ethics has spotlighted those "cases" in which the dying are completely dependent. By focusing on the most extreme cases of debilitation, the literature ignores those physically afflicted persons who are alive in psychological, social, and spiritual ways that they were not before their terminal illnesses were diagnosed, persons who are therefore most capable of participating in their own end-care decisions.

While the role of dying was being attenuated, expectations surrounding the role of being sick were becoming more clearly defined and more consistently acknowledged in our culture and were sometimes even imposed upon dying people. "Sickness" has come to mean not only a state of physical or mental deterioration but also a distinctive set of behaviors determined by social expectations of how a person in such a situation should think and act. In his classic work on the sick role, sociologist Talcott Parsons identifies how society expects the sick to respond to their condition: they are expected to assume that they will escape their undesirable condition by getting well, they are expected to depend upon medical science to achieve a cure, and they are expected temporarily to suspend themselves from routine responsibilities while on medical treatment (p. 613). If Parsons is correct in assessing the role of being sick in America, the diagnosis "sick" becomes not only a convenient label but also an underlying set of social expectations about how sick persons are to respond and be responded to by others. However appropriate these expectations may be for those with curable conditions, they may also be quite inappropriate for those who are beyond the reach of medical cure and control, and they may even be harmful.

It is important to distinguish between the sick role, which is usually characterized by a dependence on cure-oriented decisions made by medical personnel, and the dying role, which may better be characterized by the patient's active participation in care-oriented decisions. The following comparison of the duties and rights associated with the "ideal" of each role may help in understanding how the patient's relationship with medical practitioners and with his own family can be impaired when the roles are reversed or simply confused.[2]

Sick Role	**Dying Role**
Responsibilities	
1. To desire to get well	1. To desire to live well until one dies
2. To cooperate with the physician in order to be able to resume former social roles	2. To cooperate with caretakers so as to function at as high a level as physically possible
Privileges	
1. To be cared for in a dependent state	1. To participate actively in one's own care

2. This characterization of the sick role is an abridgment of T. Parsons; that of the dying role is a modification of R. Noyes and J. Clancy.

2. To be exempt temporarily from regular social responsibilities to concentrate on getting well	2. To be exempt permanently from routine engagement in the social system so as to participate in significant spiritual, familial, financial, and related life-completion tasks

One manifestation of the confusion between the dying role and the sick role is that dying patients sometimes put subtle pressure on their physicians to treat them as if cure were possible. Their physicians, trained to cure diseases and socialized to view death as the ultimate defeat, are often eager to comply. Whether the physician, patient, or those closest to the patient are primarily responsible for confusing the sick role and the dying role,[3] this confusion can be reinforced by the way our medical-care system is structured—with largely negative results. In admitting chronically ill, dying patients to acute-care hospitals, we place them in an environment in which they must be cared for by those who are trained primarily to cure. One result is that terminally ill patients may not realize the seriousness of their conditions.

It is probably not in the best interest of those who are dying to be denied the truth of their condition. In fact, we believe that failure to disclose the truth about a patient's terminal condition deprives that person of an opportunity to participate in decisions affecting both himself or herself and others. While there remains much room for discussion about how best to tell the truth, truth-telling does require "troth." And troth involves being faithful to those who are dying, not just to the cold facts about their terminal condition. The failure to tell patients that they may be dying deprives them of the opportunity to participate in decisions about their dying and violates both their moral agency and their social nature. By encouraging patients with terminal

3. The previous section suggests that this may be a chicken-or-egg debate. W. May comes down rather hard on physicians for accepting the impossible role of acting as though what they do to and for the patient can always prevail over death. By adopting the military metaphor, he claims, they not only rationalize their cure-oriented activity but recreate the world to conform to that image (*Physician's Covenant*, 20). If doctors foster consistently lofty patient expectations, it is hardly surprising to May that doctors are blamed (and possibly sued) when health fails—as sooner or later it must. At the other extreme, R. Noyes and J. Clancy highlight the patient's role in initiating the problem: "Confronted, in an emotionally charged atmosphere, with a patient having high expectations and a family wishing 'everything to be done,' the doctor responds in an active manner. What we have begun to realize is that such treatment is often more appropriate to acutely ill persons and may unnecessarily prolong the suffering and disability of dying people" (p. 304).

diseases to cling to false hopes of cure, we prevent their personal involvement in life-completion tasks and possibly even contribute to the deterioration of their relationships with both kin and physicians at a time when trust, integrity, and open communication are the fundamental needs.

Particularly devastating are situations in which patients surmise their withering or dying but do not have the freedom to share their situation with those to whom they should be able to look for comfort and security. Even young children are perceptive enough to pick up clues of their terminal condition, and when their parents don't want to acknowledge it, they often feel compelled to play along with their parents in keeping the secret. Often the result of ignorance or mutual pretense is loneliness, isolation, feelings of abandonment, distrust, and a diminished opportunity to fulfill unfinished personal, social, and spiritual endeavors.[4] Although a host of variables—such as certainty of diagnosis, stage of the disease, and personality differences—defy giving a pat answer to precisely how the message should be delivered, it seems clear that truth-telling depends more upon manner, tone, and the quality of the relationship with the patient than it does upon the quantity or technical weight of the words used (May, *Physician's Covenant,* 141-44). In fact, nonverbal clues probably speak as loudly to the patient's condition as what is said.

The literature on the awareness of dying (e.g., Glaser and Strauss) points beyond the amount of knowledge possessed by each of the involved parties to how they jointly come to emotional terms with that knowledge. Psychologists have noted the emotional hazards that exist when feelings about one's own dying are not synchronized with the feelings of those to be left behind. For instance, the dying patient might express a willingness to die before the loved one is willing to give up hope for a dramatic recovery.[5]

The delicate complications involved in fostering an appropriate "dying role" suggest the wisdom of having institutions and personnel

4. Retrospective evidence from families whose children died from leukemia is instructive. Parents reported that even children below the age of five, despite parental attempts to shield them from the seriousness of their condition, gave evidence that they knew of their own impending death. Researchers go on to speculate that "the children who were perhaps the loneliest of all were those who were aware of their diagnosis but at the same time recognized that their parents did not wish them to know. As a result, there was little or no meaningful communication" (Binger et al., 319).

5. Beginning with R. Fulton and J. Fulton, a growing body of literature indicates that the anticipatory grief of survivors, like the preparatory grief of dying patients, has both adaptive and maladaptive possibilities for both survivors and patients. For a brief overview, see B. Backer et al., especially pp. 261-65.

trained in and devoted to the distinctive needs for care that the dying experience. This is one reason to support the hospice movement, a point that we will make at the end of this chapter.

Of course, being willing to distinguish between the sick and dying roles does not, in itself, lessen the clinical difficulties in diagnosing a patient's condition or determining a patient's prognosis. But the very real empirical uncertainties in deciding whether a patient is dying should not be confused with or magnified by an unwillingness to face or discuss the probability of that patient's death. Indeed, what we have said earlier about informed consent (Chapter Two) and uncertainty in medicine (Chapter Four) implies that both the uncertainty of prognosis and what to do in the face of it should be discussed openly with patients and their families. We now turn to some main considerations that are relevant to such discussions.

General Principles

A starting point for Christians thinking about life-and-death issues is acknowledgment of the biblical truth discussed in Chapter One—that life as God created and intended it is a gift that is good. God's intention for humanity is life and flourishing, not death and disease. The resurrection of Jesus is the guarantee that God's intention is not ultimately thwarted by the Fall. Its evil consequences, however, do persist in the not-yet character of earthly existence.

The good of human life cannot be reduced to biological existence. Although the latter is a fundamental value in that it is necessary for what makes human life good, it is not sufficient to make life good. As we discussed in the first three chapters, what makes human life fundamentally good is caring relationships—relationships with God, with other people, with creation, and with ourselves. When the possibility for these relationships is irreversibly lost or is overwhelmed by the very technology used to sustain biological life, then the latter no longer serves the good that God intends for human life. Although the promise signified in Christ's resurrection does not imply that death is no longer an enemy, it does imply that in some circumstances there can be enemies worse than the death that will inevitably come. Unlike death, these enemies — isolation, alienation, unbearable suffering, the extravagantly wasteful use of psychological, medical, and financial resources, and so forth—can still have a powerful sting.

As imagers of God, persons are cloaked in a sanctity which, as

Chapter Two argues, calls for a reverence that transcends social worth and yields a disposition that resists manipulating — even lovingly manipulating — the life and death of persons. The considerations we have outlined will help us to answer the question of when medical treatments should or should not be used to extend human life.

One popular strategy for sidestepping the question of how far medical treatments should go is to reduce the substantive question of *what* should be done to the procedural question of *who* should decide. In Chapter Three and elsewhere we have argued that patients are givers and hearers of reasons and are not simply responsible by themselves for decisions about themselves. They are in relationship with family members and medical professionals who are also givers as well as hearers of reasons and whose lives and identities are being shaped by their responses to both the needs of and conversations with their patients. The personal autonomy of a patient is important, but we cannot deny our relational and interdependent nature in exercising autonomy. Even if we grant that a patient should be the primary decision-maker about whether a life-extending technology is to be used or withheld, a patient is hardly well served if the dialogue about what is the *best* decision breaks down and the patient is told, "It is *your* decision."

When patients and those caring for them try to reach consensus on treatment decisions, a distinction is often made between ordinary and extraordinary means. Some have suggested that the use of traditional, medically customary, commonly available means is morally obligatory, whereas the use of out-of-the-ordinary, exotic, medically experimental, and innovative means is morally optional. If one could sort each type of treatment into one of these two categories, decision-making would be simplified, but the difficulty with this approach is obvious: it is arbitrary to base the morality of using a treatment on how long it has been available or on how often the need for it arises.

To avoid this difficulty while still making use of what seems a plausible and important distinction, many thinkers define *ordinary* and *extraordinary* (or heroic) in terms of treatments whose costs are proportionate or disproportionate to the good that they accomplish. Gerald Kelly defines them this way:

> Ordinary means of preserving life are all medicines, treatments, and operations, which offer a reasonable hope of benefit for the patient and which can be obtained and used without excessive expense, pain, and other inconveniences.
>
> Extra-ordinary means of preserving life are all those medicines, treatments, and operations which cannot be obtained without ex-

cessive expense, pain, or other inconvenience, or which, if used, would not offer a reasonable hope of benefit.[6]

Under this definition, there are two necessary conditions for a treatment's being ordinary: it must offer a reasonably probable benefit, and it must do so without excessive cost. Likewise, there are two sufficient conditions for a treatment's being considered extraordinary or heroic: if it is either excessively costly (even if beneficial) or offers no reasonably probable benefit (even if cheap and easy), it is extraordinary.

This definition of types of treatments would allow one to classify few if any treatments as always ordinary or always extraordinary. The classification would generally depend on a cost-benefit judgment that would be relative to the particularities of each different situation. Even for the same patient, a given treatment could be beneficial at one point and cease being beneficial at another. For example, giving penicillin to fight pneumonia would usually be ordinary treatment, but it could be extraordinary if given to a patient in great pain who will die soon even if pneumonia does not provide an earlier and easier death. In this case, the use of a respirator would also be extraordinary, but often respirators are an effective and comparatively inexpensive (and therefore ordinary) treatment for patients on the way to a cure.

Covenantal compassion and stewardship should make Christians sympathetic toward using such criteria as "excessive expense, pain, or other inconvenience" in determining whether a medicine or treatment should be used. But Christian discernment is required, because these criteria are subject to individual experience and interpretation, and because they are not immune to the cultural relativity of values and beliefs. Moreover, the criteria do not necessarily require Christian virtues or the marks of Christian discipleship, which should influence our decisions and which imply that there are benefits of expressing care that transcend a narrower cost-benefit calculus.

However, to admit that no definitive interpretation exists to establish beforehand what does and does not constitute excessive expense or pain or what does and does not contribute to human flourishing in each particular situation is not to be left directionless. We believe that the following guidelines for making decisions about whether and when medical treatments should be used are grounded on the biblical principles about life and death that we outlined in Chapter One and summarized at the beginning of this section.

6. This definition, taken from Kelly's *Medico-Moral Problems* (p. 129), is widely used. See, for example, P. Ramsey (*Patient*, 122) and T. Sullivan.

1. A Christian need not regard the mere prolongation of biological life as intrinsically beneficial.

Someone in an irreversible unconscious state is deprived not only of being in meaningful relationship with his or her own body and with other persons, but also of the opportunity of acknowledging a personal relationship with God—the very essence of what makes life good. Furthermore, the mere prolongation of physical life in such a case can be financially, emotionally, and physically costly to others.

2. A Christian need not strive to endure irremediable and intense suffering when it eclipses the good of relationships with God, self, and others.

Pain can be of such magnitude that it severs the integral and natural relationship patients have with their own bodies, the meaningful relationship they have with others, and their ability to acknowledge and pay attention to God's care. We do not wish to deny or to minimize the fact that God's grace is sufficient to convert physical suffering into a catalyst for and conduit through which such Christian virtues as patience, trust, and gratitude are expressed. In fact, suffering can be an experience through which discipleship can be demonstrated and God's faithfulness can be expressed, as the sufferer identifies with the one who became vulnerable to suffering to the point of dying on our behalf. Yet, while both Scripture and human experiences confirm that saints, through their physical suffering, can be powerful witnesses to the faith, it does not follow that acceptance of every kind of suffering is a prerequisite for faithful Christian living or dying. Furthermore, Scripture does not promise that suffering will increase faith. The ultimate hope and reality of the Resurrection are not that we may endure suffering well but that we may ultimately experience the abundant life, a life which we gain by passing through physical death. Physical death that ends intense and prolonged suffering, although an evil, is not the worst enemy. In fact, it can provide a transition to ultimate well-being. It is in these terms that we believe it is possible for the Christian to actually give testimony to his or her belief in eternal life by requesting that the dying process not be artificially prolonged.

3. Christians should not be devastated by the state of dependency that sometimes characterizes sickness and dying.

An underlying biblical truth which bears on how we choose to live and die is that we mutually depend on each other. Such interdependence is rarely acknowledged in a culture in which individualism and self-assertiveness are deeply entrenched values and in which dominating others and simply being "in charge" are highly prized.

Patients who are led to believe that their dignity is obliterated by the negative features of their physical affliction must be reminded that our dignity is irrevocably embedded in who we are: imagers of God—that is, special and unique creatures designed to represent God. Covenantal ethics allows no person to treat another or to be treated either as a totally self-determining agent or as a mere object. To be whole, every person—irrespective of role, social station, and physical circumstances—needs others. Not only do patients-as-persons need doctors-as-persons, but doctors-as-persons need patients-as-persons. Thus our human nature becomes for all of us an opportunity to cultivate our humanness by simultaneously serving and being served—in our sickness and in our health.

4. End-care decisions Christians make for themselves must not be grounded exclusively in how these decisions affect them personally.

The fact not only that life is a gift which is good but also that we are by nature socially interdependent disallows any claim that it is an individual's exclusive prerogative to define or dictate the terms under which life is no longer worthwhile. Furthermore, Christians mandated to implement the love ethic should not restrict their considerations of "inconvenience" just to themselves or their circle of loved ones and acquaintances. Rather, in the face of limited economic, social, and medical resources, we are called to consider the impact that our being treated has on others. These others include not only our immediate kin and community but our Third World neighbors as well. Thus inequitable distribution of medical and health resources both in our own country and abroad offends principles of justice and stewardship.

We believe that taking the preceding principles seriously will lead to a stronger emphasis on the role of dying than is commonly seen in the secular world. Although most of us will not welcome death when faced with it, or at most will welcome it reluctantly,[7] we believe that Christians may use their own dying as an exceptional opportunity to give their Christian identity and conviction definitive and final human form. Realizing that our creation in God's image makes us self-conscious choice-makers and recognizing that God's gift of life is good, Christians must seek to do God's will in the way they die as well as in the way they live.

If fear of physical death is not the Christian's overriding concern, it seems reasonable to expect the Christian community to take a lead in acknowledging the importance of the dying role. Consequently, we might

7. John McEllhenney goes further, acknowledging death as a gift of God when seen in the light of Christ's resurrection. He regards death in the face of prolonged dying as "a conquered enemy who is now to be greeted as a friend" (quoted by Wennberg, "Euthanasia," 287).

expect Christian patients to be active participants in decisions that affect the way they die. For instance, willingness to forego a medical treatment in order to be more alert while dying is a legitimate choice of a terminally ill Christian, even if it means that he or she will die a bit earlier than would otherwise be the case. Christian patients who are terminally ill may also be reluctant to insist on heroic means—treatments which would only prolong their dying—in the hope that by their refusing such treatments, others might be able to avail themselves of scarce medical resources.

Those struggling with a specific difficult case might be frustrated by the generality of the preceding principles. Even if one wholeheartedly accepts them, it is not clear what they imply for a given case with its almost infinite number of interrelated variables. We offer two observations in response to this frustration. First, principles serve as a compass; they help us negotiate difficult terrain. They also act like a light, illuminating what is under scrutiny. But they do not work like a mathematical formula or a categorical rule, specifying the exact action to fit each situation. Second, we believe that moral discernment is a communal task in which Christian patients, professionals, and other concerned individuals engage in dialogue, a dialogue that must include both mutual support and constructive criticism. This chapter is a part of that dialogue.

Questions of Competence

Suppose we agree that treatment decisions should result from covenantal dialogue among patients, medical professionals, family, and loved ones. At least two problems can arise. First, there can be disagreement. When disagreement reaches the stage of legal push and shove, the courts in both the United States and Canada tend to give the final say to the patient (sometimes within guidelines established by legislatures). As long as dialogue has been sincerely tried, we see no better alternative than allowing a competent patient to have the final word. But a second problem is that the competence (and therefore the autonomy) of the patient is often in question. As we noted toward the end of Chapter Two, illness is not something superimposed upon the otherwise normal person; it can affect one's cognitive and affective faculties in such a way that one cannot think clearly, and it often leads others to wonder whether what they are hearing from the patient is the authentic thinking of the person they know or whether the patient is still his or her "normal" self. Perhaps family members and medical professionals sometimes judge competence by whether or not the patient agrees with their own conclusions, but no such high-handedness is required to call into serious question the competence of many patients.

Competence is not always an all-or-nothing matter, of course. What follows is a classification scheme (adapted from Richard Momeyer) that distinguishes between different types or degrees of competence, yet claims neither completeness nor mutually exclusive categories.

- The Essentially Competent: Those whose ability to participate in decisions is and remains intact when they are confronted with a medically tragic condition. Certainly a large number of persons who are sick and dying fall into this category.
- The Partially Competent: Those with *diminished* ability or yet *undeveloped* ability to participate in decisions when confronted with a medically tragic condition. This would include many growing children who are in the developmental process of becoming fully competent, withering adults who may progressively develop senility, and some persons who are retarded.
- The Intermittently Competent: Those with *sporadic* ability to participate in decisions when confronted with a medically tragic condition. This would include some persons afflicted with psychic and mental disorders, some withering adults, and in a general sense all of us, since we are more capable of making rational decisions at some times than we are at others.
- The Potentially Competent: Those with *temporary* inability to participate in decisions when confronted with a medically tragic condition. This would include infants whose prognosis indicates they will mature to the age of discretion, as well as some persons whose impoverished social environment has impaired their ability to make independently responsible choices.
- The Never Competent: Those who *never have had nor ever will have* the ability to participate in decisions when confronted with a medically tragic condition. This would include human beings who are severely and profoundly retarded, human beings who are anacephalic, and the like.
- The Formerly Competent: Those who have *lost* the ability to participate in decisions when confronted with a medically tragic condition. This would include human beings with severe mental disorders as well as those who have entered into a state of permanent unconsciousness.

In many cases those who care for patients cannot escape the awesome responsibility of making decisions on their behalf. In some cases the surrogate decision-makers have no opportunity even to ask what the patient would request if he or she were competent. But in other cases, the values and even the explicit wishes of a formerly, partially, or intermittently competent patient can be an important influence in the decision. Sometimes the desires of the patient can be so clear and explicit that the surrogate decision-makers become, in effect, delegates for carrying out the priorly expressed decision of the patient.

How can one best provide for good decision-making when grave illness threatens? Many think that the living will is an excellent way to communicate one's values and desires with respect to one's dying so that even if one becomes incompetent, one's (previously stated) decisions play a significant role in treatment decisions.

The Living Will

A Critique and a Model

The living will seeks to state one's viewpoint regarding death and dying and to specify what one wants done or left undone when one's physical condition deteriorates beyond the cure, control, or even palliative care of medicine. Thus it is an attempt to give guidance and direction to both the medical community and one's own support community.

The increasing popularity of living wills must be seen in the context of a mechanized society in which medical technology has the potential of being a threat as well as a benefit for a growing number in an aging population. We here acknowledge the inherent dangers of technology not in order to diminish the accomplishments of medical science in either diagnosis or treatment but rather to warn against overtreatment in situations that are beyond medical control or cure. Such overtreatment is usually the result of a certain mind-set, sometimes referred to as "the technological imperative," meaning that if it *can* be done, it *should* be done, that if the techniques and equipment are available, they ought to be used. This threat is exacerbated in an urbanized society in which a personal relationship with one's primary-care physician has been eclipsed by impersonal relationships with specialists who are often strangers. A living will can prevent the introduction of high technology and its attendant specialists in the aggressive treatment of conditions for which, medically speaking, there is no hope.

We believe that living wills can also be useful in making the role of dying a more active role again, in contrast to the role of being sick, which (according to Talcott Parsons) is a more passive role. The living will recognizes that there is a form of autonomy that is morally justifiable, one that not only permits but even requires that we weigh alternative courses of action and that we deliberate on moral issues. If humans are created with the ability to be reflective choosers, they are, we believe, morally responsible for the choices they make—or fail to make—both in how they live and in how they die. Because we are responsible moral agents and because we are able to share meanings through symbols and thereby to think about future events, we are compelled to consider our stance on medically tragic events that may occur to us in the future—including those that may involve us after we are no longer competent to make moral choices. Deciding ahead of time what we think is right for our dying days will affect not only us but also others, for, created as we are in God's image, we are intrinsically social creatures.

We believe that the concept of the living will is consistent with Christian faith and practice, although particular versions or justifications of it may not be. Creating a living will can be viewed as an opportunity we have as God's image bearers to witness to others by making responsible plans for our dying as well as our living. (This responsibility might also include estate planning, funeral plans, personal wills, and so on.) Because it forms and informs the decisions made about medical treatment, a living will provides an opportunity to express such Christian principles as love, stewardship, and justice.

Such Christian principles stand in judgment of the spirit which appears to be the driving force behind the many model living wills now vying for attention. As might be expected in a pluralistic society, the declarations and directives in most ready-made, ready-to-endorse living wills represent a rather minimal set of "common values," which can be appealed to even by those inclined to confuse freedom with the license "to do one's own thing," based on a narcissistic definition of autonomy. Even the titles of some of these documents suggest underlying premises antithetical to Christianity. Many states (including California, the pioneer in living-will legislation) have passed "*Natural* Death Acts" (italics ours). While it is true that in our human condition there is something *natural* about death, we must be careful not to confuse the state of our existence after the Fall with God's creational intention for human life. Death as we know it—which is psychologically, socially, and physically wrenching—is not part of life as God created it; it is a part of our fallen human condition and not really *natural.* Other states have "Right to Die" acts, which by their titles might leave the impression that the *right* is ultimate and therefore must be honored, without any consideration of the morally weighty distinction between allowing a patient to die and actively killing that patient. The morality of the means of achieving the right is not suggested by the label. Still other states have adopted the "Death with Dignity" cliché,[8] which implies that death is preferable to any kind of losing face because one has become totally dependent, mentally disturbed, or physically uncomely. However, despite the unfortunate implications sometimes caught in the label "Death with Dignity," we do believe that there is dignity in making decisions (as moral agents) about our dying, if these decisions are made with Christian principles in mind.

Not only the titles but also the contents of many of the current models of living wills are incompatible with a Christian witness. We are not sympathetic, for example, with the following quotation from an early version of the living will by the Euthanasia Education Council: "I do not fear death as much as I fear the indignity of deterioration, dependence and hopeless pain." It appears to regard dependency as a basic evil rather than as a condition of relationship to God and each other that is intrinsic to our very created nature. A more flagrantly secular spirit of autonomy is embodied in Marya Mannes's *Last Rights,* once a best-seller in the United States, in which she demands that "measures be taken to end my life should I fall victim to . . . any accident or disease resulting in vision too impaired to see or read, or in total deafness. . . . And if [there is] a difference of opinion among you . . . I beg that one of you provide me with the means to take my own life" (pp. 149-50).

Having acknowledged that secular values permeate the readily available living wills, we have attempted to compose a sample document incorporating Christian principles, which is, we hope, free from secular underpinnings. Box 10.1 represents our attempt.[9]

---

8. We judge this to be a currently fashionable but inappropriate cliché for reasons best expressed in P. Ramsey's "The Indignity of 'Death with Dignity.'"

9. Although the document is markedly different in tone, content, and structure from most existing living wills, those familiar with existing models will recognize phrases and ideas taken from the following sources: the California Natural Death Act, Concern for Dying, Christian Affirmation of Life, the Christian Living Will, and Directions for My Care (in Bok, "Personal Directions"). It should also be noted that the living will used as an example in this chapter is personalized and therefore has some built-in hazards if regarded as a model simply to be signed by another. A true model document should have many additional clauses in it to fit particular situations of particular individuals and instructions for deletion of those parts that aren't pertinent. For instance, women of child-bearing age should consider a standard pregnancy clause such as the one contained in the California Natural Death Act: "If I have been diagnosed as pregnant and the diagnosis is known to my physician, this directive shall have no force or effect during the course of my pregnancy." Or one might wish to include a preference for home care over acute hospital care, such as the following variation of a provision in a recent Concern for Dying living will: "I would prefer to live out my last days at home or hospice rather than in an acute-care hospital if it does not jeopardize the chance of my recovery to meaningful and sentient life, if it is medically feasible in terms of palliative care, and if it does not impose an undue burden on my family." Beyond the issue of how complete to make one's living will is the necessity of keeping it viable and current, aligned with changes in self and society as these occur.

BOX 10.1

MY LIVING WILL

TO MY FAMILY, FRIENDS, PASTOR, AND PHYSICIAN

As a Christian, I believe not only that we are the Lord's both in living and in dying (Rom. 14:8) but also that, through the power of Christ's resurrection, death is swallowed up in victory (1 Cor. 15:54). Just as biological death is certain, so is the faithfulness of God in death as in life. As one who believes that Jesus Christ has overcome the ultimate state of death for his followers (alienation from God and from each other) by his participation in the physical event of death on the cross, I wish to be responsible in dying as well as in living, being comforted by the fact that death does not annul my life but translates it from history to eternity with God.

Having this assurance, I implore all those responsible for my care and knowledgeable of my condition to be totally honest with me in the event of my terminal condition, so that I may participate responsibly in decisions and preparations that surround my dying, especially as these have bearing on family and friends I leave behind.

If in any situation other than an emergency situation (where initial care or treatment is needed to stabilize and assess my condition) I am found to have an incurable injury or disease certified to be terminal by two physicians (where the application of life-sustaining procedures* would serve only to artificially prolong the moment of my death and where the attending physician determines that my death is imminent), I request that such procedures be withheld or withdrawn and that I be permitted to die. Furthermore, if two physicians certify that the indications are clear that I have lost entirely the ability to interact symbolically with others—as in an irreversibly insentient (e.g., advanced Alzheimer's disease) or irreversibly comatose state—and that I have no reasonable chance of regaining that ability, I do not wish my mere biological existence to be prolonged indefinitely by artificial means.

I am not asking that any affirmative action be taken to end my life. Death is, after all, an enemy that negates God's gift of human life. I believe that God's intention for human flourishing is reflected in the gift of life. However, when it is no

---

*By "life-sustaining procedures" I mean medical interventions that utilize mchanical or other artificial means to sustain or supplant a vital function. Specific measures of artificial life support that I refuse in the face of impending death or irreversible coma (unless their primary function is to make organ donation possible or to alleviate physical pain or distress) are these:

a. Electrical, chemical, or mechanical resuscitation of my heart when it has stopped beating

b. Nasogastric, orogastric, or parenteral feeding when I am paralyzed or unable to take nourishment by mouth

c. Mechanical respiration when I am no longer able to sustain my own breathing

longer possible for me to interact with God's creation and my fellow creatures, death can be a release, a transition to an eternal reward made possible by Christ's death. Therefore, I ask that my dying not be unreasonably prolonged when, in the face of impending death, advanced insentience, or irreversible coma, the maintenance of my physical existence becomes an unjustly heavy burden for my family and/or an unfair monopoly of medical resources. As a person created in the image of God (and thereby representing God), I ask that the expenditures of scarce human, financial, and medical resources be made with due consideration to the needs of other human beings, who are also made in the image of God. In this spirit I also freely donate for transplant any organs that may assist others in living a fruitful life. Life-support systems may be used in order to achieve any such transplants.

Following Christ, I do not necessarily regard physical or mental suffering as an indignity, and I gratefully acknowledge that Christ not only suffered and died for me but also participates in my suffering. On the other hand, I do not consider suffering an essential component of Christian dying. Acknowledging Christ's willingness to accept the vinegar, I regard relief from intense suffering as a meaningful ministry of mercy to me. Therefore, I ask that drugs be administered to me as needed to relieve terminal suffering, even though this may hasten the moment of my death.

Let my death be consonant with the dignity with which God has endowed me, and may the dignity of those who minister to me be enhanced by their active care and compassion for me in my dependent state.

This request is made voluntarily, thoughtfully, and prayerfully while I am of sound mind and in good health and spirits. I intend this document to be morally binding and carried out to the extent permitted by law. I request those who care for me to honor its intent, which is in part to relieve them of some of the responsibility of this decision. I take this responsibility in dedicating my life back to God who gave it.

In the event that I become incompetent or otherwise become incapacitated as a decision-maker, I hereby designate _____ _____ to serve as my agent in interpreting the intent and contents of this will. This person knows the values to which I am committed and will weigh my incompetence, suffering, and dying in the context of Christ's victory over death. Should it be impossible for this person to serve, I authorize _____ to substitute as my agent. If neither can serve, the line of authority shall proceed in the order of persons listed below the agents. I have discussed my desires concerning terminal care with them and trust their judgment on my behalf.

Signed: _____   Date: _____

Witness: _____

Witness: _____

I have discussed with each of the following persons not only the above provisions but also the reasons behind them. By their signatures they acknowledge their concurrence and support:

_____   _____

First Designated Agent   (Relationship to Patient)

_____   _____

Substitute Agent   (Relationship to Patient)

_____

Pastor

_____

Family Physician

Advantages and Possible Disadvantages of a Christian Living Will

A living will can serve the patient, the patient's family and friends, members of the medical profession, the community in general, and the Christian community in particular.

On a personal level, a living will permits people unencumbered by pain, depression, medication, or other debilitating accompaniments of serious illness to actively participate in making decisions about the treatment to be given them when they do become mortally ill.

A living will can benefit family and friends by preventing or relieving feelings of betrayal and guilt that can accompany the request for "no code" (no resuscitation) orders or the decision to refrain from using heroic measures when such restraint is morally justifiable. When the wishes of the no-longer-competent patient are either unknown or not clearly stated, the anxiety of loved ones can otherwise easily result in attempts to do everything possible to delay the moment of physical death (Bok, "Personal Directions," 367).

As far as care-givers are concerned, a living will can counter the pressures a medical-care delivery system places on medical staff to engage in death-prolonging procedures. It is not difficult to imagine how a coercive ethos can be fostered by governmental incentives or disincentives, insurance reimbursement policies, a hospital's policies, administrative convenience, professional and personal needs, and, not incidentally, threats of malpractice suits. For good and understandable reasons, technology is most concentrated in acute-care hospitals, precisely where it can intervene and bring back to well-being many whose lives hang in the balance. Unfortunately, technology can also merely prolong dying, and the health-care reimbursement system in the United States has probably fostered this regrettable practice by offering better insurance benefits to families of patients in acute-care hospitals than to families of patients in facilities that offer less-skilled care.[10] A living will can prevent care-givers in an acute-care institution from using acute-care techniques on a dying person.

The living will makes it less necessary for medical practitioners to speculate about patients' underlying values and what end care they would desire. It can temper medical practitioners' fear of legal action for not using the maximal therapeutic measures, obviate their having to make "no-code" decisions on an ad hoc basis, and eliminate the possibility of their having to assume the role of arbitrator, mediator, and advisor in those situations in which family members waver on the appropriate course of treatment or nontreatment to be taken.

The general community benefits from the living will in at least two ways. The entire community benefits when medical personnel in acute-care hospitals are free to do what they should do best—treating their treatable patients aggressively—rather than devoting their primary efforts to attending terminally ill patients. Eventually the general community can also benefit when its members are reminded about values higher than self-interest and different from merely prolonging life, values witnessed in the carrying out of a Christian's living will.

For the Christian community, of course, living wills become opportunities not only to acknowledge that life is a created and creative gift of God but also to recognize the reality of death, which shall come to us all. The good news for Christians is that through Christ's resurrection the separations caused by biological death have been overcome and ultimate well-being in relationship to him and to others is achieved.

The foregoing advantages of a living will are not meant to imply

10. In any case, such a policy has provided an incentive for families to keep dying patients in acute-care hospitals, where bills have been more fully covered than they might be if patients or their loved ones would have opted for chronic-care facilities. This situation has been complicated in turn by a new reimbursement system initiated by the government and aimed at controlling costs in the delivery of hospital services (see Fox and Lipton). By establishing a formula for hospital reimbursement based on a specified maximum length of stay for each ailment category (beyond which reimbursement stops), a different kind of incentive can arise—namely, for the hospital to "dump" patients before their allotted hospital time is expended, in which case the hospital realizes a profit from the insurers.

that such a will is a panacea that neatly packages all death-related problems and solves the knotty moral dilemmas that surround tragic cases. In fact, before anyone considers adopting any one of a number of existing living wills for personal use, he or she should pay attention to a number of issues and concerns that these wills generate. The possible disadvantages of living wills affect the same groups as do their advantages: the patient, the family and friends, medical professionals, the general community, and the Christian community.

One possible disadvantage for the patient with a living will is that he or she may receive less care than the patient with no living will because a hospital has decided, either formally or informally, to "dump" patients with living wills in favor of treating those who desire acute care.[11] This situation would be particularly tragic for those patients not fortunate enough to be able to avail themselves of the care-giving resources of hospice, home, or high-quality chronic-care facility.

A second possible disadvantage of a living will is that those asked to sign it as witnesses, agents, or professionals may not themselves agree on such weighty matters as treatment and nontreatment. While a strong case can be made that arriving at end-care treatment decisions in the company of one's support group is not only covenantally appropriate but also advantageous, it is possible that reaching consensus on such an emotionally charged issue may be difficult. The writer of the sample living will in Box 10.1, by simply assuming that there would be consensus among those asked to sign the document, made no provision for conflict resolution in the event that consensus could not be reached. Every writer of a living will should address that problem if there is any possibility of its damaging the will's effectiveness.

A third possible disadvantage, one that especially affects the medical community, is that, by relieving medical professionals of legal vulnerability for undertreating, a living will may subject them to the prospect of liability for overtreating, particularly in an era in which claims of patients' rights and patient autonomy are being pressed and validated in legislative and judicial quarters. And liability questions aside, a living will may tend to reduce the question of what *should* be done to the procedural question of exactly what the patient signed his or her name to, no more and no less, although at the time of signing the document he or she was

---

11. This concern is expressed as follows by the President's Commission: "A patient who chooses to forego aggressive therapy may have trouble finding emotional or material support. . . . Turning down aggressive care may leave no justification for acute-care-hospital level of reimbursement, prompting the hospital to press for discharge" (*Deciding*, 103).

not aware of the many variables that would be involved in the actual situation. Related to this difficulty is the inevitable difficulty of interpreting a living will at a time when the patient is no longer personally capable of assisting in getting behind the words to their intended meaning.[12]

It is conceivable, too, that living wills could have a negative impact on a community in general. For instance, the medical community may assume (sometimes erroneously) that those who have not made living wills want their biological existence prolonged to the last possible moment, irrespective of their terminal, comatose, or insentient state. This may mean a prolonged dying for those without the education, resources, or enthusiasm for writing a living will.

A weightier concern for the community in general is the possibility that the public mind may erroneously equate selectively *allowing to die* with carte blanche *permission to kill*. Vigilance is in order lest permitting the withholding of treatment out of respect for the values of one who wishes that his or her dying not be prolonged (a morally justified act) *appears* by analogy or extension to justify some other practice that is not morally justifiable.

Since law has a symbolic moral force in society, some believe it best not to press for formal support for living wills at this time. On the other hand, law can also provide restrictive barriers that may someday become necessary in the United States to protect vulnerable patients against overly aggressive medical interventions. For the Christian, any appeal to the law as ultimate smacks too much of reducing the issue to a procedural one of rights rather than showing regard for others with

12. The need for such interpretation follows from several related factors that inevitably characterize such a document. For one thing, words by their very nature are abstract, categorizing as they do entities that are not identical. For instance, the living will found in Box 10.1 uses the concept of "imminent death." Questions inevitably arise: How imminent? In whose estimation? Furthermore, the fact that a living will must anticipate events that have not yet occurred makes only limited specificity possible. In addition, medical prognosis is somewhat imprecise and uncertain regarding the individual case, not only because of the subjective element that enriches the medical art but also because it relies on science, which deals in probabilities. Looked at from the prospective patient's viewpoint, any attempt to anticipate future contingencies must also take into account personal and technological changes that may occur. But how can we envision the particularity of the future when we have seen how treatments formerly regarded as "heroic" are now viewed as routine and ordinary? A final confounding element is the fact that laypersons who write living wills lack the technical knowledge to make refined diagnostic or prognostic distinctions. This has prompted some physicians to draft very specific and technical instructions such as the following in their own living wills: "In the event of a cerebral accident other than a subarachnoid hemorrhage, I want no treatment of any kind until it is clear that I will be able to think effectively. . . . In the event of subarachnoid hemorrhage, use your own judgment in the acute state." This example is found in the context of a discussion on certainty and specificity of diagnosis (Veatch, "Choosing," 10).

whom we are in covenantal relationship. Law may better serve as a framework for dialogue than as a specific directive here. The living will in Box 10.1 looks for only minimal protection from the law; it is rooted primarily in a sense of community, requiring the concurrence and support of significant others. Since we believe that covenant relationships as expressed in a sense of community are the truly Christian orientation, we doubt the wisdom of making laws about an individual's attempt to anticipate a future disability if such laws would rigidly bind family or physicians to act as if they had no choices about a patient's end care. No statute should require families and physicians automatically to implement a person's previously made choice for allowing death without at least some regard for their own current personal misgivings and interpersonal distress. Periodic reaffirmation of the living will on the part of all signatories can possibly best accomplish the covenantal spirit in which such a will should exist.

The Christian community may be concerned over the fact that living wills, by focusing on what is not to be done, thereby neglect any consideration of the cultivation of Christian virtues in the face of suffering and imminent death. Living wills do not give much guidance to medical personnel on *how to care;* neither do they speak to the meaning of suffering nor how, in handling it, the Christian patient can witness to the reality of God's presence in the valley. But, then, that is not their purpose.

Allowing to Die and Killing

Whether one is deliberating about the contents of one's own living will or thinking through the awesome responsibility of participating in life-and-death decisions for a patient or family member, one cannot avoid the fact that medical technology has the potential to be either friend or foe—a friend when it relieves suffering or prolongs meaningful life, a foe when it artificially prolongs one's dying or alienates the dying from family, friends, and self.

Of course, the uncertainties inherent in fallible diagnosis and prognosis make it difficult in a given instance to say whether the technology used in a proposed therapeutic intervention would be friend or foe. Probability is all that finite imagers of God have to go on, although often the probability of a given prediction can be so high that it is beyond a reasonable doubt. And on life-and-death matters, as on all others, we believe God requires of his imagers not omniscience but cautious reasonableness.

Let us assume that we are confronted with a case in which it seems beyond reasonable doubt to the decision-makers that a given technology or therapeutic intervention is not a friend and is quite likely a foe. Perhaps it merely prolongs an unconscious dying or maybe even increases the suffering of conscious dying. In such a case, is withdrawing the treatment the moral equivalent of withholding it? And if both withholding and withdrawing a treatment can be justified, can one also justify intentionally killing the patient, since the very considerations that prompt withdrawing a medical treatment (such as stopping useless suffering) seem even more forthrightly served by intentionally hastening death? Which practices can we recommend, which ones can we tolerate or cooperate with, and which ones must we refuse to tolerate?

Allowing to Die by Withholding Medical Means

We believe that it is sometimes morally acceptable to allow those in tragic medical situations to die by deliberately withholding medical means. For example, if the medical means of treatment can reasonably aim at no more than prolonging the patient's physical life in the face of permanent unconsciousness, or if the terminally ill patient suffers from an anguished and lingering dying, we recommend withholding such treatment. We are speaking here of medical conditions in which the advanced stages of disease or the known results of severe injury are correctly seen as the primary cause of death. In such cases, in which death is not intended but merely foreseen as a side effect of withholding useless (and therefore extraordinary) treatment, it is appropriate to regard the cause of death to be not the omission of treatment, but the terminal disease. To use medical means aggressively in such circumstances, sometimes even against the patient's will, can make such intervention both artificial and cruel, a violation of the integrity of the patient's life narrative no matter how customary or traditional the medical means. This point is illustrated in the following case:

> A doctor aged sixty-eight was admitted to an overseas hospital after a barium meal had shown a large carcinoma of the stomach. . . . By the time the possibility of carcinoma was first considered, the disease was already far advanced. . . . The patient was told of the findings and fully understood their import. In spite of increasingly large doses of pethidine, and of morphine at night, he suffered constantly with severe abdominal pain. . . . On the tenth day after the gastrectomy, the patient collapsed with classic manifestations of massive pulmonary embolism.

Pulmonary embolectomy was successfully performed in the ward by a registrar. When the patient had recovered sufficiently he expressed his appreciation of the good intentions and skill of his young colleague. At the same time, he asked that if he had a further cardiovascular collapse no steps should be taken to prolong his life, for the pain of his cancer was now more than he would needlessly continue to endure. He himself wrote a note to this effect in his case records, and the staff of the hospital knew his feelings. His wish notwithstanding, when the patient collapsed again . . . he was revived by the hospital's emergency resuscitation team. His heart stopped on four further occasions during that night and each time was restarted artificially. (Beauchamp and Childress, 263-64)

We must admit that this is an extreme case and that it can be misused to elicit the sort of indignation that might attempt to justify withholding medical means in unlike cases where selfish motives, emotional overload, or morally questionable reasons intrude. But we hope there is agreement that the actions taken in the illustrative case ought not to be defended on Christian principles. The actions would more likely be defended by appeal to the false god of vitalism, which teaches that biological life is not just the necessary condition for what makes human life precious but is itself a priceless commodity that must be preserved at any cost. Or perhaps the actions might be defended because no one could be absolutely certain that death was imminent or because extraordinary measures and heroic suffering can serve as noble symbols of God's grace in the valley of death. In this chapter we have already given our reasons against such defenses. And we have given reasons to cooperate with stewardly requests not to use expensive medical means to prolong dying, especially when money devoted to life-extending technologies greatly exceeds that devoted to cost-effective community health and nutrition programs.

Our argument is not that withholding medical treatment is always permissible or tolerable. The Baby Doe cases remind us that sometimes treatment is withheld that is not excessively costly in terms of either suffering or economics and that could contribute not just to the biological life but also to the psychological flourishing of the patient. To withhold such ordinary treatment — treatment that would readily be given to other infants—because the infant has Down's syndrome, for example, is a conscious omission that intends the death of that infant—an infant, moreover, whose image-bearing capabilities were already developing.[13]

---

13. We do not mean to impugn the motives of all parents who withhold ordinary treatment from their infants. Their motives may derive from selfishness or from the

Such acts of omission are sometimes the result of the tendency to think of all cases of withholding treatment as "passive euthanasia" and to think of acts of commission as "active euthanasia." If one thinks that the former but not the latter is morally and legally permissible, one may be willing to omit actions on the grounds that the resultant harm is nature's course or God's will, whereas one would be unwilling to commit any action that would hasten death. Indeed, this viewpoint has been attributed—incorrectly, we think—to the American Medical Association and has been cited as the reason for allowing Down's syndrome infants to starve to death (for lack of a simple operation that would allow food to be digested) and also as the reason for prohibiting the merciful killing of these infants that have been condemned to die (Rachels).

We think the terms "active euthanasia" and "passive euthanasia" should be avoided because their use often leads to inappropriate decisions. Such thinking is flawed because it misconstrues the viewpoint we (and probably the American Medical Association) are arguing. We believe that intentionally causing death is generally wrong, and that one can intentionally cause death through commissions, such as giving a lethal drug, and through omissions, such as withholding care that is beneficial and is not excessively costly. At the same time, we believe that without intending death one may perform acts of either omission or commission that one can see will result in an earlier death. Many of one's actions—such as wearing out one's tires when one drives or disappointing Smith when one hires Jones instead of Smith (Sullivan)—have results that one can foresee but does not intend. In the medical context, when it is extraordinary treatment (namely, that which is useless or excessively costly) that one is withholding, one's intention can and should be to avoid inflicting useless or too costly treatment on a patient. One can foresee but not intend the earlier death as a side effect of the omission, a side effect one might try to avoid if one could do so without inflicting the extraordinary treatment. But it is hard to see how one could

---

"perfect baby" syndrome, but they may also derive from protectiveness or compassion. Yet good motives are not sufficient justification for actions. The highly publicized Baby Doe rules are intolerant of withholding treatment when doing so amounts to discrimination against infants who are handicapped. This intolerance we applaud. But sometimes the handicap itself is linked to medical conditions that seem to require extraordinary and even cruel medical intervention, as when an infant is born with a spina bifida condition that has severe complications. In such cases, withholding treatment is not necessarily discrimination against infants who are handicapped; it can be a recognition of the tragedy that medical intervention can do more harm than good to a dying infant. Society should be very careful about using the strong arm of the law to intervene in very complicated, value-laden medical decisions.

withhold ordinary treatment (namely, that which is beneficial and not too costly) without intending the foreseen death, a death one could easily prevent without causing harm (Sullivan). So we believe that in withholding extraordinary treatments one does not necessarily intend to hasten death even when one foresees and allows it, but that in withholding ordinary treatments one does intend to kill.

We do not claim that our position is without difficulties. Sometimes it is hard to separate what one intends from what one merely foresees.[14] And we have already noted that the ordinary/extraordinary distinction is based on a value-laden weighing of costs and benefits that is unique to each case and that can be influenced by extraneous considerations. But we do believe our position is defendable against the logical version of the slippery-slope argument which maintains that the justification for withholding some treatments also justifies withholding any and all treatments.

Allowing to Die by Withdrawing Medical Means

Since one can act by omission (conscious refraining) as well as by commission, we do not see any intrinsic moral difference between withholding or withdrawing medical treatment. The moral evaluation of either action depends instead on such things as intention and the impact of the treatment that is withheld or withdrawn, rather than on whether physical movement is involved in the action that permits an earlier death. Indeed, we believe physicians may sometimes give a pain-killing medicine even though they foresee that it will hasten death. The critical question would be whether the person giving the medicine intends to relieve a patient's suffering by killing the patient with a fatal dose. However, one need not *aim for* death even if the amount of medicine required to relieve suffering does hasten death; one would avoid hastening death if one could do so without permitting intolerable suffering. So, as far as its intrinsic moral standing is concerned, an overt

14. One common way to defend the distinction between what one intends and what one foresees is the "principle of double effect." This principle teaches that one may perform an action that one knows has both a good effect and an evil effect if and only if (1) the action in itself is good or at least morally indifferent, (2) the agent intends only the good effect while the evil effect is merely foreseen—allowed but not sought, (3) the evil effect is not a means to the good effect (both effects must follow from the same action), and (4) there is a proportionality or favorable balance between the good and evil effects. This principle is controversial, but, as our examples illustrate, something like it is presupposed in many of our actions. For discussions of this principle and related ideas, see R. McCormick and P. Ramsey's *Doing Evil to Achieve Good.*

action that is motivated by the sort of reasons we endorsed in the preceding section and that is aimed at removing extraordinary treatment or relieving intolerable suffering is the same as an omission that hastens death without intending it.

But there are some external differences between omissions and commissions that imply different morally relevant consequences. Withdrawing treatment is often a more open, visible, and dramatic act than withholding it, and this fact, besides having psychological consequences for medical personnel, allows a greater range of interpretations and misinterpretations by the patient, loved ones, the public, and the legal system. This fact perhaps argues for more caution about withdrawing treatment than about withholding it. A covenantal community must be concerned not to undermine mutual trust and not to desensitize people about actions that can symbolize abandonment or uncompassionate cost-benefit analysis. On the other hand, if medical personnel find it significantly harder (legally or psychologically) to withdraw treatments than to withhold them, they may become overly cautious and predisposed to withhold the very treatments that could save lives, fearing that once a treatment begins it cannot be withdrawn even when it turns out to be extraordinary treatment. Our considered judgment is that withholding and withdrawing treatment should not be viewed as significantly different either legally, morally, or psychologically, but we respect the view that the symbolic difference between them creates a moral difference. Some of those holding the latter view believe that the symbolic dimension of withdrawing *nourishment* raises an especially troublesome question.

Is Withdrawing Nourishment a Special Case?

While there appears to be a growing consensus that terminal and unconscious patients are not always best served by the continuation of all medical treatments and that withholding and withdrawing such treatments have moral similarities, the question of deliberately withdrawing nutrition and fluids remains unsettled and unsettling. Whether artificial means of nourishment and hydration should be classified as extraordinary treatment (and therefore should be optional in tragic cases of terminal disease or permanent unconsciousness) is still a matter in moral, legal, and philosophical ferment.[15]

15. For an overview and evaluation of some of the prominent reasons given for and against withholding and withdrawing such treatments, see J. Lynn and J. Childress's "Must Patients Always Be Given Food and Water?"

Those who do not condone the withdrawal of nourishment and hydration regard food and water as natural and universal needs shared by all humans and not as artificial or extraordinary treatment restricted to patients. For them, the act of sharing these essentials of life is also a socially rich symbolic act expressing community and interdependence, expressing life itself. Withdrawing nourishment, they argue, signals abandonment rather than care or concern for each other. Moreover, withdrawing nourishment inevitably results in death, which seems to put it in a different category from withdrawing a respirator, which (as in the Karen Quinlan case) can be compatible with the indefinite continuation of life. Some have claimed that the certainty that death will result from the withdrawal of nourishment and hydration implies that death is intended and not merely foreseen as a side effect. Sometimes the claim is also made that dehydration and starvation have not only distressing but also painful effects on the dying patient.[16] It has even been suggested that the option to withdraw nourishment can provide an agent with a publicly condoned means for unjust killing (e.g., as a cover-up for previous malpractice).

On the other hand, those who regard withdrawing such treatment as ethically justifiable are inclined to stress the invasive and, for the conscious patient, the painful nature of artificial means used to achieve nourishment (e.g., nasogastric "forced feeding"), its frequent failure to achieve either personal well-being or medically defined well-functioning, and its failure even as a gesture of caring when the pain and distress of the treatment are disproportionate to the possible benefits. It is true that food and water are universal needs, but so is oxygen. What is not universal is the technologically invasive way of providing these needs. It is the latter point that leads some thinkers to classify both artificial respiration and artificial nourishment as extraordinary treatment when they provide no personal or medical good. Furthermore, it is not clear that the certainty of death after the withdrawal of artificial nourishment implies that the death is intended and not merely foreseen. In some cases it seems certain that withdrawing artificial respiration will result in death, but that certainty in itself does not morally distinguish the action of withdrawing artificial respiration in those cases from withdrawing oxygen in cases where death is expected but less certain.

16. The evidence on actual effects of such discontinuation appears to be inconclusive. There is some reason to believe that the comatose do not experience hunger and thirst and that dehydration and lack of nourishment sometimes allow dying patients to be more comfortable and sometimes aggravate the conscious patient's discomfort. See R. Dresser and E. Boisaubin's "Ethics, Law, and Nutritional Support" and J. Zerwekh's "The Dehydration Question."

Moreover, many of our actions have inevitable deleterious side effects that we do not intend (e.g., polluting the air somewhat when we drive). So when artificial nourishment provides no detectable benefits but does cause various sorts of hardships, one can argue that withdrawing it signals covenantal concern, not abandonment.[17]

We conclude, then, that withdrawing artificial feeding should sometimes be permitted and even recommended. Our toleration for and cooperation with it, however, require the satisfaction of two important provisions: (1) safeguards must ensure that the welfare of the terminally ill or permanently unconscious patient is the primary consideration, and (2) appropriate means must be used to minimize the negative psychological side effects. For some, however, these provisions may seem infeasible. The possibilities for abuse and the powerful symbolic nature of withdrawing what is universally accepted as necessary to sustain physical life make us respect the stand of those who find it morally impermissible to cooperate in acts of withdrawing artificial means of providing nourishment.

Suicide and Mercy Killing

The vast majority of North Americans now survive a whole spectrum of infectious diseases and health hazards that in previous generations took their toll early in life. The hazards are now at the other end of the life span, where afflictions accompanying the degenerative diseases are a growing threat as the population ages. Those very health measures that have rather effectively prevented our early demise from infectious diseases have increased our statistical chances and those of our loved ones of becoming afflicted with medical conditions (such as Alzheimer's disease) in which human flourishing is progressively diminished as physical and mental debilitation increase. As the population continues to age, such conditions can be expected to become more prevalent despite the application of medical means (and sometimes with their "assistance"). Often patients' self-consciousness about their own desperate condition is a part of the burdensome tragedy they experience, as they envision a bleak future both for themselves and for those they love. Does such a condition ever justify intervening in one's own or another's death trajectory?

Consider the following case. A sixty-one-year-old husband and

17. An evaluation of recent legal decisions on these matters is found in J. Paris and F. Reardon, and in the study entitled *Life-Sustaining Technologies and the Elderly* by the Office of Technology Assessment.

father of four married children is diagnosed as having two severe diseases, each having a predictably consistent downward trajectory. One is causing progressive deterioration of his mind/brain, already causing some dizziness, memory loss, inability to speak clearly, and sporadic, unpredictable, and bizarre behavior. There are already signs that his behavior will become robotized or at best trainable only by means of conditioning, signals causing a general foreboding as he faces both his and his family's future. The other disease is a terminal physical condition involving progressive physical dysfunction and some pain, which has been medically diagnosed and confirmed but has not yet debilitated him physically. In his lucid moments he grasps the gravity of his condition and understands the prognosis—basically an irreversible death trajectory with predictably increasing pain and dysfunction until he will likely choke to death. He is still aware not only of the love and affection bestowed on him by close kin and fellow church members but also of the trying circumstances in which his condition places those who love him.

This case illustrates that sometimes even if patients resolve to avoid any extraordinary medical care, they may still face a long, painful, and debilitating dying that may be psychologically and financially very costly to them and those who care for them. No wonder there are highly publicized cases (and probably many more unpublicized ones) of people taking their own lives or the lives of spouses and loved ones when they are withering and dying in such conditions. We respect some of the motives and reasoning that lead to such suicides and mercy killings, but the following considerations lead us to urge a disposition of uncooperation with and intolerance toward them.

The first consideration against mercy killing appeals to our earlier point (p. 31) that the love which persons show to one another must be conditioned by the awe appropriate toward imagers of God. Persons are clothed in a sanctity that limits even the ways in which they may be merciful to each other. When we approach imagers of God, we approach "holy ground," and we express our reverence by what we refuse to do as much as by what we are willing to do. Benevolent deception, manipulation, or killing of God's creatures that are not persons is sometimes appropriate and even required, but such acts are neither appropriate nor required in the case of those creatures created in God's own image, who have a calling from God that only God can decide is fulfilled. (The exception accepted by most Christians is deception, manipulation, or killing of aggressors in the defense of other innocent human life.) Both the refusal to inflict extraordinary treatment and the refusal to kill are expressions of reverence toward God's imagers. And both the willingness to inflict extraordinary treatment and the willingness to kill betray an overly manipulative attitude toward them. Therefore, we think that those who would extend human life by any means and those who would intentionally end it display an inappropriate attitude toward God's gift of graciously creating God's own imagers.

This is a hard doctrine, and it is important to see why some Christians may disagree with it. We already agreed that one may act in a way that intends to relieve suffering while foreseeing but not intending that death will be hastened. We think that, for persons in covenantal relationships, intentions are very important and that different intentions can give actions different moral significance even when the foreseen results are the same. Obviously, those who restrict the moral significance of actions to their consequences—such as utilitarians—would disagree. Moreover, even if we maintain the distinction between what one foresees and what one intends, it is often difficult to separate them, especially in cases of terminal illness. When a murderer shoots someone, not only is the motive evil; there is also no foreseeing of imminent death apart from a knowledge of the murderer's intention. In the mercy killing of one terminally ill, however, not only is the motive benevolent, but the imminent death is already foreseen apart from the merciful intention to hasten it. It might be argued that in such a case one is merely cooperating in an exceptionally active way with God's will or nature's course. Surely, one might claim, God would not blame us for killing a friend who is burning to death while trapped in a wrecked car, and, one might argue, mercy killing to eliminate the intolerable suffering of someone terminally ill is in the same moral category.

We respect this position, but we disagree with it. First, most cases of terminal illness are not analogous to burning to death, either in terms of suffering or in terms of the imminence of death. And we have already argued that one may give whatever treatment is required to relieve intolerable suffering—short of intending to kill the sufferer—while foreseeing but not intending that death will be hastened. Moreover, people are all mortal, and we fear that justifying the benevolent killing of those who are dying can too easily justify the benevolent killing of other mortals, even those who are not yet dying. The dying are still living, after all; they are distinguished from the rest of us by having contracted the condition that will likely kill them in the indefinite future. But it is not clear that this distinction will prevent the logical slippery slope we fear, the slope that begins with the justification of mercy killing for those terminally ill (in order to prevent needless suffering) and ends with the justification of mercy killing for those not terminally ill.

Another consideration we urge against mercy killing appeals

to the empirical form of the slippery-slope argument. (The two forms of this argument are explained on pp. 75-77.) The differing gravity of various situations leads us to wonder if all acts of mercy killing are equally condemnable. Certainly the quality of mercy is more apparent in some acts of killing than in others. In fact, those that are done in the most tragic of circumstances, where an individual's deteriorating condition while dying is indistinguishable from torture, might elicit a measure of empathy in us as fellow human beings. Who cannot empathize, for instance, with Roswell Gilbert, whose love for his wife of fifty years apparently prompted him to end her suffering by ending her life as she lay dying from Alzheimer's disease compounded by advanced osteoporosis. Nevertheless, we believe society should remain intolerant of the practice of mercy killing because we fear the moral erosion that tolerance of it could cause.

Our fear of slippery-slope momentum is based upon the fear that practices which cause or allow physical life to be shortened may eventually have negative side effects upon our delicate social fabric, which still affords at least minimal protection to the lives of even the most vulnerable.

That worry, of course, is not necessarily limited to mercy killing but can be applied as well to a decision permitting someone to die, even if that decision is consistent with the patient's wishes and our guidelines. Such permission, it is argued, can contribute to the eventual erosion of community because it is a precedent, no matter how small or how seemingly innocuous. From it could evolve a mind-set that ultimately would allow those in positions of social power to actively eliminate the powerless, those defined as being a burden to the rest of us. The ultimate spectre is that power wielders — being tacitly encouraged or at least not restrained—may kill those whom they deem unworthy, be they aged, retarded, deformed, or otherwise lacking in the attributes a secular society uses as its current standard. We must also be soberly reflective about the possibility that a permissive attitude may eventually make us individually and collectively incapable of shuddering when innocent and viable life is not adequately protected.

Does consistency then compel us to be as intolerant of allowing death as we are of mercy killing? Certainly the impulses of those who resist allowing death for fear of slippery-slope consequences are compatible with those Christian motivations that resist whatever social forces erode the awe and respect due life as a gift of God to those created in God's image. To fail to protect the lives of others as neighbors is to violate our obligation to a creator God who not only entrusted us with the lives of persons but also holds us responsible for the welfare of others with whom we are interdependent. Yet the question remains whether permitting permanently unconscious and terminally ill patients to die will lead to the flagrant abuse some predict. It is our judgment that the guidelines we have specified as necessary preconditions for withholding or withdrawing artificial means are sufficient to guard against widespread abuse and certainly against anything as flagrant as the nightmare of the Holocaust.

Recall that our position specified that it is only extraordinary treatments which may be withheld or withdrawn and that death may not be the intention—even the merciful intention—of the care-giver. We admitted that it is sometimes difficult to distinguish extraordinary from ordinary treatments and to separate what one intends from what one merely foresees. But, despite these difficulties, we believe that the psychological and social character — and therefore the consequences and risks—of the practices we accepted are distinguishable from those of the practices that clearly intend to cause the death of patients. The moral hazard of tolerating the injection of a lethal drug into a patient's veins, for example, is that even if it is sometimes justifiable, once people overcome the natural psychological barriers against killing and get used to doing it in narrowly restricted cases, there is a real possibility that the practice will spread to less restricted cases. Eventually an ethos could evolve that would condone killing oneself or others whenever, as the saying goes, the flame is not worth the candle. "The problem is that these decisions in the extreme cases [begin] to legitimize a logic and soon a set of priorities that [take] on a momentum of their own" (Appelbaum and Klein, 26). Unfortunately, some decisions that may be morally compelling in certain individual cases can slide into loose and dangerous public policy.

Related to this point is a special concern about the effect of mercy killing on the medical profession. Many medical personnel have long recognized that when disease has overmastered patients, the goal of their caring must shift from restoring health and maintaining life to comforting patients and controlling pain. In other words, wise practitioners know that, in treating terminal patients, they cannot strive for the primary good of medicine—preserving a healthy life; they must instead strive for another good—relief of suffering. But to ask them to directly contradict their primary good (and not merely to cease pursuing it) in order to achieve another good seems to strike at the very heart of their identity and character. We think it would be unfair for society to ask and unwise for society to encourage medical professionals to incorporate into their traditional calling the willingness to be hired mercy killers. We earlier suggested that patients should be assured that medical personnel are willing to stop inflicting useless and painful treatment; patients should not feel trapped in a system that inexorably pushes for its own aims while ignoring their welfare and autonomy. But patients should also be assured that those who know when to surrender to the enemy are not really double agents, collaborating with the enemy just because sometimes there are worse enemies. We fear that the traditional trust between patients and medical professionals, which serves as the foundation for effective medicine, will be undermined if physicians and nurses incorporate mercy killing into their calling. The uses of such benevolence in a fallen world have too often been abused.

The point just made applies even to the family and friends of terminally ill or irreversibly withering patients. Anyone contemplating intervention in another person's death trajectory must be reminded that not only do our attitudes and character influence our acts, but, reciprocally, our acts influence our attitudes and our character. The moral rightness or wrongness of such intervention must be judged, therefore, not only in terms of the patient's condition and the likely responses of others to the act, but also in terms of the impact such intervention will make upon our personal sensitivities to and care for the dying person. Most dying people are mentally and emotionally aware and need our presence, our active care, our support, our promise not to abandon them. They give opportunities for the healthy to demonstrate personal care and to grow by learning from the dying through caring for them. Accordingly, any guideline or practice that gives even the appearance of "care-lessness" to the dying or diminishes our desire to attend to those who suffer can threaten our own character as care-givers.

The slippery-slope argument rightly cautions us that noble intentions or motives do not in themselves justify mercy killing. We would not want to deny that some exponents of it are well intentioned. Nor would we deny that mercy killing can be motivated solely by love. Rather, we acknowledge the possibility that even acts of love can have negative effects on public policy when they are undertaken without regard for the awe and respect that are due God's gift of life. Even well-intentioned efforts—like those of the Hemlock Society—favoring rational suicide in the face of advanced terminal illness can be hazardous. Derek Humphrey's manual entitled *Let Me Die Before I Wake: Hemlock's Book of Self-Deliverance for the Dying* can appropriately be characterized as forthrightly advocating euthanasia as an act of love and humane caring, but its danger is in its failure to recognize that even pure motives and noble intentions are not sufficient (as human nature and human history bear testimony) to stem the abuse to which euthanasia can be put by those whose motives and intentions may be self-serving.

Although it is true that the envisioned dangers of the slippery-slope argument have been neither confirmed nor refuted, our knowledge of human nature and human history is sufficient to make us concur with Richard McCormick's statement of resistance to more permissive norms:

> The risk . . . is simply too great. There are enormous goods at stake and both our past experience of human failure, inconstancy, and frailty, and our uncertainty with regard to long-term effects lead us to believe that we ought to hold some norms as virtually exceptionless . . . this is the conclusion of prudence in the face of dangers too momentous to make risk tolerable. ("The New Medicine and Morality,"320)

If law is to function in the arena of dying, as indeed it must in a sinful world, let it be used to nurture a disposition toward life and caring for those who are dying. Granted, official policies and statutes against killing and bureaucrats who administer them can come down too hard on those who, for morally weighty reasons, intervene in another's dying process. What is most needed is a spirit in the criminal-justice system that will enable prosecutors and judges to make wise decisions by balancing the need to maintain the legal and moral force of the law with the need to be merciful to those who are more legally than morally vulnerable.

The Covenantal Base of Caring

In the face of death and dying, the Christian community is tied together by shared faith and shared fellowship. On the one hand, our shared faith bears witness to the fact that sickness, disease, and death are not the ultimate enemy. In his divine nature, Jesus demonstrated his power not only over sickness and disease by healing the sick, but also over death by rising victorious over the grave. Yet, on the other hand, our shared faith acknowledges that death and its ravaging effects are dreadfully real and not to be taken lightly. In his human nature, Jesus demonstrated his vulnerability to the severing of human relationships by weeping at the death of his friend Lazarus.

The shared fellowship that ties the Christian community together, grounded as it is on an acknowledgment that we were created to be social creatures, leaves no room for Christians to abandon fellow image-bearers who are dying. Rather, it gives opportunity for supporting them and their loved ones in the face of painful affliction and loss of function. As noted previously, our commitment to provide care—or our failure to do so—not only reflects but also inevitably affects our attitudes about what it means to be a member of a community.

In the face of sickness, dying, and bereavement, covenantal caring can be expressed in a multitude of ways. Whatever the manner of its expression, its essence is its readiness to find ways to meet the physical, psychological, social, and spiritual needs that each of us has and that are intensified in the face of death and dying (Saunders). Especially in the face of the loss and the threat of loss that accompany terminal illness, the Christian community must be aware and persistently caring.

But what does Christian caring come to? Basically it is a response of affiliation and sharing with fellow human beings that is grounded on gratitude for God's work of creating us as social beings, relating to us despite our weakness, and promising eternal life to those who believe in his divine power over the wages of sin, which are death. For members of the Christian community, that faith is represented in attitudes and actions which embrace others and their needs as opportunities to serve. Christian care-givers try to ease pain by using medical means, to quiet fears imposed by sickness and dying, to meet the social needs of those too often abandoned in their affliction, and to acknowledge the reality of the Christian faith through words and gestures that testify to the faithful presence of God in the valley. In caring for others, care-givers demonstrate their gratitude to God, who created, sustains, and preserves us by the power of love in the very midst of human afflictions.

Medical practitioners are strategically positioned to give concrete expression to our commitment to care for the vulnerable. The dependence of the ill and the dying upon medical practitioners provides doctors and nurses with opportunities beyond the minimal moral obligations of human community. The moral obligations that arise in the face of the loss and the threat of loss that accompany sickness and death are far more demanding. In their covenantal capacity, Christian physicians and nurses, imitating their heavenly Father, can respond to a patient's vulnerability (including inequity, uncertainty, and imposed intimacy) as an occasion to exercise greater responsibility than mere contractual arrangements can require. Granted, the expression of Christian caring in the face of suffering unto death is not always distinguishable from acts of concern by those who do not profess Christianity. Nevertheless, gratitude for our God—who, as one who shared the suffering of fallen human creatures, has chosen to relate to us in sustaining and redeeming love—can provide not only an incentive for the Christian medical practitioner but also a comfort that has the power to transcend the relief of physical or mental symptoms for the Christian patient.

We do not mean to suggest that mere pious words are an effective antidote for deep human suffering. Medical treatment has a very significant role to play in covenantal caring. In the face of deep physical affliction, the powerful medical treatments and medications that the medical practitioner is uniquely equipped to administer are truly gifts from God for correcting or alleviating the physical and mental malfunctioning that cause sickness and disease.

But, in the face of the dependency that accompanies dying, does medical treatment exhaust our opportunities or responsibilities to care? Whether the immediate goal of medical treatment is prevention, cure, or control over the forces of disease, treatment must be motivated by care for the patient. And we must acknowledge that there are other types of care besides technical care. In fact, the special opportunity that medicine has to express caring also allows for unfaithfulness to covenantal relationships. There are occasions when the application of medical technology can fall short of the kind of caring required by a covenantal ethic; sometimes the application of medical technology may actually constitute a sophisticated form of abandoning a suffering, terminally ill patient. Our acknowledgment that there is no final escape from our finitude and that some forms of suffering cannot be relieved by medical technology does not relieve us of our responsibility to care, but it does allow us to limit and restrain careless technological meddling in a patient's living out his or her final days. The community that defines care solely in terms of technology is unfaithful to those sick and dying who are beyond the reaches of medical cure and control.

As suggested in Chapter Five, while the physician must not intend death by practicing hospitality toward it, neither must the community encourage the physician to practice hospitality toward suffering or intend human life without flourishing (as in an irreversible coma). When resisting death by medical technology can promise neither the restoration of a capacity for human relationships nor the relief of pain, then the physician may allow death its apparent and inevitable victory, and the community should support the physician's decision. It is especially at such a time that the dying patient needs the caring support of the broader covenantal community. The fact that dying persons often fear isolation and abandonment more than death itself (Saunders) may be seen as an indictment of the covenantal community. Those with physically chronic and degenerative conditions provide an opportunity for members of the Christian community to model a selfless kind of care, a ministry that transcends everyday encounters or mere contractual obligations.

For the Christian in the covenantal community, allowing death when medical intervention is no longer efficacious is the opposite of abandoning the patient. As Paul Ramsey reminds us, it is ceasing to do what was once called for (treatment to cure) in order to do what is now called for—active, empathic caring (Ramsey, *Patient*). In the face of imminent death, the single-minded pursuit of physical life can be an impediment to caring when it pre-empts the patient's simple but profound need for communal support and the personal presence of loved ones in the valley. Leonard Weber sums this up effectively: "The positive meaning of 'allowing the patient to die' is the attempt to provide for a peaceful death in the midst of family, rather than having a patient die alone because the family may interfere with the staff's fight to keep death at bay. Actually, a good case can be made for initiating this type of care for patients earlier than is usually done" (p. 12).

We believe that the hospice movement—founded upon Cicely Saunders' recognition that the dying person has interrelated physical, psychological, social, and spiritual needs—can be an impressive example of Christian caring. Hospice care attempts to minimize as much as possible the isolation, anxiety, fear, and pain associated with incurable illness; to assist the patient in maintaining relationships with others as long and as comfortably as possible (for instance, by controlling pain); and eventually to lend support to survivors in bereavement. Although current hospice programs are not always grounded on explicit Christian principles, and although implementation of the hospice programs sometimes falls short of the original hospice concept,[18] the hospice movement can teach us much about communal care in the face of death and dying.

The scope of Christian caring must be broad enough to reach beyond the patient to those who must make the difficult, often rending end-care decisions. It is particularly incumbent on the Christian community to support key participants in end-care decisions, especially medical practitioners, who are frequently called upon not only to participate in some of life's most difficult decisions but also to be present when others retreat.

Christian caring requires continued affiliation with, compassion toward, and a readiness to forgive even those whom we judge not to have adequately protected the gift of life. It elicits encouragement and tangible support for those who have chosen to sustain and nurture the personal life of the vulnerable, including those on whom society has imposed such labels as "defective," "handicapped," and "abnormal." And Christian caring also requires actively engaging—and sometimes challenging—the structures of society so as to break down the great physical, psychological, and social barriers that obstruct the path of those per-

18. That programmatic implementation of the hospice concept (when compared with conventional medical care) can fall short of lofty expectations is apparent from the results of the American National Hospice Study. Also see R. Kane et al.

sons, including parents and children, who are called upon to bear sacrificially some of life's heavy burdens without much social support.[19]

19. Patrick and Carol Berger put the challenge this way: "If Christians are to have any credible input into the euthanasia debate, they are going to have to bear more witness to the care of the old, the dying, and the unsuccessful" (p. 588).

11   AIDS and Care[1]

The central agenda for this book has been to express our faith in God in the context of the new powers of medicine and to suggest what faithfulness to God requires of those who provide and of those who use medical care. We started with certain convictions about God and about the human creatures who image God. Then we examined the place of such convictions in a pluralist society and the relationship of such convictions to the way we understand medicine and its tools. Next we considered some of the moral questions prompted by the new powers of medicine—questions about the allocation of resources, about technologically assisted reproduction, about abortion, about genetic control and counseling, and about appropriate care for the dying. Now, in this last chapter, we turn to a disease that has reminded us all that, despite its extraordinary new powers, medicine is not as powerful as we may have supposed.

That disease, of course, is acquired immunodeficiency syndrome, known as AIDS. It has so far proved resistant to medical intervention, and it may very well prove to be the severest test yet to the faithfulness of Christians. It is less than a decade since the first cases were

1. During the 1985-86 study year, the Calvin Center for Christian Scholarship team discussed the many topics covered in this book. We also regularly discussed acquired immunodeficiency syndrome (AIDS) and the ethical issues surrounding it as we witnessed the rapid and dramatic unfolding of many new details and developments of this mysterious new disease. But because of the tentativeness of these new discoveries and the remaining uncertainties about AIDS, we chose at that time not to specifically address the issues surrounding AIDS in our original manuscript. During further manuscript preparation over the last two years, however, it became apparent that this would be a serious omission. Consequently, in the fall of 1988, the team wrote Chapter Eleven, applying the principles set forth in Chapters One through Ten to AIDS in the light of the best scientific information available. It should be noted that the team did not have an opportunity to discuss the morality and theology of homosexual behavior. Therefore, this chapter focuses on AIDS as a disease and says no more than is necessary about homosexuality either as orientation or as practice. The data in this chapter will change as the medical community further defines the disease and its treatment, but we believe the Christian principles that we articulate will enable all of us to respond appropriately as Christians to AIDS.

diagnosed, but already millions of people are infected with the virus, and the "null hypothesis"—which postulates that all those infected with the virus will eventually succumb to AIDS—has not yet been challenged by any convincing counterevidence (Lemp, 56). Medicine seems relatively powerless against the disease. Public response has been mixed, confused, and fearful—in part because of the perception of medicine's powerlessness. A society that thought it had death on the run has discovered again what it suspected all along but tried desperately to deny: human beings are mortal, and ultimately medicine is powerless against mortality (Snow, 14). The response of the church has been no less mixed, confused, and fearful (Shelp and Sunderland), but it is our conviction that the Christian faith has resources with which to care for and nurture those with AIDS. Indeed, it is our conviction that faithfulness to God both requires and provides guidance for such care.

Our agenda for this final chapter, then, is first to describe the disease and then to discuss the appropriate human and Christian responses to it, which we do primarily by restating some of the affirmations and conclusions of previous chapters as they bear specifically on AIDS. Thus this chapter will provide something of a summary of our work—and surely something of a test for it.

The Disease: AIDS

Nicole Burk does *not* have AIDS. She is the only member of her family who does not. Her father, Patrick, recently died from AIDS. A hemophiliac, he contracted the *human immunodeficiency virus* (HIV) through a blood transfusion before the blood supply was routinely screened for HIV antibodies. Nicole's mother, Lauren, contracted the virus from Nicole's father before he knew he was infected, and now she has AIDS. And Nicole's little brother, Dwight, contracted the virus from his mother, either during pregnancy or through breast-feeding, and has now died from AIDS (Redfield and Burke, 91).

The Burks' sad story is a dramatic but not an isolated tragedy. Patrick and Dwight are just two of the 46,348 Americans in the United States who have died from AIDS as of December 31, 1988 (Centers For Disease Control, 229); Lauren is just one of the 1 to 1.5 million living Americans already infected with HIV (Heyward and Curran, 75). And the estimates for the future are chilling. The Surgeon General of the United States projects that in this country alone "an estimated 270,000 cases of AIDS will have occurred [by the end of 1991], resulting in 179,000 deaths within the decade since the disease was first recognized" (U.S. DHHS, *Surgeon General's Report*, 6). But AIDS is not limited to the United States; the world-wide statistics are even more chilling. Globally, the estimates are that over 250,000 cases of AIDS have already occurred, that 5 to 10 million people are already infected with HIV, and that by 1993 over one million new cases of AIDS can be expected (Mann et al., 82).

Clearly, AIDS is epidemic, even pandemic — affecting great numbers of people over a wide geographical area. Yet it was less than a decade ago, in 1981, that health-care practitioners on both the East and the West coasts of the United States first noticed a startling increase in the occurrence of several otherwise rare infections, including a pneumonia caused by the protozoan *Pneumocystis carinii* and a cancer called Kaposi's sarcoma. Ordinarily, these rare infections were seen only in elderly persons and in people whose immune systems were suppressed (such as cancer patients and transplant recipients taking immunasuppressive drugs). But in most of these new cases, the persons were young homosexual men. They were diagnosed as having a disease that destroyed their immune systems. The disease was soon called *a*cquired *im*muno*de*ficiency *s*yndrome, or AIDS—so named because it was acquired rather than inherited, and the principal feature in its victims was the gradual destruction of the body's immune system.

Health-care researchers began a concerted effort to identify the natural history of this new disease. What causes AIDS? How is the disease transmitted? What are its symptoms? How does AIDS progress in patients and how rapidly? What ways are available to control the disease? Can it be cured? These and many other questions were almost immediately asked, but in 1981 there were no answers to any of these questions, just a fearful and eerie suspicion, soon borne out, that people with a compromised immune system do not live very long.

A great deal of research has been done since 1981. Laboratory researchers have worked to identify the causes of the disease. Epidemiologists have analyzed population data in an effort to determine the modes of transmission and the demographics of AIDS. Medical researchers have struggled to develop cures and looked for ways to alleviate the symptoms of AIDS in those affected. Within the decade, all three groups have made remarkable—even unprecedented—progress in characterizing this disease. But there has been no progress in changing its outcome: AIDS leads to death. For those dying of AIDS, the remarkable progress has not been progress enough.

The Human Immunodeficiency Virus (HIV)

It is now known that AIDS is the last stage of an infection by a virus called the human immunodeficiency virus, or HIV. This virus infects a population of human white-blood cells called T4 lymphocytes.[2] Initially the virus appears to stimulate the host's immune system. Over the course of six weeks to a year, the infected person's immune system responds slowly by producing HIV antibodies. Within three to eight years the virus slowly destroys T4 lymphocytes as it replicates within these cells (Redfield and Burke). Since these cells are essential for a well-functioning immune system, their destruction leaves a person susceptible to myriads of infections. Many infections that normally would be effectively fought off by the human immune system now become life-threatening.

HIV affects the infected person through the T4 lymphocytes; the disease is communicable because HIV is not confined to these lymphocytes. As the virus replicates, the progeny viruses are released into body fluids—particularly into blood, semen, and vaginal fluids, and perhaps breast milk. It is unclear just how long the virus can survive outside a T4 lymphocyte, but it is known that the virus can survive only briefly (seconds or minutes) apart from body fluids.

HIV Transmission

Despite its deadly effects on infected persons, HIV on its own is a very weak virus. Because it cannot survive outside human body fluids for more than a few seconds or minutes, it cannot be contracted by just being in the same room or by swimming in a swimming pool with someone who has AIDS; it isn't caught like a cold through airborne viruses, nor can it be transmitted by a handshake or by insects or pets. There is still no known instance of a family member's becoming infected with AIDS through casual, everyday contact with another family member who has AIDS—even when eating and drinking utensils, toilet facilities, razors, toothbrushes, combs, towels, and clothing are shared (Heyward and Curran, 80; U.S. DHHS, *Surgeon General's Report*, 21). Nor is there any case of AIDS in which kissing is known to be the mode of transmission.

HIV is transmitted within a narrow range of behaviors: it has

2. For further information on the human immunodeficiency virus, readers are referred to Gallo and Montagnier, Haseltine and Wong-Staal, Essex and Kanki, and Weber and Weiss.

been transmitted by sexual intercourse in its many different forms and varieties (homosexual, bisexual, and heterosexual; particularly anal, vaginal, and perhaps oral). It has been transmitted by careless intravenous drug use and by transfusions of infected blood or blood products, including coagulation factors.[3] And it has been transmitted from mother to developing fetus or newborn infant, primarily across the placenta. Only a few cases are known to have resulted from breast-feeding. In short, transmission requires close, intimate contact with infected body fluids via penetration of the skin or exposure of the mucous membranes of the person about to be infected.

The epidemiological evidence accumulated in this decade indicates that of all adults in the United States diagnosed as having AIDS, 63 percent are homosexual or bisexual men, 19 percent are heterosexual intravenous drug users, 7 percent are homosexual or bisexual intravenous drug users, 4 percent are heterosexual men and women, 3 percent are recipients of blood or blood-product transfusions, 1 percent are people with hemophilia or other coagulation disorders,[4] and 3 percent are victims of the infection from an undetermined source. Children represent the fastest-growing category of AIDS patients (Heyward and Curran, 78). As of April 22, 1988, 934 cases of AIDS in children under thirteen years of age had been reported to the Centers for Disease Control (Rogers). Of all children in the United States diagnosed as having AIDS, approximately 78 percent are born to mothers with AIDS or at increased risk for AIDS, 13 percent are recipients of blood or blood-product transfusions, 6 percent have hemophilia or other coagulation disorders, and 4 percent are victims of the infection from an undetermined source (Heyward and Curran, 78). Infection via breast milk is thought to be very rare ("HIV Risk").

The epidemiological evidence indicates, however, that HIV has been transmitted in two significantly different patterns (Mann et al.).

Throughout the Western Hemisphere, western Europe, Australia, and New Zealand, the pattern has been that HIV infections occur

---

3. The Red Cross and some pharmaceutical companies prepare some essential components of blood from outdated donor blood. These can be used to treat patients with blood deficiencies. Persons with bleeding disorders such as hemophilia can be treated with blood-clotting factors purified from human blood.

4. The blood-product categories include individuals who received infusions of blood components that were contaminated with HIV; nearly all of these incidents occurred before the national blood supply was routinely screened for HIV antibodies. There is a general agreement that a theoretical risk still exists because of (a) the six-month "window" period shortly after infection when no antibody is present and (b) false negatives. A recent report examined thirteen cases of transfusion-associated AIDS from blood that had tested negative (Ward et al.).

with greatest frequency among homosexual or bisexual males and urban intravenous drug users. Although initially low, heterosexual transmission of HIV is increasing. The ratio of infected males to infected females in these areas is still on the order of 10 to 1 or even 15 to 1 (because the infection is being transmitted principally by homosexual males). Because initially so few women were infected, the incidence of babies and children infected with HIV was also small. However, as women become a larger percentage of those infected with HIV, the number of infected babies and children will increase. Approximately 30-50 percent of the children born to infected mothers will develop the disease (Falloon et al.).

In contrast, throughout much of Africa and some Latin American countries, the principal pattern of infection occurs among heterosexuals, and the ratio of infected males to infected females is approximately equal. Because so many women have been infected, many more babies and children have also been infected. Within the central African countries of Congo, Rwanda, Tanzania, Uganda, Zaire, and Zambia, HIV is so prevalent that it is estimated that 5 to 20 percent of the sexually active age group is infected (Mann et al., 85).

In other countries (in eastern Europe, Asia, the Middle East, North Africa, and the Pacific), HIV infection is still not very prevalent. Most cases occurring here are isolated cases and appear to be traceable to persons from these areas who have traveled to parts of the world where HIV is prevalent and who either have engaged in sexual contact with infected individuals there or have obtained contaminated blood products (Mann et al., 84).

Stages of HIV Infection

The natural history of HIV infection is still being clarified through many careful studies. Various clinical centers have attempted to use different clinical criteria for distinguishing between progressive stages of the disease. Initially, HIV infection was divided by gross symptoms into three stages: an asymptomatic stage, followed by AIDS-related complex (known as ARC), followed by the final stage of AIDS. For the layperson, these categories are helpful. For the clinician, however, a better diagnostic scheme was essential. It has been provided in the seven-stage classification system developed by several researchers at Walter Reed Army Hospital (Redfield and Burke).

In the first stages of HIV infection, most people have no symptoms whatsoever. Presently, tests are incapable of detecting the virus itself; they detect only antibodies to HIV. Until these antibodies appear, which typically takes anywhere from six weeks to a full year after initial infection, infected persons are in Stage 0. During this initial stage, those infected may infect others, but they have no way of knowing that they are infected. When persons test positive for the presence of HIV antibodies, they are classified as being in Stage 1. The test, however, is given only when persons know they are at risk for HIV infection. Accordingly, unless people know they are at risk, the first inkling they have that something is wrong may be chronically swollen lymph nodes, which is an indication of Stage 2. This stage may last from three to five years. With the onset of Stage 3—which lasts, on the average, about eighteen months— the number of T4 lymphocytes begins to plummet. The beginning of Stage 4 is identified by a measurable loss of immune function, as judged by several skin tests. Stage 5 is characterized by a seriously impaired immune system, which usually manifests itself in many different kinds of viral or fungal infections and/or ulcers. As the immune system continues to decline, patients develop opportunistic infections (for example, *Pneumocystis carinii*, Kaposi's sarcoma, toxoplasmosis, cryptosporidiosis, cryptococcosis, histoplasmosis, and cytomegalovirus). These mark the last stage, Stage 6, or AIDS.

AIDS (or Stage 6 of HIV infection) is debilitating, painful, and ultimately lethal. Infected individuals in this stage become very dependent upon others for care. As the last vestiges of their immune systems fade, persons in this stage must be protected even from healthy individuals, from whom they are at great risk of picking up infections, because an infection that is harmless in healthy individuals may be fatal to persons with compromised immune systems. In some cases the virus also attacks the nervous system and causes damage to the brain, damage that may manifest itself in memory loss, indifference, loss of coordination, partial paralysis, and/or mental disorder. It appears that AIDS is inevitably fatal; it is a downward trajectory of dying. The time between diagnosis of AIDS (Stage 6) and death varies; current statistics indicate that 50 percent of patients die within eighteen months of entering this stage, and 80 percent die within thirty-six months (Mann et al., 82).

Many questions remain. Once infected, does every individual progress from Stage 0 to Stage 6? How much does this progression vary from individual to individual? On the average, it takes eight to nine years to progress from Stage 1 to Stage 5 (Mann et al., 82). Can early treatment delay or arrest further development of the infectious process? Initially it was thought that perhaps 30 percent of patients with ARC would develop AIDS. In the past several years, that figure has now climbed toward 50 and even 60 percent. The pessimistic prediction is that without effective treatments, the progression from one stage to the next may be inevitable. The cautiously optimistic prediction is that with the discovery of treatment and the provision of early treatment, progression from stage to stage can at least be delayed appreciably.

HIV Testing

As we have pointed out, it is still not possible to test directly for the presence of HIV—only for the presence of HIV antibodies. In 1985 several tests were established that can quite accurately identify persons whose blood has HIV antibodies. Presumably these antibodies are present in the blood only if the person's immune system has been exposed to and has reacted against an HIV infection. (It is possible that someone could receive HIV antibodies through a blood transfusion, but—except in very rare circumstances—only if the blood was not screened for antibodies. Similarly, it is possible that the baby of an HIV-infected mother may have antibodies from the mother in his bloodstream for several weeks or months after birth or as long as he is breast-feeding.)

The most common HIV test is a two-step test (Selwyn, 143) that can be performed on a small sample of blood. The first step consists of an *enzyme-linked immunosorbent assay*, called the ELISA test. Since March 1985 this test has been performed routinely on all donated blood that will be used for blood transfusions or purification of blood products. The test is also performed for individuals who suspect that they are at risk of being infected with HIV. The ELISA test is both very sensitive and very specific; yet, since it is not 100 percent sensitive and specific, it will sometimes give false negatives (indicating that someone who is infected is not) and false positives (indicating that someone who is not infected is).[5] Blood that tests positive in the ELISA test is not used for blood transfusions or blood products. Because of the implications of a positive test, blood that tests positive is usually retested. The Western blot test is used for subsequent analysis. It is even more sensitive and specific (and expensive) than the ELISA; it uses an electrophoretic process to separate HIV components and measures their reactivity against HIV antibodies. Only after a blood sample tests positive in both the ELISA test and the Western blot test is a person notified that he or she is HIV positive.

Because HIV testing is normally requested only by persons at risk for HIV infection and because the results of the tests have serious

5. It is important to note that the chances of false negatives affecting the blood supply are very small and that there are not yet any documented cases of AIDS contraction via screened blood products.

implications, HIV testing must be accompanied by appropriate counseling, both beforehand and afterward, for the benefit of the individuals being tested. The testing must also be accompanied by safeguards to ensure complete confidentiality; if it is not, those who should take the test will avoid it.

It is important to note that HIV testing does have shortcomings. A negative test does not rule out the possibility of HIV infection, since most people will not form antibodies (which the test detects) until about six weeks to a year *after* infection. Furthermore, in areas where AIDS is not very prevalent, and among people with no symptoms and no risk factors, a positive test is more likely to be a falsely positive test than an accurate indication of actual infection. In other words, HIV testing will never detect all those who are infected, and some uninfected people will falsely test positive (Task Force on Pediatric AIDS).

Medical Treatments for HIV Infection

There is no known cure for HIV infection or AIDS. But as with many other diseases, early diagnosis permits early treatment of the symptoms. These treatments appear to be modestly effective in increasing life expectancy. One of the more effective treatments is azidothymidine (AZT), also known as zidovudine, a drug shown to both increase the survival time and improve the quality of life of AIDS patients (Yarchoan, Mitsuya, and Broder). This drug works by interfering with replication of the virus. Unfortunately, AZT can also be quite toxic, particularly to bone-marrow cells. Thus treatment with AZT requires careful monitoring of its side effects. Another drawback is expense: the estimated cost of treatment with AZT for a single patient is $8,000 per year. As long as the drug treatment was experimental, many insurance carriers refused to pay for it. Now most insurance companies will pay for AZT treatment, but one in five AIDS patients is without insurance, and 40 percent of the people with AIDS are covered by Medicaid(Fineberg, 134)—and are therefore being treated largely at the public's expense.

Research continues in the hope of finding a cure, but in the absence of a cure, many researchers are investigating the possibility of a vaccine against the disease (Matthews and Bolognesi). Vaccines are usually developed by means of one of two strategies: either by giving the person an intact but inactive virus or by giving the person parts of the virus believed capable of eliciting an effective immune response. The first strategy is not believed to be a good one for HIV, since even attenuated viruses carry a low risk of transmitting diseases rather than stimulating the immune defense against them. In the case of HIV, then, a vaccination could cause death, because the HIV virus is usually fatal. Even if HIV involved no higher proportion of risk than other viruses, the severity of the risk is too great. The second strategy carries fewer risks in theory but demands more work—work to isolate prospective antigens and research to test their abilities to elicit an appropriate immune response. Initial efforts have been discouraging for several reasons. First, the virus is not easy to grow. Second, there is good reason to believe that HIV exists in several slightly different forms, which means that a single vaccine would be effective for only some HIV forms. Furthermore, the virus is probably capable of changing its form sufficiently to escape the immune system without losing its deadly potential. Third, when a vaccine is finally ready for clinical testing, the testing process is time-consuming. Because of these complications, medical authorities are cautioning that any vaccine is probably not going to be available until the turn of the century.

Prevention of HIV Infection

When cures are unknown and treatments for a disease are palliative at best, prevention remains the best option. How can HIV infection be prevented most effectively?

HIV is transmitted among adults principally by sexual relations. Presently, most persons infected with HIV in North America are men who have had sexual relations with other men (homosexual) or with both men and women (bisexual), but this majority will decline as heterosexual transmission increases. The more sexual partners one has, either male or female, the greater the risk of HIV infection. Prostitutes and other sexually promiscuous persons are at greatest risk for becoming infected with HIV and for transmitting it to subsequent partners; sexually faithful persons in a monogamous relationship have virtually no risk of being infected by HIV through sexual intercourse.

Sexually transmitted HIV can be prevented by faithful commitment in a monogamous sexual relationship. If neither partner is infected at the start of such a relationship and neither becomes infected by any other mode of transmission, the partners cannot become infected through their sexual relationship. For those who do not make such a commitment, there is no absolutely "safe" sexual relationship. However, the risk of transmitting HIV through sexual relations can be significantly reduced through the use of condoms. Such "safe sex" is safer than unprotected promiscuous sexual intercourse, yet even condoms, although highly effective, can fail, and thus carry some small risk. To be effective against HIV, condoms must be used from start to finish during intercourse, must be used every time, must not be composed of animal membranes (HIV can penetrate membranes), and must not leak.

Prevention of blood-transmitted HIV infections requires vigilance in four areas. First, society must maintain an HIV-free blood supply for transfusions and blood products. Donations from at-risk persons must be aggressively discouraged, and samples of all donated blood must be tested for HIV antibodies—as they presently are—via the ELISA method. HIV cannot be contracted by donating blood. However, HIV can be transmitted by receiving HIV-contaminated blood. Since 1985, when it became routine to screen the national blood supply for the presence of HIV antibodies and to aggressively discourage high-risk persons from donating blood, the risk of receiving contaminated blood by transfusion has become minimal (Zuck, Fisher). Until then, blood products such as coagulation factors given to persons with bleeding disorders could contain the virus.

Second, those health-care practitioners routinely exposed to blood and blood products must be encouraged to wear protective gloves and clothing to minimize exposure of their mucous membranes and any cuts and abrasions they might have to contaminated blood. This special risk exists for health-care workers who, in the course of their work, may accidentally be sprayed or spattered with HIV-contaminated blood (e.g., during surgery, labor and delivery, emergency-room trauma, dental hygiene) or stuck with a blood-contaminated needle. The risk is relatively low: estimates are that fewer than 1 in 200 incidences of accidental needle-sticks with an HIV-contaminated needle (or accidental exposure of mucous membranes to contaminated body fluids) result in HIV transmission as measured by a subsequent HIV-antibody test (James Allen). Nevertheless, adequate precautions should be taken.

Third, intravenous drug users must be educated about the risks of using intravenous drugs and the dangers of sharing needles, syringes, and drug doses. Intravenous drug use accounts for most blood-transmitted cases of AIDS. Perhaps because of ignorance or neglect, or because of the enormous expense of illegal narcotic drugs, or because of the lack of access to clean syringes and needles, or because of a combination of these factors, many intravenous drug users share needles, syringes, and doses of drugs. When injecting the drugs into a vein, the user confirms that the needle is in a vein by drawing back on the syringe plunger and watching for venous blood to flow into the syringe before injecting the dose. If the user is sharing the dose with other people, all subsequent users receive not only their portion of the dose but also some of the first user's blood, which may be contaminated.

Fourth, prevention of maternally transmitted HIV infections across the placenta during pregnancy, during labor and delivery, or (rarely) through breast-feeding can be achieved only by effective education, counseling, and screening. Ideally, women at risk for HIV infection should be tested for HIV antibodies before becoming pregnant. Unfortunately, women who have put themselves at greatest risk for HIV infection have neglected to make or have refused to make wise choices regarding sexual relations and/or intravenous drug use; in these cases there is little cause for optimism that such women will become concerned about HIV infection in anticipation of becoming pregnant. It is more likely that health-care practitioners and society in general will be confronted with the issues of how best to provide prenatal and pediatric health-care services for infants with AIDS. By 1991, some have estimated, 10,000 to 20,000 children will be infected. Care for these children will be expensive, especially since many will have mothers who are also sick and dying from AIDS. Outpatient care alone for these children could cost $100 million. Most of these cases will fall on the already overburdened health-care delivery systems in our inner cities (Oleske, Conner, and Boland).

The Response: Care

The sad story of AIDS is not fully told in an account of the natural history of the HIV virus. The personal histories of those infected with HIV are often made sadder still by the responses of the healthy.

If it is true that "perfect love casts out fear" (1 John 4:18), might it also be the case that true fear destroys capacities to care? That people respond to AIDS in fear is not hard to understand; AIDS is an infectious and deadly disease. But when fear leads family members to shun other family members with AIDS, or doctors and nurses to abandon AIDS patients, or Christians to condemn AIDS sufferers, then fear has cast out care. That sad story has been too often true (Shenson, 34). There are horror stories of stigmatization, abandonment, and persecution in response to AIDS.

We call upon the Christian community to tell a different story — indeed, to live the story we love to tell, the story of "perfect love" which "casts out fear." Such love is not learned from an abstract principle, whether it be the principle of beneficence or the principle of equal regard; it is learned from a life story, the story of Jesus. There "the love of God was made manifest among us" (1 John 4:9). No abstract principle can cast out fear, but the love of God can nurture both courage and care. Perfect love can cast out not only fear but the instinct to abandon and condemn that is prompted by fear. God did not abandon us, after all; God did not simply leave us to our condemnation. God cared, and God bore the cost of caring. That is the story Christians love to tell. And that is the story Christians must learn to live—even in response to AIDS. That, indeed, is the "commandment we have from him, that he who loves God should love his brother also" (1 John 4:21). If anyone says, "I love God," yet hates—or abandons or neglects or shuns or condemns —his brother with AIDS, he is a liar (1 John 4:20). The truthfulness of our claims to love God is tested by our faithfulness to God, and faithfulness to God is tested in one way by our response to those infected with AIDS.

Faith in God and Faithfulness in Response to AIDS

In the opening chapter we expressed our faith in God and drew certain inferences that guided our reflections about the faithful use and practice of medicine. Those same affirmations and conclusions can direct our reflection about an appropriate response to AIDS.

God is the creator, we said; and so we criticized both idolatry and dualism (pp. 3-7). AIDS has reminded humankind of the limitations of medicine and of medical technology. But in response to AIDS we are sometimes tempted to make an idol of our own life and health. Life and health are good gifts of the creator, and we must receive them with gratitude and protect them with care. But we must sometimes also be ready to put them at risk for the sake of God's cause and our neighbor's good. In response to AIDS we are also sometimes tempted to reduce the embodied person with AIDS to the disease we fear and to care for that person only for the sake of managing that disease. When we succumb to such a temptation, we nurture fear and the responses prompted by fear; succumbing to that temptation may lead to a future in which society attempts to control and eliminate AIDS by controlling and eliminating those with AIDS (Harris). Dualism thus threatens to cast out care.

Our affirmation that God is the creator did not prevent us from acknowledging the reality and strength of evil. In a world God created good, we said (pp. 7-8), there are still real evils: death and sickness—and AIDS—among them. Evil entered the world as a result of human sin. AIDS, too, has entered the world as a consequence of human sin, and some persons who have contracted it have acted sinfully. But we do not stand with those who make a connection between sickness and sin in order to judge and condemn the victims of AIDS. In a 1988 Gallup poll of registered voters, 42.5 percent of those surveyed agreed with the statement that AIDS is God's punishment for immoral behavior ("Times Mirror"). Such a conclusion ignores the fact that many victims of AIDS are infants, ignores stories like that of the Burk family, ignores the observation that "if there is a divine judgment on unrighteousness, we may take God's word for it that there is also perhaps more severe judgment on self-righteousness" (Plantinga, "Justification," 16); such readiness to condemn is unlike God, who provides for human creatures in spite of sin and finally redeems them. And faithfulness to that God in response to AIDS will be disposed not to condemn and judge the sick but to care for them.

God is the provider, we said (pp. 8-15); God's care is the world's constant companion. We did not then in response to suffering—and we do not now in response to the suffering of AIDS—attempt to provide a tidy theoretical theodicy by construing all suffering as justifiable as either punishment or training (pp. 9-11). In the first chapter—and now again—we simply call attention to a Roman cross and to the innocent Jewish teacher who hung there. There one sees in all its horror that evil is real and powerful in this world, and there one sees in all its mystery that God's care is this world's constant companion, that none suffers entirely alone, that God suffers with all who suffer, including those who suffer from AIDS. Faithfulness to God the provider—also in response to AIDS—means to care; it means "com-passion" even and especially when we cannot cure. Faithfulness to God the provider will always join respect to care (pp. 12-15), will cherish and celebrate the embodied integrity of patients and acknowledge the restraints that patients' freedom may impose upon the effort to do good for them (or for others).

God is the redeemer (pp. 16-26), and we read God's cause in the ministry and resurrection of Jesus. In his healing ministry Jesus signaled the future reign of God and the future victory over the power of death and demons and sin. It is important to say once again in the context of AIDS that God's cause is life and health, not death and disease. AIDS reminds us of the "not yet" character of our life and medicine. AIDS reminds us that people still suffer, that people still die sometimes premature and horrible deaths. AIDS reminds us of the limits of medicine, that medicine is not messianic. But in the context of AIDS, the ministry of Jesus reminds a watchful people to nurture the powers of medicine to heal the sick and — in the absence of such powers — to continue to struggle hopefully against unnecessary suffering, to share faithfully in Jesus' compassion for those who suffer, and to be present and to care lovingly for those who cannot be cured.

In his healing ministry Jesus disowned (p. 20) the putative connection between sin and sickness. He rejected the question about whether one was born blind because of his sin or his parents' sin; instead, he simply pointed to the power of God to heal and made that power felt. A watchful people will follow Jesus by not allowing any putative connection between AIDS and sin to distance them from the sick: they will not allow any such connection to induce them to renege on their obligations of solidarity with the suffering, or to refuse to be present with them and to care for them. A watchful people will be disposed not to condemn but to cure, and failing that, at least always to care.

Relying on the account of Luke, the physician, we also called attention to the fact that Jesus was the Christ, the one "anointed . . . to preach good news to the poor" (Luke 4:18; pp. 21-23). It is God's cause to bless the poor, and faithfulness to God demands justice for them and evokes a special concern for them. That is important to say again, because the poor and others at the margins of our society are especially affected by AIDS (Curran et al., 610). It is noteworthy, for example, that in the United States 25 percent of the people with AIDS are black, and 13 percent of the affected adults and 20 percent of the affected children are Hispanic (Curran et al., 611). Those who would be faithful to God and watch for God's future should not use such statistics to further stigmatize the victims of AIDS or to renege on the obligation to care for them; those who would be faithful will use such statistics to show that a social concern about AIDS must be joined with a concern about poverty and the despair, disease, and death it brings.

The commitment to justice and the concern for the poor that belong to faithfulness are obviously relevant to questions about allocation that are raised anew by AIDS—an issue that we will give fuller attention in subsequent discussion.

Imaging God: Persons with AIDS and the Response to AIDS

In the second chapter we turned our attention to the human creatures who are created in God's image and who are called to image God. We noted the controversies about when embodied human beings begin to be image bearers of God and when they cease being image bearers of God, and we gave our own best judgment about such matters (pp. 34-51). The point to underscore here is that there can be no controversy about whether the person with AIDS images God.[6] The person with

---

6. Of course, there are still controversies about whether or not a fetus infected with the HIV virus by its mother has begun to image God, and whether or not a patient

AIDS is to be seen and treated as an image bearer of God, and that fact has some profound implications.

Because people with AIDS are image bearers of God—fallen like the rest of us, but image bearers still like the rest of us—they have a special moral status. We may cite again the powerful words of Calvin—still more powerful in this particular context—as he advises us to "look upon the image of God in them, which cancels and effaces their transgressions, and with its beauty and dignity allures us to love and embrace them" (quoted on p. 30). But the special moral status of image bearers of God evokes not just an embracing love but also a reverential and deferential awe; it is the special moral status of "sanctity" (p. 31). It is especially important to emphasize the sanctity of people with AIDS, because a variety of factors conspire to put them at risk of being controlled and eliminated in an effort to control and eliminate their disease: the fear of the deadly disease, the costs of caring for those with HIV, and the social stigmas so easily attached to many of those affected (Harris, 147). In an upcoming section we will discuss sanctity and its bearing on both mercy killing and the allocation of resources.

Because all persons, including those with AIDS, are image bearers of God, they deserve to be treated with respect as choice-makers, as "givers and hearers of reasons" (p. 32). Accordingly, the second chapter drew attention to the moral significance of autonomy and informed consent (pp. 57-66). The guidelines developed there can be specifically applied here. Persons at risk for AIDS or with AIDS should not have their freedom arbitrarily diminished. They should not be subjected to tests without their knowledge and consent, nor should the results of such tests be disclosed without their consent. Therapies—including experimental therapies—should ordinarily be undertaken only when informed consent has been given. Of course, every person's autonomy is limited by the duty not to harm another. Thus a person infected with HIV may not deliberately put another person at risk of contracting the infection without that person's consent. This limit to autonomy justifies mandatory blood testing of donated blood and programs to secure a safe public blood supply for transfusions and a safe organ supply for transplants. It justifies prohibiting persons at risk for HIV infection from donating organs or blood (just as we prohibit persons with flu or hepatitis and persons who have traveled to countries where malaria is endemic from donating blood). It justifies disclosing the results of a test to the sexual

with AIDS who has permanently lost consciousness has ceased imaging God. The point is that AIDS is irrelevant to the determination of whether a human being images God.

partner(s) of the person infected with HIV. But the very narrow range of transmissibility of the disease does not justify recommendations to quarantine persons affected with HIV.[7]

The balance to be struck is one that preserves and protects both the autonomy of those infected with HIV and the health of others (Sunderland and Shelp, 46; Merritt). In the context of the fear of AIDS and the stigmatization of many of its victims, that balance will be hard to strike or preserve unless we are keenly aware that as imagers of God AIDS patients deserve to have their choice-making capacities respected. But this is not to condone all possible choices. The notorious AIDS victim who consciously chose to infect others made a morally reprehensible choice.

However, in the second chapter—and throughout the book— we also acknowledged that a myopic focus on autonomy can provide only a minimal account of the moral life. If the minimal nature of that account is not acknowledged, the result may be a distorted vision of the moral life. We do not image God simply as autonomous and independent individuals. We image God also in community (pp. 32-33), in interdependence upon one another. The second chapter develops this notion with special reference to persons with disabilities (pp. 56-57); here, perhaps it is enough simply to say that we image God in community with people who have AIDS. Christian convictions cannot vindicate the "rights" of the healthy to withdraw from the obligations of community with the sick, including those sick with AIDS. If we see persons with AIDS as imagers of God with us, as fallen imagers of God like us, as imagers of God alongside us in a world still under the power of suffering and death, then we will find the resources to image God's care for the most vulnerable—indeed, to care for those the world counts as "least," out of the conviction that such care is rendered, as our Lord said, unto him, the true image of the invisible God.[8]

7. It is worth observing that, because their deficient immune systems make them vulnerable to opportunistic infections, AIDS patients run a risk of contracting infections from healthy people that will prove deadly to them—a risk that is much greater than the risk of HIV infection posed to those who have casual contact with AIDS patients.

8. The reference, of course, is to the parable of the last judgment (Matt. 25:31-46). Among the several acts of love listed is "I was sick and you visited me." The verb translated "visited" also means "to care for" and could be used to refer to a "physician's medical visitation of a patient" (Amundsen and Ferngren, 109-10).

Covenantal Fidelity: Responding to AIDS in a Pluralistic Society

In the third chapter we described more theoretically the notion of covenantal ethics that shapes our examination of moral questions in the use and practice of medicine. We took note of its affinities with and differences from the main alternatives in ethical theory in the West. The affinities of this notion with other ways of thinking about morality give us hope that some of our arguments will be convincing not only to other Christians but also to other members of our pluralist societies. Some of the differences give us hope that we and other Christians can make a distinctive contribution that will influence the thinking about and the responses to these issues. This is worth noting again in this chapter, because the response to AIDS must include both the heroic faithfulness of those Christians whose love casts out fear, and the social policies and programs that honor both the obligations of community to help (or at least to do no harm) and the rights of individuals. We pictured covenantal responsibilities on a spectrum (p. 92), with minimal but legally enforceable responsibilities at one end and heroic faithfulness to God on the other end. The point here is that the response to AIDS must cover the whole spectrum. The Christian community must both laud the heroic voluntary efforts of some of its members (and of some heroic Christian communities) to express God's care for those with AIDS and commend social policy designed to protect the rights of AIDS patients to health care and within health care. The Christian community cannot be satisfied with either alone.

The third chapter distinguished between "the inclusive covenant" and "special covenants" (p. 88) and called attention to the special goods and standards that belong to particular communities and relationships. Medical professionals participate in such a special covenant, and that covenant is relevant to their response to patients with AIDS.

The Character of Medicine and the Duty to Treat

The refusal of some physicians, nurses, and dentists to treat AIDS patients is one of the most painful symptoms of the fear of AIDS (Shenson, 34). The number is probably small, to the credit of health-care practitioners (Arras), but the issue is important, and our account of medicine in the fourth chapter bears on it.

There we construed medicine as a practice (pp. 102-8), as a profession (pp. 109-13), and as a calling (pp. 113-15), and the relationship of physician and patient as covenantal (pp. 116-22). As a practice and as a profession, medicine is committed to a certain good—namely, health or at least palliative care for those who are sick. This commitment entails certain obligations necessary to attain that end, not the least being the obligation of treating sick persons who seek medical care. In order to pursue that good and to meet those obligations, those in medicine must strive to meet certain standards of excellence in both their work and their character. AIDS does not change that, but it does remind us that among the standards of excellence necessary to honor the commitment to healing and caring for the sick is the virtue of courage.[9]

In 1847, when the AMA was organized, its first code stated that "when pestilence prevails, it is their [physicians'] duty to face the danger, and to continue their labors for the alleviation of the suffering, even at the jeopardy of their own lives" (cited in Arras, 14). In 1987 the AMA renewed that commitment and obligation in response to AIDS: "A physician may not ethically refuse to treat a patient whose condition is within the realm of the physician's current realm of competence solely because the patient is seropositive" (cited in Freedman, 24). We commend that statement of professional responsibility and think it is required if medicine is construed as a practice and a profession, as a moral enterprise and not simply as a marketable commodity.

As a calling, medicine is a form of discipleship, and as such it is marked by a readiness to care, to cure if possible, but never to neglect or abandon, and surely not to neglect or abandon those who need help most sorely. Jesus healed the sick, blessed the poor, was a friend to the despised, ate with sinners, and shared the suffering of fallen human creatures, and medicine as a calling follows him. The cost of discipleship is still not cheap. Faithful disciples know that they are not the Messiah and that there are limits to the human resources of both energy and compassion; but faithful disciples also know that they are not above their teacher (Matt. 10:24), that sometimes for the sake of God's cause and the neighbor's good, they may have to put their own life and health at risk.

And there is a risk. It is folly to deny it. But it is also folly to exaggerate it. Within health care, transmission of HIV can take place by needle-stick accidents and, rarely, by blood splashing. But compared

9. In a remarkable essay, Abigail Zuger and Steven Miles make this point in stunning fashion. They acknowledge that the professional tradition is spotty—that both the Greek physician Galen and Thomas Sydenham, "the English Hippocrates," fled from patients with epidemic diseases, for example—but they argue that an understanding of health care as a moral enterprise (rather than simply as a right or a contract) sustains a duty to care for AIDS patients. See also J. Arras.

with the risk of being infected with hepatitis B by such occurrences, the risk of being infected with HIV is very small (James Allen). The risk of acquiring hepatitis infection after parenteral exposure to the blood of someone with hepatitis B is 30 percent; the risk of acquiring HIV infection after similar exposure to the blood of an HIV-infected person is 6 percent (James Allen). The risk can be made smaller still by carefully taking the recommended precautions. The risk is small and can be made smaller —but it is nevertheless real. As of February 1988, at least eight health-care workers had acquired AIDS (Arras, 17). And although the probability of being infected is small, the consequences of infection are very great. The consequences include not only suffering and dying, but suffering and dying from a disease that has a social stigma attached to it. If we expect medicine to honor its commitment to caring for and healing the sick, then surely medicine can expect gratitude and honor for its heroism from the broader community. Instead, however, some physicians report that being an "AIDS doctor" elicits not praise but its own stigmatization (Arras, 18-19). If, as Stanley Hauerwas says, "medicine as moral practice draws its substance from the extraordinary moral commitment of a society to care for the ill" (*Suffering Presence*, 13), then the lack of a supporting ethos in a supporting community will gradually erode the commitment of medicine to the good of caring for and healing the sick in accordance with the standards of excellence — including courage—that are necessary to honor that commitment. Then it will not be medicine that is to blame for the failure to treat, but society that is to blame because of its failure to care. The church has an opportunity and an obligation to support and sustain medicine's duty to treat by being a community ready to take certain risks for the sake of imaging God's care for sinners.

The duty to treat an AIDS patient is probably not legally enforceable (T. L. Banks; Annas, "Legal Risks"). It is not a minimal contractual obligation; one does not legislate courage. But that duty can be supported and sustained by the acceptance of medicine as a practice, a profession, and a calling in a society that envisions itself as one community, composed of both those who are healthy and those who are not.

Technology, Tragedy, and AIDS

The relevance of tragedy to AIDS is obvious. AIDS is a "sad story," the first sort of tragedy we contemplated in Chapter Five (pp. 124-25). At this point medicine has few tools to intervene in the sad story of AIDS —and none to give it a happy ending. But researchers continue to work to find new tools to care for AIDS patients. This is a task that is motivated by compassion, and we pray that it yields new "powers to intervene purposefully to forestall death and to restore health" (p. 125). But researchers can be the "flawed heroes" of the AIDS story; the story of "the flawed hero" was the second sort of tragedy we considered in Chapter Five (pp. 125-32). The researcher's crusader-like devotion to a good end can blind him or her to the injustice of certain means. A case in point is the proposal to test potential AIDS vaccines in some African countries because of the high percentage of heterosexuals infected there. An AIDS vaccine would be a very great good, and utilizing such populations in African countries makes some economic sense (because the test subjects would require relatively low compensation), some scientific sense (because of the ease of gathering a sufficient number of test subjects), and even some moral sense (because the greater risk of exposure makes the additional risk of the experimental vaccine proportionately smaller and the possible benefit of immunity proportionately larger). But for all that, such experiments risk injustice. The tragic flaw is apparent in researchers' willingness to disregard the difficulty of obtaining genuinely informed consent in a culture that is unfamiliar with research concepts like randomization and that holds non-Western concepts of disease and of the individual's relation to the community. The tragic flaw is apparent in researchers' willingness to choose research subjects on the basis of their easy availability and compromised ability to refuse to participate. The tragic flaw is apparent in researchers' willingness to allocate the risks of research to poor populations although they are unlikely—precisely because of their poverty—to share in the benefits should the research be successful. And the tragic flaw is apparent in researchers' willingness, for the sake of the experiment, to withhold counseling regarding behaviors that increase risk (Barry; Christakis). None of this suggests that experimentation to develop tools to intervene against AIDS and its spread should not be carried out or that it is impossible to conduct a morally satisfactory experiment in an African country; on the contrary, research is morally important. But the good end of knowledge and power against AIDS must not blind us to the injustice of certain means to attain it. Researchers must resist the temptation to be crusaders. If they don't, that too is a tragedy, the story of flawed heroes.

The treatments we already have and those we may yet develop are certain to confront us with the third sort of tragedy considered earlier: Sophoclean tragedy, the colliding of goods and the gathering of evils (pp. 132-36). In treatment using AZT, for example, the two evils that sometimes gather and cannot both be avoided are the advancement of AIDS without AZT and the toxic effect of AZT on bone-marrow cells.

Careful monitoring of AZT use can increase its beneficial effects and minimize its harmful effects, but sometimes trade-offs are necessary, and the trade-offs are usually tragic. The cost of AZT confronts us with Sophoclean choices of another kind—not choices about the treatment of one patient but choices about who will get treatment when not all can have it.

In searching for and researching ways to intervene in the sad story of AIDS, it is important that we acknowledge that new tools will not eliminate tragedy of the Sophoclean sort. AIDS has reminded us of our mortality and of medicine's powerlessness against it; no new tool against AIDS will provide an escape from our mortality. AIDS is also reminding us of the limits of our resources, and no new technique is likely to rescue us from finite funds. In the context of our acknowledged mortality and the finitude of our resources, we should search and re-search not only for new technologies but also for ways to respond in other than technological ways to this threat to human life and flourishing, to care even when medicine cannot cure (p. 134).

How to allocate resources for AIDS and how to care for those dying of AIDS are issues to which we will shortly return, but we have said enough to preface those remarks with the observation that there are no easy answers in a Sophoclean tragedy or in the trade-offs that are sometimes part of medical care (p. 135).

The fifth chapter also called attention to another story, the glad story of an unflawed hero in whose reign all goods cohere, the story of Jesus (pp. 136-43). The story of Jesus is not a tragedy, but neither does it deny the tragic features of our lives and our medicine. It points us *beyond* tragedy to God's grace and future, but it is beyond *tragedy* that it points us. So Christians pray and work for the development of technologies that may make it possible to intervene against the sad story of AIDS but without extravagant and idolatrous expectations. Christians hope and trust and invite others to hope and trust—ultimately, in God's grace and future. The glad story of Jesus and of the triumph of God that Jesus announced can sustain and nurture care—indeed, the patient love that casts out fear—in response to the sad story of AIDS, even in the absence of medical technologies or in the face of their failure to cure (p. 138).

The story of an unflawed hero reminded us, we said, that the rest of us are still sinners (p. 139). There are not two societies, one righteous and the other wicked, one powerful and the other optionless, one well and the other sick—or one that is righteous, powerful, and well, and another that is wicked, optionless, and sick. In the story of this Jesus —the perfect one who took upon himself the sins of the world, the wounded healer, the Lord who is a servant — there are resources to renew both a sense of community and the efforts to express it with care and respect.

The gospel, finally, does not provide easy answers to what are currently insoluble questions; it does not deny the "not yet" character of our medicine and of our existence as it watches for God's coming sovereignty. But in response to AIDS, watchfulness can sustain and nurture essential virtues in a people and in medicine: *truthfulness, humility, gratitude* for opportunities within our limitations to serve God's cause, *care* even for those who don't amount to much as the world counts worth, *respect* for the integrity of embodied people made in God's image, and, indeed, *courage* to make the ambiguous choice in the certain confidence of God's forgiveness and to make the right choice in the carefree confidence that casts out fear (pp. 142-43).

Scarcity and AIDS: Personal, Public, and Professional Responsibilities

We began the sixth chapter by acknowledging the financial crisis in medicine (pp. 144-50); AIDS will only make that crisis worse. The Surgeon General of the United States has projected that in 1991 "an estimated 145,000 patients with AIDS will need health and support services at a total cost of between \$8 and \$16 billion" (U.S. DHHS, *Surgeon General's Report*, 6). That enormous figure must be kept in perspective: the annual health-care bill in this country was projected to top \$500 billion (James, 41), so the cost of health and supportive service for AIDS patients would increase the bill by only 1.5 to 3 percent—a figure that perhaps sounds more manageable. Nevertheless, some hard choices are going to have to be made—and have already been made. In 1985 the U.S. government, unprepared for the AIDS epidemic, took \$126 million from the funds that had been appropriated for health programs for Native American and rural populations in this country in order to fund programs for AIDS (Levine, 26). And in 1986 the government reappropriated \$55 million from the Heating and Energy Assistance Program for Low-Income Families in order to help fund the trials, manufacture, and distribution of AZT (Levine, 26).

The point here is not that these choices were wrong, although one may ask whether it is fair to put the burden of paying for AIDS on the backs of the poor. Rather, the point is that choices like these were and are necessary. We have limited resources, and this scarcity makes tough allocation decisions necessary. There are other claims on our resources besides health care (pp. 145-46), including claims like keeping the homes of the poor warm in wintertime. Moreover, there are competing claims on our resources *within* health care (p. 147)—AIDS is not the only disease. And even with respect to AIDS our resources are assailed by competing claims for education, prevention, research, primary care, acute care, hospice care, chronic care, and so on. Such hard choices about allocation sometimes necessitate the still harder choices about who will receive the scarce new drug, the only bed left in intensive care, or the potential and potentially scarce vaccine (p. 148).

It is scarcity that makes these decisions necessary, but it is sanctity that makes them tragic (p. 148). In the sixth chapter—and again here—we reject any attempt to deal with allocation decisions that denies either scarcity or sanctity (pp. 148-49). There is no eliminating the tragedy of such choice, but that does not mean there are no intelligent and appropriate responses to the financial crisis. In the sixth chapter we suggested that individuals should take seriously their responsibility for their own health (pp. 150-56), that public officials should exercise careful stewardship of resources (pp. 156-62) and allocate limited resources fairly (pp. 162-70), and that physicians should act with integrity in the midst of tragedy (pp. 170-75). As AIDS has made the financial crisis of medicine worse, so too it has made these responsibilities even more pressing.

It is important to underscore again in this context the position we took in Chapter Six on personal responsibility for health. Prevention is the best medicine available for AIDS, and it is clear that prevention is largely a matter of personal responsibility.

As previously noted, HIV is transmitted by a narrow range of behaviors. The principal mode of transmission is by sexual intercourse with an HIV-infected person (male or female). The principal means of prevention is simply to avoid such intercourse. Sexual faithfulness—whether in homosexual relationships or in heterosexual relationships—virtually eliminates the risk of HIV infection through sexual intercourse. The famous seven rules for health (p. 152) should be amended to include an eighth rule: Do not be promiscuous. It is simply not prudent, and it is morally wrong. That said, it is important to note that the risks of promiscuous sexual behavior can be reduced—but not eliminated—by avoiding sexual partners known to be at risk for AIDS, by avoiding partners whose history and status are unknown, and by using condoms.

The second major mode of HIV transmission is careless intravenous drug use. Sharing needles or syringes or dosages is simply not prudent. The rules for health should also include a rule against the recreational use of drugs. The wisdom of the street might very well be that life in the fast lane of drugs and promiscuity can be deadly.[10]

We call upon individuals to exercise responsible stewardship of their health simply on the basis of prudence. But we also would remind people of their responsibility to others. Those who are infected with HIV or know themselves to be at risk for HIV have a responsibility not to put others at risk. We call upon them to refrain from sexual intercourse and from sharing needles. Both prudence and responsibility to others, then, should prompt individuals to take personal responsibility for their health in response to AIDS—and so, as we said, should piety (p. 153). Persons are responsible to God, finally, for their stewardship of God's good gifts, including the gifts of life, health, and sex.

This call to personal responsibility in response to AIDS is not inconsistent with compassion. Indeed, if we do not see people as image bearers of God and therefore as responsible givers and hearers of reasons, we also will not see them as deserving of respect and care. But it is important to repeat again and emphasize in response to AIDS what was said in Chapter Six: we must not use the failure to accept responsibility for personal health to condemn the victims of disease, to distance ourselves from the "irresponsible sick," to deny our solidarity with the suffering, or to renege on our obligations to care for them (pp. 155-56). It is also important to repeat and emphasize a related point: that staying well can be made harder or easier by the community in which one lives (pp. 155-56).

We call again upon physicians to fulfill the role of teachers, to provide information, and to engage in the delicate but deliberate task of transforming the habits of their patients (p. 154).

We call again upon the government (p. 154) to make it easier for persons to take responsibility for avoiding AIDS. That effort should surely include educational programs and preventive programs. We commend the work already being done in screening blood for transfusions and organs for transplants in order to secure a supply uninfected by HIV. We commend the voluntary HIV testing and counseling programs for those at risk for AIDS, including the provision of condoms and sterile needles as a part of such programs.[11] We call upon the government to

10. We should also mention here that health-care workers should take responsible and reasonable precautions whenever there is the possibility that they will be exposed to blood or other body fluids. The recommendations of the American Hospital Association and the Center for Disease Control should be followed.

11. The counterargument that providing condoms and sterile needles only encourages promiscuity and drug abuse is not without merit, but it can be met by paying careful attention to the context within which condoms and needles are recommended or

make it easier for people to stay healthy by initiating programs to combat the poverty and prejudice which so often lead to such despair that recreational drugs seem to be the only "savior."

Finally, we call upon churches to nurture the capacities of people to exercise personal responsibility. We call upon churches to speak clearly and candidly about the risks of AIDS and to speak no less clearly and candidly about the Christian moral vision of "good sex." Briefly, we understand "good sex" to be neither a technology of pleasure-seeking nor merely a romantic quest for intimacy, but the "one flesh" union of a man and a woman that gestures the commitment and covenant stated in vows and carried out in fidelity (p. 194).[12]

Some, like Dan E. Beauchamp, claim that this vision is part of the problem, that it has created a religious prejudice against homosexuality and has sponsored a legal moralism which impedes public-health efforts to reduce homosexual promiscuity ("Morality"). There is much that churches can learn from Beauchamp's critique, including much for which they need to repent. Nevertheless, it is our conviction that to keep the Christian vision of "good sex" alive and to articulate it cogently are no small part of the churches' service to AIDS prevention and no small part of the churches' faithfulness to God. So we call upon churches to continue to speak of the way they see human sexuality in the light of God's creative and redemptive purposes, but we also call them to speak of their vision in ways that demonstrate some appreciation for the understandable rage against the church and the legitimate suspicion of the church which some homosexuals have because of the way Christians have used and applied that vision to shun and stigmatize homosexuals.

We suggest two revisions in the way churches have sometimes applied their vision, two revisions that would enable churches to re-

---

provided. Ron Sider (p. 14) draws a striking contrast between a TV advertisement featuring a glamorous young woman who says she wants love but doesn't want to die for it and a TV ad in which someone ravaged by AIDS says candidly that safe sex requires fidelity, but if you want to play Russian roulette with your life, then please use condoms. The first ad glamorizes promiscuity; the second surely does not.

12. Obviously we cannot develop here a full or even adequate account of a Christian sexual morality. We cannot deal fully or even adequately with the basis for it or questions concerning it. To interested readers we commend the following: Lisa Cahill, *Between the Sexes;* Margaret Farley, "Sexual Ethics," in *Encyclopedia of Bioethics;* Lewis Smedes, *Sex for Christians;* and Stanley Hauerwas and Allen Verhey, "From Conduct to Character—A Guide to Sexual Adventure." Concerning the biblical materials, see Barry Bandstra and Allen Verhey, "Sex; Sexuality," in vol. 4 of *The International Standard Bible Encyclopedia;* and Victor Paul Furnish, *The Moral Teachings of Paul.*

spond more cogently to Beauchamp's criticisms. First, while we caution churches against the "no fault" sexual morality of Beauchamp, we would also caution churches again (pp. 92, 101) against attempts at legally enforcing their particular vision of the good sexual life. The danger of Beauchamp's view is that it reduces sexual morality to the minimal standards of mutual consent and doing no harm. Those standards are legitimate and important, but if their minimal character is not acknowledged, they distort the moral life. The danger of the other view is another form of the tragedy of the flawed hero: churches have sometimes let a good end blind them to the injustice of certain means in attempts to legislate a sexual morality.

Second, while we caution churches against giving up their vision of "good sex," we also caution them against applying it prejudicially and oppressively against homosexuals. We agree with many Christians who say that the distinction between heterosexual intercourse and homosexual intercourse should not be a matter of moral indifference to churches, but we would also insist that the distinction between promiscuous intercourse (whether homosexual or heterosexual) and intercourse within a relationship of faithfulness (whether homosexual or heterosexual) may also not be a matter of moral indifference to churches. Even as churches refuse to condone homosexual intercourse, they should recognize that faithfulness—also an important aspect of "good sex"—can be present in homosexual love as it can be absent in the promiscuity of some heterosexuals and the serial polygamy of those heterosexuals who marry and divorce every few years. And with respect to the prevention of HIV infection and AIDS, faithfulness is most important.

The Christian vision of "good sex" may eventually play an important role in prevention and in enabling individuals to take responsibility for their own health. But it is likely to play that role only if churches are not prejudicial in their application of that vision and also care for those who are already the victims of AIDS.

Chapter Six discussed not only personal responsibilities to preserve health but also public responsibilities to exercise stewardship of resources (pp. 156-62) and to secure an adequate level of health care for all members of society (pp. 162-70). The scarcity of resources in our battle with AIDS may not be denied, and that scarcity makes efficiency a morally legitimate and important concern. But scarcity does not allow us to deny the sanctity of all persons, including AIDS patients, whose well-functioning and well-being may be contingent upon health care, and that sanctity prohibits us from allowing efficiency to have a moral monopoly on our concern. That point was important in our attempt to suggest priorities for health care (p. 165), and it is important now in our attempt to suggest priorities for AIDS care. An "adequate level" of health care surely includes access to a primary care-giver (pp. 164-165), because medicine is one way in which members of a society express care for one another. We underscore this point for those with AIDS. An adequate level of health care also surely includes access to programs that provide protection against unnecessary health risks (p.165), because medicine, like police protection, contributes to the protection of life and health. Again, we underscore this point with respect to AIDS. An adequate level of health care also includes, "as appropriate to age and condition," those medical and rehabilitative services "that effectively restore or maintain normal functioning" (p. 165), because medicine, like education, secures a range of opportunities. This point, too, must be reiterated with respect to AIDS. We may ask, however, whether AZT, which only temporarily alleviates symptoms, belongs to this "adequate level" of health care and whether the "condition" of AIDS patients minimizes a legitimate claim to this medical service. We acknowledged, after all (p. 165), that only "if resources permit" should treatment of established diseases for which there is no radical cure be included in an adequate level of health care, and expensive procedures of unproven benefit were even lower on our allocation list. Having raised this point, however, we acknowledge that there are some societies where scarcity prevents AZT from being included in the health care to which their citizens are entitled, but we do not think the United States and Canada are among them (p. 169). Moreover, when AZT is one of the few even minimally effective medical measures against AIDS, its importance as an expression of care and as an affirmation of the sanctity of AIDS patients prohibits efficiency from monopolizing our attention in allocation. Our best hopes against AIDS are prevention and research, and both should be given priority in allocation decisions, but they should not monopolize our concern to such an extent that the statistical patient or the future patient makes it impossible for society to care—and to care medically—in a meaningful way for the real patient who is sick now (p. 161). These are hard choices, tragic choices, where goods collide and evils gather. We acknowledge that to fund AZT therapy almost certainly means less money for other therapy or research or programs.

It is important, finally, to recall our conclusion (p. 169) that hospice care for the dying and at-home nursing care for the chronically ill belong to an adequate level of health care. That conclusion applies also to those chronically ill with AIDS and those dying from AIDS. Medicine is, after all, a gesture of care for and presence with another in the midst of tragedy (including the tragedy of not providing the "best" care because it is expensive and marginally and/or doubtfully beneficial), not a way to deny tragedy.

In response to the increasing scarcity caused by AIDS, we continue to call for societies to provide an adequate level of health care for every member of the community, including the person with AIDS, and to discern what is included in that level of care not simply on the basis of efficiency but also on the basis of justice and sanctity and the character of medicine.

Children, Abortion, and AIDS

In the seventh, eighth, and ninth chapters we turned our attention to the questions of making babies and aborting fetuses and controlling the genetic inheritance of children. Children are also affected by AIDS. In fact, children are the fastest-growing category of AIDS patients in the United States. Nearly all of them receive HIV from their infected mothers through blood exchange in the uterus or during birth. As the population of infected women grows, so will the population of children with AIDS. They will be born already suffering their way to their deaths at age three or four.

This is a sad story, and our response to it should begin with a tear, with a lament, with a cry of complaint to God. When tears are shared in a community of faith, it is sometimes possible to work our way to the certainty that God hears our cries and to hope that God will yet bless the children—in spite of suffering and death and AIDS—for God is faithful to God's own cause, made known in Jesus. And while we cry and hope, while we watch and pray for God's good future, the community of faith may, through its care, at least bear witness to the God who suffers with those who suffer and grieves with those who grieve.

In Chapter Seven we talked of children as "gifts of God" (pp. 197-200). This notion should nurture a disposition in parents and in the community to welcome and cherish even children born with AIDS. To receive and welcome a child born with AIDS "as given" is itself a gesture of "uncalculating nurturance" (pp. 199-200). The obligations of parental care for such a child "as given" should not be disowned because the child is imperfect and doomed to suffering and death, but neither do the obligations of parental care include making any and every medically possible intervention in the desperate hope that the child can yet be made perfect or spared, "as though the imperfect materials themselves had to be surpassed for anything good to come of the life" (May, "Parenting," 154). Uncalculating nurturance of a child "as given" requires not an anxious effort to cure where there is no cure but a compassionate effort to care for the child while he is dying. That kind of care will surely include carrying and caressing and comforting—and sometimes saying no to desperate technological efforts to "save" the child.

The discussion in Chapter Nine about procreative decisions made in cases where there is a genetic risk to any future child (pp. 251-55) may also serve as a guide for procreative decisions by those who know they are infected with AIDS. There we commended decisions not to have children "when the probability of a genetic condition is high and where the magnitude of the harm caused by the genetic condition is great" (p. 255). AIDS is not a genetic condition, but the probability of the mother with AIDS infecting her child during pregnancy is great,[13] and the magnitude of the harm caused by AIDS is enormous; therefore, we recommend that those with AIDS choose not to have children. To help women with HIV see the wisdom of this choice and carry it out effectively, there must be voluntary screening programs, educational and counseling services, and funding for voluntary sterilization.[14]

Even with good programs and services to enable women infected with HIV to voluntarily prevent pregnancy, some of these women will become pregnant and face the question of ending the pregnancy by aborting the fetus. Our consideration of abortion in Chapter Nine also determines our response to abortion in the context of AIDS. Because we are not convinced by arguments that the fetus is an actual person at conception or implantation, we do not equate abortion with murder, but because of our argument that the fetus is a *potential* person at conception or implantation, we view abortion as a grave moral matter requiring serious justification (Chapter Two, pp. 34-47; p. 208). Further, because we are convinced that faithfulness to God requires a disposition to care for the vulnerable and to welcome them into our fellowship and community even if they have no legal "right" to it, we refuse to reduce the moral question of abortion to a legal question of the rights of the fetus, and we suggest (as the story of the good Samaritan suggests) that even when a fetus possibly infected with HIV is initially perceived as a threatening stranger, treating such a fetus as a neighbor will usually enable us to see it as one (pp. 208-23).

However, this disposition to welcome nascent life—developed and nurtured by Christian convictions and the Christian story—does

---

13. According to P. Ferrieri, as many as 50 percent of the children born to infected mothers will develop AIDS.

14. We oppose nonvoluntary screening programs and, of course, nonvoluntary sterilization.

not justify legal prohibitions against abortion (pp. 228-33). Moreover, the disposition to welcome nascent life is sometimes overwhelmed by other moral features of a particular situation. In our view, abortion is never to be celebrated, but it is sometimes tragically indicated. We mentioned some kinds of tragic circumstances in which we would regretfully recommend an abortion and/or cooperate with it (p. 226), and some of these circumstances are surely relevant to cases in which women with AIDS are pregnant. We said, for example, that "we would sadly but strongly recommend abortion when a woman's carrying a fetus is a serious and undeniable threat to her life" (p. 226) and that we would cooperate with abortion when there is a "significant threat to life or health" (p. 226)—and some pregnant women with AIDS are put in jeopardy by their pregnancy.

We said we would "recommend abortion in those rare cases in which life would inevitably be short and subjectively indistinguishable from torture" (pp. 227, 247-51). AIDS may be another such rare case to be set alongside the genetic conditions we have talked about; this is an empirical question that will be answered only after careful treatment and evaluation of the living and dying of those born with AIDS. In any case, until an accurate diagnostic test for HIV infection of the fetus is developed, we cannot recommend abortion for fetuses at 30 to 50 percent risk for AIDS. However, we think the risk is great enough and the harm momentous enough for Christians to cooperate with abortion under these circumstances, at least when the decision is made with sensitivity to the covenantal presumption against eliminating suffering by eliminating the sufferer.

We also said we could cooperate with abortion in cases in which the future life of the fetus would be too burdensome for the woman to bear alone and there is also very limited willingness or very limited ability of other members of society to help bear the burden (pp. 228, 250). Sadly, such is sometimes the case for pregnant women infected with HIV, and we can think of circumstances in which we would cooperate with a woman's decision that abortion is a tragic necessity. At the same time, we call upon society to support programs and services for women with AIDS and for their children that will make the choice not to become pregnant a realistic possibility, and that, should pregnancy occur, will make the choice not to abort a realistic possibility. Sharing tears and suffering, bearing one another's burdens of grief, can be a beginning for healing— if not for a child afflicted with AIDS, at least for a society divided by it. Our sharing of laments and burdens, when done in community, may finally turn into confidence in the God who would bless children in spite of death and suffering and AIDS, into hope for God's grace and future, and into the comforting assurance that even now and until then God suffers with those who suffer, grieves with those who grieve.

Dying of AIDS and Covenantal Caring

Finally, we come to death. The person with AIDS is dying, and our response to that sad fact is guided by the reflections throughout this book, but especially those in Chapter Ten. Much of that chapter—indeed, most of it—could simply be repeated in the context of discussing AIDS; short of that, we will at least underscore some points in response to AIDS.

The chapter began by calling for a distinction between the sick role and the dying role (pp. 268-73). This distinction has almost been obliterated by the tendencies of medicine to deny its own limits and the tendencies of patients to have extravagant expectations. But AIDS has reminded us of both human mortality and the limits of medicine; it has shown the reality and the importance of the distinction between being sick and dying in ways no argument could. Even so, some—care-givers as well as patients—refuse to acknowledge that they are "overmastered by their diseases": some patients refuse to shift their focus from getting well to living well until they die, and some care-givers refuse to shift their focus from curing their sick patient to caring for their dying patient. We hope for a cure and for the coming of "the great physician," but in the meantime we call people to acknowledge and to honor the role of dying.

Earlier we said, "The dying are still living, after all" (p. 299). That point seemed too obvious to stress before, but we should emphasize it in response to AIDS. Many have been ready—indeed, eager—to assign patients with AIDS the dying role, but doing so has sometimes been another attempt to distance them from the rest of us, to separate them as "the dying" from us, "the living," to dissolve the bonds of community among all the mortal living. The truth about AIDS and about the limits of medicine should not be denied, but neither should the simple truth be denied that those dying of AIDS are still living and still deserve the care and respect due living image-bearers of God.

In response to AIDS it is necessary to underscore the sanctity (pp. 274-75) of AIDS patients. This sanctity, this deferential awe and reverence due AIDS patients as image bearers of God, requires care, to be sure, but it also guides and directs that care. Sanctity entails—as we can extrapolate from our earlier discussion (pp. 298-99)—both a prohibition against intentionally killing a person with AIDS and a prohibition against intentionally inflicting extraordinary treatment upon someone with AIDS against that person's will.

The first of these entailments may simply be repeated and emphasized: mercy killing and suicide (pp. 297-303) are prohibited as responses to AIDS. A doctor may risk death in order to achieve some great good or to avoid some great harm for the patient, or a patient may risk death to achieve some greater good or to avoid some greater harm, but death itself may not be intended. Death may be accepted as a foreseeable consequence of a human action (or omission) that intends some other great good or the avoidance of some other great harm, but the death of one still cloaked in sanctity may not be directly intended.

The second of the entailments also needs to be underscored: no "extraordinary" treatments may be imposed on AIDS patients against their will. We described "extraordinary" treatment (pp. 275-76) as that which is judged to be "excessively costly (even if beneficial)" or which offers "no reasonably probable benefit (even if cheap and easy)" (p. 276). Sanctity—and the respect it evokes for the AIDS patient as a giver and hearer of reasons and as a responsible choice-maker—requires not only that extraordinary treatments not be used against the patient's will but also that the patient's judgment about what counts as "extraordinary" be respected. However, we have not before and we do not now reduce morality to respect for autonomy or reduce the relevant moral questions to the procedural question about who should decide. The relational and interdependent nature of human selves should make us attentive to the possibility that, by saying some treatment is not "worth it" (and so is extraordinary), a patient with AIDS may really be saying, "I'm not worth it." And we should also be attentive to the possibility that the AIDS patient is saying "I'm not worth it" because medical professionals or family or friends or society has been saying (or the patient has at any rate been hearing them say), "You're not worth it." Sometimes the patient's refusal of treatment is really an attempt to raise a valid question: "Do you think I'm worth anything?" Accordingly, refusal of treatment should not be immediately accepted by family and friends (Chapter Two, p. 66). Conversation about the treatment should continue, and some care, including some medical care, may be necessary and indicated in order to continue the conversation and to determine whether such a refusal of treatment is really a veiled expression of feelings of desperation and guilt, of dependence and abandonment (Marzuk). Sometimes, however, continuing conversation will not provide a reason for the patient to collaborate in the treatment; sometimes the patient really means what he has said. In such circumstances treatment may not be imposed upon the patient without violating the patient's sanctity.

It is important to note, however, that AIDS sometimes renders a patient "incompetent" or at least only "partially competent" or "intermittently competent" (p. 280). It is not uncommon for people with AIDS to develop dementia. In such cases, of course, a surrogate decision-maker will have to make choices about medical treatment. Ordinarily, the "next of kin" or a spouse would be called upon to make such decisions. But some AIDS patients may be alienated from their "kin" and not want them or trust them to make decisions about their treatment. Or some AIDS patients may have a lover with whom they have a relationship analogous to that of spouse in a heterosexual marriage and to whom they would entrust such decisions, but the lover has no legal standing to become the surrogate decision-maker. In such cases it is especially important that those infected with HIV draft or use a document like the living will (see Box 10.1; pp. 284-86), which gives directives and designates an agent to determine their care when they are no longer competent. Such a document is the extension of the person's autonomy, and it should be respected.

Care for those who are dying from AIDS must include more than merely medical care. The dying person has needs that no medicine can touch — psychological, social, and spiritual needs. The person dying from AIDS needs relief from a sense of isolation and abandonment and relief from anxiety and fear as well as relief from pain. The one dying from AIDS needs to restore and maintain not only certain physiologic processes but also certain relationships with others. For these reasons we urge communal and church support for hospice programs (p. 306).

In response to AIDS the church may not abandon the AIDS patient to medicine nor the medical practitioner to science. The church has resources to nurture and sustain both the dying and the healer. It has resources in a story of perfect love that casts out fear—resources to cast out the fears of abandonment and death, to cast out the fears of infection and the failure to cure. It has resources in a story it loves to tell — resources for learning to love courageously and caringly—as Christians watch for the one who is to come, the one who commanded the way of love.

As the church faces what may be its severest test of faithfulness, it may find wisdom for responding in an old story that the rabbis used to tell.[15]

The sages asked, "Where shall we look for the messiah? Will he come to us on clouds of glory, robed in majesty and crowned with light?"

Rabbi Joshua ben Levi wondered too, and he put the question to the great Elijah. "Where shall I find the messiah?" he asked.

"At the gate of the city," Elijah replied.

15. Babylonian Talmud, Sanhedrin 98a, cited by K. Rosemann, 141.

"But how shall I recognize him?" Rabbi Joshua wanted to know.

"He sits among the lepers," was Elijah's reply.

Rabbi Joshua, astonished by the reply, protested, "Among the lepers? What is he doing there?"

"He changes their bandages," Elijah replied. "He changes them one by one."

Appendix A: Balancing Christian Compassion and Clinical Detachment

Kurt Kooyer

Christians have long known that health-care professionals treat complete persons and not simply diseases. We also know that our Christian identity calls us, even in our professional capacity, to treat all persons with whom we have contact as whole, unique individuals,[1] created in the image of God. Accordingly, we sometimes feel that we must invest the same love, compassion, and caring in each of our patients as Christ does, through his saving power, in each of us.

John Calvin points out that it is God's image we must embrace in our fellow man (*Institutes* III.vi.6). Correspondingly, it is only *after* recognizing this image that health professionals may see the organic malady which the imager has acquired. Patients, therefore, should never be identified as "cases" or "fractures" or "MIs." Neither are they GOMERS (Get Out of My Emergency Room), "dirtballs," or undesirables. Patients must be perceived as psychological, social, and spiritual creatures as well as physical creatures and recognized as image bearers worthy of all the dignity and respect God bestows on each individual. Since patients are deserving of our caring, understanding, and compassion, it seems clear that God expects us to invest ourselves personally and emotionally in each patient to the best of our abilities.

1. Secular society has become aware of the importance of recognizing all dimensions of the patient and has recently challenged the traditional biomedical orientation toward health and illness. This is evidenced by the systems-oriented biopsychosocial model championed by George Engel (43-60) at the University of Rochester as well as by the LEARN guidelines proposed by Elois Berlin and William Fowkes (934-38) at Stanford University. The LEARN guidelines are designed to aid the health practitioner in diagnosing and treating patients. The practitioner must Listen to the patient's perception of illness, Explain his or her perception of the illness, Acknowledge and discuss the similarities and differences of these perceptions, Recommend treatment, and Negotiate agreement.

But all Christian health-care practitioners are also aware of the phenomenon of clinical detachment as practiced and even recommended by many health-care professionals, and they are faced with trying to reconcile or choose between the rational, objective state in which human compassion and emotion are withdrawn and the Christian obligation to invest oneself personally in the lives of those who need health-care services. Three observations need to be made that will challenge the notion of complete personal investment and suggest that there may perhaps be room for clinical detachment in Christian health care.

The first observation is that complete emotional investment in each patient is physically quite impossible. Health-care practitioners work long hours, see many patients in short periods of time, and are expected to make quick, accurate diagnoses. The demands upon them are high, and, consequently, not only do they often find it difficult to give each patient the attention, understanding, and compassion deserved but also, as a result of trying to do so, they are often forced to neglect their families' needs and even their own personal needs. Under these conditions, attempts at complete emotional investment are quickly met with defeat and frustration.

A second observation is that, when crises arise in a medical context (and they often do), it is undeniably advantageous for health-care professionals to remain as objective as possible. Although emotional involvement is seemingly dictated by compassionate investment in patients, an outpouring of emotions, especially those emotions that hamper lucid thinking and physical coordination, is anything but beneficial in a life-or-death situation. Therefore, in crisis situations, clinical detachment *is* in the best interest of the patient and at these times must be not only tolerated but welcomed. Furthermore, Christian health-care professionals who develop feelings of shame or guilt as a result of experiencing clinical detachment need to realize that those emotions, though perhaps unavoidable, are indeed unwarranted.

A third observation to be made involves the notion that Christian investment of oneself, emotionally and compassionately, involves dealing with the psychological and sociological aspects of patients. However, because medical training emphasizes physiological mechanisms and diagnoses rather than behavioral sciences, most health-care professionals are not the qualified therapists their profession sometimes calls them to be. Certainly more than a little knowledge—and more than intuition—are required to deal effectively with all aspects of a human being. A liberal arts education may give a health professional the insight to recognize the psychological, social, and spiritual natures of the whole person, but it does not equip him or her with all the essential knowledge required to effectively counsel a patient in those areas. In fact, attempts at counseling, no matter how well-intentioned or wholehearted, can be not only unproductive in terms of expense and progress toward healing but even potentially detrimental to both patient and health-care practitioner (Hilfiker, 56). Simply stated, health-care professionals should not try to be all things to all people, for it is quite possible that this "complete investment" can result in more harm than good.

In short, although our Christian identity calls for unconditional compassion and unlimited selflessness and seemingly *refutes* the appropriateness of clinical detachment, the impossibility of complete emotional investment, the undesirability of subjectivity in times of crisis, and the limited counseling skills of health-care practitioners indicate that effective health care sometimes *warrants* clinical detachment. Christians must recognize that a proper balance between compassion and objectivity is integral to appropriate patient care and that "total emotional investment," though well-intentioned, is potentially more dangerous than laudable in a health-care system.

Appendix B: Health-Care Delivery in Great Britain, the United States, and Canada

Ken Faber and Scott Vander Linde

Introduction

The study of health-care systems has developed into a fascinating area of research.[1] Mechanisms of funding for health care, delivery of services, and administrative structures have all come under the critical eye of medical economists. These studies are often international in scope, as the health-care systems of several countries are being compared with one another. The obvious hope of these studies is that they will assist countries in assessing the strengths and weaknesses within their own health-care systems. Sharing this knowledge will also contribute to the betterment of all health-care systems globally, as similar issues and constraints are beginning to affect the evolution of each system.

What follows is a modest attempt at comparing the health-care systems of Canada, Great Britain, and the United States. The first part of this appendix presents a short history and some characteristic features of each system; the second part deals with problems found in each

1. Since completion of this appendix in July 1986, a series of articles and an editorial have appeared in *The New England Journal of Medicine*, largely confirming and elaborating upon the points made herein (Inglehart, "Health Policy Report," 202-8, 778-84, 1623-28; Relman, "United States," 1608-10). In addition, further policies have been proposed within each system described. The policies have been developed in response to patient concerns, reimbursement levels, and general allocation questions. This highlights the necessity of looking ahead in the health fields, and should not detract from the purpose of this article: to introduce the reader to the major issues continuing to shape health policy in each of these health-care systems.

system. The intent is not to provide an in-depth critical analysis of the three systems but to give the reader some general information regarding each system, with the hope that the discussion of problems within each system demonstrates that neither a free-market medical system nor a socialized medical system offers an ideal solution to the problem of health-care delivery.

History

Great Britain

The history of national health insurance in Great Britain begins in 1911 with the establishment of the National Health Insurance Scheme.[2] Originally this insurance, obtained through employment, gave rather restricted coverage. For example, dependents of insured persons were excluded from coverage, and benefits were applicable only to a limited number of maladies. In 1942 the Beveridge Report, with the help of a favorable social climate, recommended that the entire population of Great Britain have access to a limited amount of health care. John Jewkes, an economist at Oxford, credits this report with creating among British people an irresistible desire for a comprehensive national health service. The shift from minimum health services for some to comprehensive services for all occurred in 1944 with the publication of the White Paper on health services. The development of a health service that provided the best medical facilities to everyone regardless of the patient's ability to pay was perceived by the British citizenry as a natural progression from the health system outlined in the Beveridge Report (Jewkes and Jewkes, 3). The White Paper eventually became the blueprint for the formation of the National Health Service (NHS) in 1948.

The NHS is basically a hierarchy of government officials overseeing the work of health practitioners in government hospitals and clinics and in home care. Although the system is centrally organized, local authorities tend to the daily affairs of the individual hospitals. The hospitals are staffed by salaried physicians known as consultants (equivalent to specialist physicians in North America).

---

2. Information on the history and structure of the British health-care system was drawn from the following sources: Aaron and Schwartz; G. Berlyne; Day and Klein; R. Deardon; Drummond and Mooney; Jewkes and Jewkes; A. Lindsay; Mooney and Drummond; Simmons and Marine; M. Spicer; A. Williams; Yule and Mooney.

Consultants, although essentially employees of the state, may also pursue private practices, treating patients who may have purchased private health insurance in addition to state-provided insurance to avoid queuing for some national health services. Such patients are treated either in private hospitals or in government hospitals in beds allotted for private care when the NHS was first formed.[3] Recently there has been a heightened interest in private care, as evidenced by the increased number of beds available for private health care. In 1979 there were 6,758 such beds; by 1985 the number had risen to 10,174 (Day and Klein, 1291).

Compared with other nations, Great Britain has been highly successful in moderating total health-care expenditures. In proportion to the total amount of goods and services produced domestically (GDP, Gross Domestic Product) in 1984, Great Britain spent 5.6 percent on health care, whereas Canada spent 8.4 percent and the United States, 10.7 percent (Schieber and Poullier, 117). Important to Great Britain's successful record are the institutional role of the general practitioner and the explicit budget restrictions placed on national health expenditures.

Within the NHS the general practitioner (GP) oversees patient entry into the health system. In health care this role is often referred to as the "gatekeeper" role. All patients enroll in the NHS register at the office of the GP of their choice. From their GPs patients can expect to receive all primary-care services, including education about preventive health maintenance and treatment of minor ailments not requiring hospitalization. GPs are reimbursed on a per-capita basis for the patients they serve. In the event that a patient requires more specialized care than can be provided in the office, the GP can refer the patient to a consultant at one of the local hospitals. This is a routine matter for many diagnoses requiring specialty care. However, aware of the limited resources at the hospital level for services such as open-heart surgery and hip replacement, the GP may refrain from referring some patients because the high level of care needed is not economically feasible or because the waiting list is too long to benefit the patient in the near future. Therefore, the GP is instrumental in controlling the allocation of some health services.

Explicit budget restrictions within the National Health Service also help to explain its moderate total expenditures. The primary source of funding for the NHS is general income-tax revenue. Additional funds

3. Although there are a number of private hospitals in Great Britain, one can also find within most of the NHS hospitals a number of private or "pay-beds." The pay-beds were a concession granted to the medical profession when the NHS was formed to keep open the option of private care. Access to pay-beds requires payment of a specified sum of money that in turn is placed in the general funds of the hospital.

come from endowments that were in place before the establishment of the NHS and from "pay-beds" specified for private care. Recently, charitable contributions have been directed toward medical research rather than toward the provision of health-care services, since the populace generally regards provision of health care as a governmental responsibility.

As part of its budget deliberations each year, the British Parliament allocates health-care funds from general revenue to the Department of Health and Social Services (DHSS). Health-care allocations are generally based on the amount received by the DHSS the previous year, with an additional adjustment to compensate for inflation. The DHSS has the responsibility of distributing these funds to the fourteen governmentally defined health-care regions. The fourteen regions then divide the funds among the 192 individual districts, which are responsible for maintaining hospitals, providing care, and paying health-care practitioners. Britain averages roughly one hospital per district.

Once the budget has been determined and allocations have been made to the districts, health officials and hospital administrators know exactly how much money they may spend during the year on the patients in their districts. They also know that they will need to make decisions regarding the distribution of certain types of expensive care. In addition, if they upgrade diagnostic equipment or facilities for their hospitals, they realize that in future budgets there may be USS funding available for equipment in other districts or hospitals. The discipline of budget restrictions, therefore, forces difficult decisions about health-care allocation upon all involved in the system.

The United States

Whereas health care in Britain is essentially office based, the United States health-care system is directed toward hospital care.[4] Paul Starr, in his book *The Social Transformation of American Medicine*, presents an interesting picture of how health care became primarily hospital based. One of his most striking examples is found in the development of medical

---

4. Information on the history and structure of health-care delivery in the United States was drawn from the following sources: Aaron and Schwartz; F. Abrams; American Medical Association, "Report of the Council"; R. Blendon et al.; Council on Medical Service, "Closing the Gaps"; Himmelstein and Woolhandler; Lohr and Marquis; N. Lurie et al.; N. Macrae; C. Oberg; A. Relman, "United States and Canada"; P. Starr; U.S. Department of Commerce, Bureau of the Census, *Statistical Abstract of the United States: 1985*; Weller and Manga; Wilson and Neuhauser.

education. In the early part of the nineteenth century, control over medical education was at best minimal and more likely nonexistent (pp. 60-65). Gradually, however, individual states began to exert more stringent control over those practicing medicine, and in some states licensing became a requirement. This brought about a reorganization in medical education that is best typified by the establishment of the Johns Hopkins University School of Medicine in 1893. Entrance into Johns Hopkins was contingent upon the successful completion of four years of undergraduate study. Students accepted into the medical school were expected —after an additional four years of study in the classroom and in hospital clinical settings—to have adequate understanding of the basic sciences and adequate exposure to hospital treatment of various diseases. To further medical education, Johns Hopkins was the first medical school to develop hospital-based residency programs for those wishing to obtain additional clinical experience. Initially the exception, medical education at Johns Hopkins eventually became the norm that other medical schools also accepted.

This approach to medical education, with its heavy emphasis on the pathophysiology of disease, helped entrench the hospital-oriented approach to health care one finds in the United States today. Scientific medical advances made throughout the first half of the twentieth century were understood by the medical profession to be most effectively implemented in the hospital. Furthering this hospital orientation, in the 1940s the American Hospital Association organized a national commission to assess the needs for hospitals in each state. The commission concluded that 195,000 additional beds were needed in the nation (an increase of 40 percent) at a projected cost of $1.8 billion (Starr, 349). This study helped move Congress toward enacting the 1946 Hospital Survey and Construction Act (known as the Hill-Burton program) to address this "national priority," which allocated $3.7 billion for construction funding over the next twenty-five years. By 1970 the Hill-Burton program had contributed significantly to the shape of our health-care system: it had added 334,438 acute-care beds, 93,749 beds for long-term care, 1,032 outpatient facilities, 520 rehabilitation facilities, 1,258 public-health centers, and 41 state laboratories (S. Jonas, *Health*, 393).

The focus on physician specialization, even among primary-care physicians, also bears out the United States' tendency toward technical, hospital-based care. Currently, 13.3 percent of American physicians are employed in general and family practices; the remainder—the overwhelming majority— are specialists with tighter hospital affiliations. When the other primary-care specialties — pediatrics, internal medicine, and obstetrics/gynecology—are included, 43.3 percent are employed in primary-care treatment (American Medical Association, *Physician Characteristics,* 19). By comparison, in Great Britain approximately two-thirds of all physicians are GPs, and the remainder are consultants, whereas in Canada approximately 50 percent of physicians are GPs, and the remainder, specialists (Metcalfe, 144).

Traditionally, access to medical care in the United States has been contingent upon patients' agreeing to pay a specified fee for the services provided by the health-care team—a fee-for-service reimbursement system. Eighty-five to ninety percent of Americans have some form of health insurance to assist them in paying for health care they require.

Health insurance in the United States comes in several private and public varieties. Private insurance is often closely connected to jobs. Employees are often able to select from insurance plans offered by their employer as a fringe benefit. Historically, the most significant private insurers have been the nonprofit Blue Cross–Blue Shield network, which was first to enter the private insurance market, and the for-profit insurers with such familiar titles as Aetna, Equitable, Metropolitan, Prudential, and so forth. The plans available to employees vary greatly from one employer to the next. The typical private insurance plan covers a large portion of hospitalization expenses and in-hospital physician expenses, with much less thorough coverage of office-based physician care. The insured often incur out-of-pocket expenses for services they receive, the total amount depending upon "copayments" and "deductibles" built into their specific plans and the type of services covered. A copayment plan requires patients to pay for a predetermined percentage of the total hospital bill. For example, if a patient's bill is $2,000 and the copayment is 20 percent, the patient must pay $400 toward the total cost. Some plans charge a deductible. For example, if a patient's deductible is $450, the patient must pay the first $450 of the bill. Therefore, even though private insurance is extensively subscribed, out-of-pocket expenses remain substantial among the privately insured. In recent years, private insurance has covered roughly 56 percent of total health expenses incurred by those participating in private plans (S. Jonas, *Health,* 317).

In contrast to the fee-for-service reimbursement arrangements traditionally characterizing insurance arrangements in the United States, private financing of health care is now moving in the direction of prospective reimbursement and contracted care arrangements. Employers are shopping for and finding less expensive insurance coverage for their employees among the "alphabet soup" alternatives to traditional insurance provision. Health-maintenance organizations (HMOs), independent physician associations (IPAs), and preferred-provider organizations (PPOs) are the most widely available and recognized. The common denominator of these insurance groups is the idea of contracted care. HMO and IPA insurers contract with hospitals and physicians to provide a blanket of services on an annual fee-per-patient basis (or, in the case of some HMOs—for example, Kaiser Permanente health plan in the western United States—the HMO directly hires physicians and owns hospital facilities). Total care is provided for this prepaid, contracted fee, but the focus is on preventive care to minimize expensive treatment in the future. By means of incentives for practitioner and patient to prescribe and use services efficiently, HMOs and IPAs discourage the superfluous use of services. Preventive care and efficient use of services assure the insurers that they will in fact be able to cover all group health expenses for the one-time yearly premium.

PPOs are insurance groups that often insure large employer groups. The size of the patient pool that the PPO represents allows it to contract with hospitals and physicians to provide services at "preferred" rates. Patients insured by a PPO have the option of receiving care from any provider they wish. However, by using a "preferred" physician or hospital, they substantially reduce copayments or other out-of-pocket expenses. This arrangement exerts pressure on providers to keep costs low in order to be able to provide services and premiums that are competitively priced in the growing marketplace of insurance providers.

In addition to private insurance plans, the government provides insurance for certain segments of the U.S. population. Those who are unable to afford health insurance and who qualify for federal cash-assistance programs (Aid for Families with Dependent Children and Supplemental Security Income) are eligible for the Medicaid program. Those older than sixty-five and qualifying for Social Security qualify for the Medicare program. The first prominent discussion of government-sponsored health care dates back to 1935 and the establishment of the Social Security Act (SSA), wherein the federal government agreed to indirectly provide funds for health care. In 1950, amendments to the SSA made the federal government responsible for providing matching grants to each state for the health care of patients on public assistance. In 1960, an additional amendment to the SSA made elderly welfare recipients eligible for coverage. In 1965, Title XVIII and Title XIX of the SSA officially established Medicare and Medicaid.

It is interesting to note that Medicare and Medicaid are the outcome of much political debate and public concern over the health-care needs of those without sufficient financial access to the U.S. health-care system. However, as the programs have evolved, many observers view them as palliative at best, providing a floor of insurance coverage that contains many cracks.

In the thirty years prior to the enactment of Medicare and Medicaid, several comprehensive national health-insurance plans appeared as bills before the U.S. Congress and as planks in the platforms of elected presidents. National health insurance surfaced again and again in the New Deal legislation under Franklin D. Roosevelt. Although a proponent of many of the national health-insurance proposals in principle, Roosevelt hesitated to give full backing to any of the proposals in practice for fear that in doing so he would compromise other legislative goals he believed were more important. When World War II was nearing its end, Roosevelt finally committed himself to making comprehensive insurance a postwar priority. Harry S. Truman carried forth that priority following Roosevelt's death. Political opposition precluded enactment of a comprehensive insurance plan prior to the 1948 election. However, comprehensive national health insurance seemed an inevitable outcome of the 1948 election, since Truman emerged a surprise victor while running on a platform that promised national health insurance if he was elected. However, public sentiment toward Truman's proposal was quashed following the election by the extensive lobby efforts of the American Medical Association and its business allies. The lobby campaign that was orchestrated was more expensive than any previously undertaken in U.S. history. (For a more detailed discussion of the history of national health insurance, see Starr, pp. 242-95.)

No major support for health-insurance legislation appeared again until the Great Society movement in the 1960s. Although Medicare and Medicaid resulted in coverage for groups seriously lacking in access to health care, their scope is limited compared with the scope of the earlier national health-insurance proposals. The programs are much like the private insurance plans, but designed for select groups, with deductibles and copayments as major features.

Additional government health programs and provisions available include veteran benefits, workmen's compensation, public-health departments, mental-health facilities, and the construction of research facilities. In total, the federal and state governments spend 42 percent of all health-care dollars (U.S. Department of Commerce, *Statistical Abstract of the United States: 1985*, 96).

In summary, health-care delivery in the United States is considerably more complex than in Great Britain and in Canada, as we will see. Access to health care comes via a patchwork of private and public insurance sources and facilities. The public programs that have emerged, however, mimic to a large degree the philosophy behind private insurance and the incentives contained therein in order to retain political viability.

Canada

The Canadian health-care system is unique in that it incorporates elements of both the British and the American systems.[5] A combination of both socialized medicine and free-market–oriented medicine has helped to form the system as it presently exists. It is possible to argue on the one hand that, since all Canadians theoretically have access to health care and since the government is the only health insurer, the system is indeed socialized. On the other hand, health practitioners in Canada are usually not paid a salary by the government and may maintain private practices in which patients may be accepted and dismissed. Furthermore, in some provinces, physicians are allowed to charge what they wish for services rendered.

Health care in Canada is a provincial responsibility as outlined by Canada's constitution, the British North American Act. Although a national health system was first proposed in 1919, it was not until 1945 that a bill suggesting a joint federal/provincial system was presented. This first proposal, modeled after the British White Paper proposal, was never developed. However, in 1955, government-sponsored health care was revived when five provinces began to offer comprehensive hospital insurance. By 1961 all the provinces had insurance for hospital care under the guarantee that the federal government would provide 50 percent of the necessary resources. In 1964, Justice Emmett Hall, in what has come to be called the Hall Report, suggested that a comprehensive health-care system should be established for all of Canada. In 1968 Hall's recommendations were realized in the Medical Care Act.

The Medical Care Act put in place a health-care system wherein each province is solely responsible for delivery of health care to its constituents but only partially responsible for providing funds. The federal government assists the provincial health services through a process called transfer payments. Prior to 1977 the federal government's contribution amounted to about 50 percent of the total health-care bill. After 1977, feeling the pinch of economic recession, the federal government enacted legislation that established its contribution to provincial health services as a certain proportion of overall growth in gross national product. The result of the new legislation was a reduction in transfer payments, which forced the provinces to make up the difference via increased taxation.

---

5. Information on the history and structure of health-care delivery in Canada was drawn from the following sources: P. Banks; *Canada Yearbook: 1985;* de Pouvourville and Renaud; H. Emson; Kane and Kane; Linton and Naylor; V. Navarro; D. Owen; L. Richard; L. Rozovsky; Shah and Farkas; H. Southall; P. Tripp; Vayda and Deber.

Each province employs its own techniques for meeting its share of the health-care budget. Alberta, for example, uses general taxation, hospital user fees, and health-insurance premiums; Quebec relies solely on funds generated by general taxation; and Ontario finances care through insurance premiums and general taxation. The provinces are also responsible for allocating the resources to individual hospitals. Every year each hospital receives a lump sum to cover all health-care expenses except doctors' fees. How a hospital decides to spend its allocation is determined by that hospital's board of trustees.

Physicians are reimbursed directly by the provincial government on a fee-for-service basis in accordance with a schedule of fees established jointly by physicians' associations and the provincial government. Physicians in some provinces may "opt out" of the provincial remuneration system and directly bill their patients. Patients billed in this manner may send their bills to the provincial health service and be compensated for the services rendered at the provincially established levels. Whether a physician is in private practice or employed by a government-operated clinic, government-insured patients have ready access to him or her. Physicians working in government clinics are either paid a salary or paid on a fee-per-patient basis, while private-practice physicians bill the provincial health service on a fee-for-service basis. In both settings, the patient does not pay directly for services rendered, but the physician is paid by the same insurer.

In summary, the Canadian health-care system is a cooperative effort of federal and provincial governments. The system is decentralized in that each province administers its own system. Furthermore, physicians are allowed to pursue private practice on a fee-for-service basis. Finally, the system effectively provides comprehensive health care to all Canadians without problems of extensive rationing and queuing.

Health-Care Delivery Systems—A Critique

Each health-care system described, regardless of its funding mechanisms, organization, and administration, is beset with problems. What follows is a discussion of three problems considered significant or potentially significant for the future of health-care delivery in one or all three countries under discussion. The three problems are stagnation, lack of patient responsibility, and funding and cost containment.

The problem of stagnation is apparent in the British system and especially prominent in the Canadian system. In the United States, citizens have numerous options from which to select a health-insurance plan, and market mechanisms tend to promote innovations rather than stagnation. In Great Britain, citizens can select from governmental and/or private insurance plans if their personal incomes permit, but in Canada there is no option other than the provincial health service. Although the uniformity of the British and Canadian systems makes them administratively efficient, they do not encourage the innovation and creativity that led to the establishment of HMOs and PPOs in the United States but instead promote a tendency toward stagnation. This stagnation may become more significant in the future as the health-care needs of society change, invariably becoming more costly.

A second problem evident historically in each of the systems has been the absence of incentives for patients to remain healthy. Health care has been viewed more as measures necessary to combat existing maladies than as means to promote current and future health. A contributing factor may be that access to care, especially in Britain and Canada, has come largely without patients' having to pay significant out-of-pocket expenses. As a result, little thought has been given to maintaining lifestyles that encourage health. Although out-of-pocket costs are more significant in the United States, the hospital-care orientation of American medicine has evidenced the same philosophy. In Britain and the United States, explicit efforts are currently being made to alter this philosophy. In Britain, preventive medicine is at the forefront of the GP gatekeeper system (Schwartz and Aaron). In the United States, preventive medicine and cost containment are goals of many HMO systems. In addition to increases in out-of-pocket expenditures via deductibles and copayments for all but preventive services, premium rebates for remaining healthy, smoker/nonsmoker premium differentials, premium differentials for fitness-program participants, and so forth are also suggested as incentives within insurance plans to make consumers take greater responsibility for their personal health.

Funding and cost control seem to be the most prominent problems experienced by health-care systems in Great Britain, Canada, and the United States. In Great Britain, inadequate funding for services, resulting in long queues for some services, is a significant problem. The decreasing number of hospital beds available in Britain reflects the funding tightness. In 1971 there were 9.1 beds per 1,000 people, but by 1980 the number had dropped to 7.7 beds per 1,000 people (Metcalfe, 142). One consequence of the decrease in the number of beds is increased queuing for elective-surgery services such as hip replacement and coronary-artery surgery (Aaron and Schwartz, 30). In an era of fiscal conscientiousness among politicians, tighter budget constraints and increased costs have taken their toll on Great Britain's health care. As one hospital administrator put it, "The first thing we've done is stop looking after buildings which then fall down. We cut cleaning, catering, maintenance. We don't replace equipment. We don't spend on capital. We stop growth. Then we cut into the muscles. We cut back services. . . . We are cutting into muscles now. The fat went three years ago" (Simmons and Marine, 323).

In an effort to control health-care expenditures, politicians in Great Britain have forced physicians to make explicit rationing decisions, especially with respect to high-cost treatments and diagnostic equipment. One most noteworthy example is the treatment of end-stage kidney disease with dialysis. The policy adopted by the British provides kidney dialysis for patients under fifty years of age who are free of any other complicating conditions, such as diabetes. If a patient fails to meet the criteria for being accepted into a dialysis program, a general practitioner will usually refrain from telling the patient that treatment is available, even though the patient needs dialysis. (In fact, it is not available to such a patient.) In this way, confrontation and stress over being refused a life-saving treatment are avoided. As one practitioner put it, "We choose not to treat those patients who are a bit crumbly" (Aaron and Schwartz, 35). Thus, in Great Britain the number of patients does not determine the budget. Rather, the budget determines the number of patients.

In Great Britain there is also a general aversion to the development of high-technology medicine. This phenomenon is fueled by the demographics of Britain, where the most rapidly increasing segment of the population is the over-65 age group. Popular support plays a significant role in determining how resources are spent, as is evident from these comments by two British hospital administrators:

> No one is going to praise us for closing an old age ward to open new heart surgery. We have to cut back on high technology. . . .

> We have two units in this hospital that are unused. One was supposed to be an isolation unit for infectious diseases . . . ; the other, a reverse barrier isolation unit . . . intended for bone-marrow transplantation. If I were to suggest we open these units before we opened the psychiatric day hospital or the geriatric hospital, we'd be torn to shreds by the Community Councils. (Simmons and Marine, 325)

It is important to British people that resources allotted for health care are spent in a manner that provides maximum benefit to the greatest number of people. Organ transplants, life-prolonging procedures, and other high-tech procedures and diagnostics are generally not believed to provide cost-effective care. Therefore, the British have mandated that life-prolonging procedures be reserved for the young, and they allot only small proportions of the total health-care budget to high-tech services. For example, Britain's rate of coronary-artery bypass surgery is one-tenth the U.S. rate; there are one-sixth the number of CT scanners available per person in Great Britain that there are in the United States, and X-ray departments take one-half as many X-rays and use one-half the amount of film per examination (Aaron and Schwartz, 28).

But there are positive aspects associated with the refusal to invest heavily in medical technology. British physicians have been fortunate enough to retain many of the interpersonal skills that North American physicians are losing. The tendency toward increased technology in Canada and the United States has caused many medical practitioners to become technicians, manipulators of instruments and observers of data. In North America, a treatment protocol is often dictated by what costly lab reports reveal, reports that often confirm the physician's suspicion. This point is made not to bemoan the use of laboratory diagnostics but merely to underscore the fact that in North America we have gradually increased our reliance on them and have, in the process, simultaneously increased costs and dulled interpersonal skills. In making their health allocations away from high-tech care, the British demonstrate that their foremost priority is providing a standard level of care for everyone in their society. Additional care is available to a limited number, especially to those with greatest ability to pay, but not at the expense of adequate access to care for each British citizen.

In summary, medical services are openly rationed in Great Britain — but limiting services is the only logical option available to the National Health System. Since British citizens will allow their government to allocate only a certain amount of tax revenues to health care, the government must respond by limiting some health services. Consequently, the British spend less than 6 percent of their total national expenditure—GDP—on health-care services.

In the United States, total health-care expenditure at nearly 11 percent of GDP appears to be sufficient to provide for all health-care needs of the population. However, the market-oriented health system is leaving startling numbers of U.S. citizens without access to health care. Those with no health insurance have increased from 20 to 25 million in the late 1970s to 31 to 37 million today (Gail Wilensky, 34-35). When estimates of the underinsured are included—the underinsured being persons likely to spend more than 10 percent of their annual incomes on health expenses despite some insurance coverage— the numbers increase to 51 million ("Council Report"). It is not the profoundly poor who lack adequate insurance; they are covered by the Medicaid program. It is, rather, the working poor; their incomes or level of assets preclude their qualification for Medicaid, but they have too little income to purchase sufficient amounts of private insurance. This problem of access is exacerbated by the cuts in federal and state health-care contributions, which have decreased hospitals' willingness to allocate money for indigent care.

Concern over escalating total health-care expenditures has acutely characterized recent health policy in the United States and in Canada. What gives rise to this concern is the increasing percentage of the total domestic expenditure that is being consumed by health-care goods and services. In the United States the percent of total domestic output spent on health care increased from 5.3 percent in 1960 to 10.7 percent in 1984. In Canada the percent of total domestic output spent on health care increased from 5.5 percent in 1960 to 8.4 percent in 1984. Just less than one half of U.S. expenditure increases and just more than one half of Canadian increases can be attributed to the greater utilization of services and to the use of equipment more expensive than that used previously (for example, nuclear resonance imaging instead of X-ray equipment). The remainder of the expenditure change is due to inflation in the prices of health-care services (Schieber and Poullier, 117-20).

Both systems have encouraged these quantity and price increases for health-care goods and services through their reimbursement systems. In the United States, until the early 1980s, insurance would reimburse up to 100 percent of charges it considered "reasonable" for virtually any test or procedure provided for insured clients. There were few incentives in this system to moderate yearly fee increases or to carefully consider the cost of tests and procedures performed relative to the gains in diagnostic knowledge or health. In fact, there was a great tendency to employ a greater number of more technically advanced techniques and procedures than may have been absolutely required. Canada faces a similar problem with overutilization of services. Since everyone is insured and individuals bear little out-of-pocket cost for services used, there is little hesitation to use the system. Thus it is not surprising that in the province of Ontario, for example, one finds more hospital beds per capita and more extensive use of the hospital beds than in either the United States or Great Britain (Vayda and Deber, 19).

In the United States, the environment of escalating health-care costs, in combination with a more general political philosophy of scaling back the size of government, led to several major health-policy changes in the 1980s. In 1981 the Omnibus Budget Reconciliation Act reduced the federal payments available for Medicaid and increased the deductible for Medicare (Lohr and Marquis, 24). In 1982 the Tax Equity and Fiscal Responsibility Act (TEFRA) introduced copayments for some Medicaid patients, allowed states to restrict eligibility criteria for Medicaid, and laid the groundwork for prospective payment schemes (Lohr and Marquis, 31). Finally, in 1983, diagnostic-related groups (DRGs) were implemented for Medicare reimbursement to hospitals. The DRG system is a prospective-payment scheme that categorizes diseases into specific groups. For example, three of the ten most commonly reimbursed DRGs are heart failure and shock, simple pneumonia and pleurisy, and chronic obstructive pulmonary disease. Thus, if a Medicare patient enters the hospital, the hospital will receive a predetermined amount of money for treating that patient, how much depending upon the DRG into which the patient's diagnosis falls. If the hospital is able to treat the patient for less money, the hospital realizes a profit, but if the patient's bill runs over the amount specified by the DRG, the hospital must absorb the cost.

The result of the legislation just discussed has been significant with regard to trends in patient care as well as trends in the overall health-care environment. Health-cost increases have not been as pronounced since the implementation of TEFRA and the DRG system. However, the reduction in the rate of health-cost increase that has occurred can largely be attributed to reductions in the use of services by select groups. It is not occurring because actual costs per day of service have been declining. For example, the number of physician visits and hospital admissions for patients younger than 65 has dropped substantially, especially for the uninsured (Freeman et al.). For the elderly, slight reductions in admissions have occurred as well as substantial decreases in the average length of hospital stay (Davis et al.). The incidence of "patient dumping" has also increased (see Chapter Six, p. 160). Dumping has in turn put additional strain on the "overloaded and underfunded resources of the public hospitals" (Relman, "Texas," 578). Much of the tragedy associated with dumping is that a proportion of the patients are transferred without being stabilized first. This subjects patients to a much greater risk of death or permanent debilitation than the risk they face if they receive treatment at the hospitals where they are first delivered. To cope with this problem, several states, most notably Texas, have enacted legislation that effectively removes a hospital's license if it practices dumping (Relman, "Texas," 578). Additionally, built into the Consolidated Omnibus Budget Reconciliation Act, implemented in 1986, is legislation addressing patient dumping. This act places the legal burden of responsibility not on the hospital but on the physician who transfers a patient because of the patient's economic status. The financial burden continues to be borne primarily by the hospital. Despite these measures, however, health statistics continue to reveal that the cutbacks in services and the new financial arrangements are having detrimental effects on the health of poor people in the United States (Lurie et al., 1268; Freeman et al.). Finally, recent health legislation, especially by establishing a cumbersome DRG system, has created an environment of competitiveness and cost containment for public and private health-care financing institutions and providers of service. The state Medicaid programs have been encouraged to experiment with HMO and DRG financing arrangements. DRG schemes have been proposed for reimbursing physicians providing specific hospital-based services—for example, radiology, anesthesiology and pathology services. Additional reimbursement proposals for all physicians providing service to Medicare patients are currently under discussion as well. These changes have precipitated cost competition among private insurers, generating the "alphabet soup" insurance alternatives described earlier.

Canada has also developed several strategies to counter the problem of escalating health-care costs. In 1977 the federal government began to limit its health-care payments to the provinces. As a result, budgets of individual hospitals are no longer open-ended, and hospitals have to ensure that no cost overruns are encountered. Both the federal and the provincial governments have also stepped up efforts encouraging preventive care, and, finally, administrative structures have been streamlined by the elimination of duplicative administrative services. In addition, provincial governments have enacted legislation limiting the number of residencies available to graduating medical students. The reduction of residencies, coupled with the pressure to reduce the number of students admitted to Canadian medical schools, is an attempt to decrease the number of high-priced specialists who can perform certain procedures. A reduction in the number of available physicians, it is hoped, will reduce the per-capita use of health-care services.

Conclusion

The real test of success for health-care systems will be felt in the future, when present demographics shift sufficiently to place additional financial burden on the already strained health-care resources of each country. Will the British respond with increased queuing and rationing or through greater reprivatization of health-care services? Will the Canadians drift to increased or decreased governmental control of health care? Will the United States establish more social programs for the currently uninsured? What innovative approaches to health-care delivery does the future hold?

The answers to these questions will come soon enough. What cannot wait for future discussion, however, is the plight of the uninsured and underinsured in the United States and the increasingly difficult access to health care for persons with low income. It is clear that access is a persistently growing problem in the United States. This problem is compounded by the fact that the leading causes of death in the United States—heart disease, cancer, and lung disease—are expensive diseases to diagnose and treat and that the United States is inclined toward hospital care, replete with expensive, technologically advanced services. The United States continues to show its unwillingness to provide this technologically superior level of care for all its citizens. Therefore, it is urgent that the United States make explicit policy decisions about what minimum level of preventive and invasive care it is willing to provide for all of its citizens and that it alter its system accordingly so that all Americans have access to a specified level of health care.

Appendix C: The State of Health throughout the World

It is very difficult to comprehend the scope of health-care problems on a national or global scale or the prevalence and distribution of health-care resources. Pictures may be worth a thousand words, but when the global population exceeds five billion people, even pictures cannot suffice. Television may intensely though briefly focus on starving children in Ethiopia, but how can it convey the fact that every day over 35,000 children die across the globe from the effects of malnutrition? What the media do best is to focus on the tragedies of individuals or relatively small groups with sudden and sensational problems. Those with recurring ailments, diseases, and tragedies are often neglected because their stories are not attached to specific names and faces and because our sensitivities too often become dulled after just a few reminders of the chronic health peril of those we do not know and may never have seen. It is typical of our fallen human nature to be morbidly curious about or indignant over the victims of airline disasters, massive poisonings in India or Cameroon, and artificial-heart experimentation while at the same time we ignore or trivialize the carnage on our highways, our own lethal toxic dumps, the ravages of malaria and schistosomiasis, and the lack of preventive medicine.

This appendix attempts to assess the health-care needs and resources of many of the major countries of the world, not through pictures but through charts and figures, the tools of demographers. It is an attempt to portray the distribution of health and health care nationally and globally. It is left for the reader to translate the quantitative data into mental pictures of the health status of people by political and geographic boundaries. There are reasons—many of them good—why we might question the validity of some of the data. (A few sample questions make the point: How similar are the criteria for being a physician, a nurse, or a dentist in Third World countries and in Canada and the United States? How does one obtain accurate figures from remote areas that lack any form of technological communication and are highly inaccessible?). But it is doubtful whether these factors would significantly alter the profile of the health of people or their access to health care.

Demographers typically use figures for birthrate, death rate, life expectancy, and infant mortality to crudely measure health care or quality of life in a population. These figures may be further subdivided according to such factors as economic class, race, ethnic background, and geographical and political (national) boundaries. Health-care resources are typically measured in two ways: by the hospital and/or general health-care expenditures per capita and by the availability of health-care practitioners per capita.

On the next several pages are tables that depict these demographic statistics for forty countries, for the fifty states and the District of Columbia in the United States, and for the ten provinces and two territories in Canada. In addition, several tables reflect the leading causes of morbidity and mortality in Third World countries, Canada, and the United States.

Table 1. Basic Health Indicators
For Various Countries of the World[a]

Countries	GNP per capita in 1986 US $	1986 life expectancy at birth (years)	1986 crude birth rate per 1,000 population	1986 crude death rate per 1,000 population	1986 infant mortality rate (per 1,000 live births)	1981 population per physician	1981 population per nurse	1985 daily calorie supply per capita
Low-income economies[b]	270	61	30	10	69	6,050	3,830	2,329
Bangladesh	160	50	41	15	121	9,690	19,370	1,804
China	300	69	19	7	34	1,730	1,670	2,620
Ethiopia	120	46	47	19	155	88,150	5,000	1,704
Guinea	—	42	46	23	148	56,170	6,250	1,731
Haiti	330	54	35	13	119	9,200	—	1,784
India	290	57	32	12	86	3,700	4,670	2,126
Mali	180	47	48	19	144	26,030	2,280	1,810
Sierra Leone	310	41	48	24	154	19,130	2,100	1,784
Sri Lanka	400	70	24	6	29	7,460	1,260	2,485
Uganda	230	48	50	18	105	21,270	2,000	2,483
Middle-income economies	1,270	63	31	9	65	4,940	1,400	2,719
Lower-middle-income economies[c]	750	59	35	10	77	7,880	1,760	2,511
Costa Rica	1,480	74	29	4	18	1,440	—	2,807
Cuba	—	75	16	6	14	720	370	3,088
Dominican Republic	710	66	32	7	67	1,440	1,240	2,530
Ecuador	1,160	66	34	7	64	—	—	2,005
El Salvador	820	61	37	9	61	2,550	—	2,155
Guatemala	930	61	41	9	61	—	1,360	2,345
Honduras	740	64	41	8	72	3,100	690	2,224
Indonesia	490	57	28	11	87	12,330	2,300	2,476
Ivory Coast	730	52	49	14	96	—	—	2,308
Jordan	1,540	65	39	7	46	1,190	1,160	2,968
Liberia	460	54	46	13	87	9,340	2,920	2,373
Nicaragua	790	61	42	9	65	2,230	590	2,464
Nigeria	640	51	50	16	104	9,400	2,690	2,139
Papua New Guinea	720	52	36	13	64	15,610	930	2,145
Philippines	560	63	35	7	46	6,850	2,640	2,260

	GNP per capita in 1986 US $	1986 life expectancy at birth (years)	1986 crude birth rate per 1,000 population	1986 crude death rate per 1,000 population	1986 infant mortality rate (per 1,000 live births)	1981 population per physician	1981 population per nurse	1985 daily calorie supply per capita
Upper-middle-income economies[d]	1,890	67	27	8	50	1,380	900	2,967
Argentina	2,350	70	23	9	33	—	—	3,210
Brazil	1,810	65	29	8	65	1,300	1,140	2,657
Israel	6,210	75	22	7	12	400	130	3,019
Mexico	1,860	60	29	6	48	1,210	—	3,126
Venezuela	2,920	70	30	5	37	1,000	—	2,485
High-income oil exporters[e]	6,740	64	41	8	62	1,380	580	3,213
Kuwait	13,890	73	32	3	19	700	180	3,102
Saudi Arabia	6,950	63	42	8	64	1,800	730	3,057
Industrial market economies[f]	12,960	76	13	9	9	550	180	3,357
Australia	11,920	78	15	7	10	520	140	3,302
Canada	14,120	76	15	7	8	550	120	3,443
Japan	12,840	78	12	7	6	740	210	2,695
New Zealand	7,460	74	16	8	11	610	150	3,393
United Kingdom	8,870	75	13	12	9	680	120	3,148
United States	17,480	75	16	9	10	500	180	3,682
East European nonmarket economies[g]								
Czechoslovakia	—	70	14	12	14	350	130	3,473
USSR	—	70	19	10	30	270	—	3,332

[a]data compiled from the World Bank, *World Development Report: 1988* (New York: Oxford University Press, 1988), pp. 222-87.

[b]category includes Afghanistan, Benin, Bhutan, Burkina Faso, Burma, Burundi, Central African Republic, Chad, Ghana, Democratic Kampuchea, Kenya, Lao PDR, Lesotho, Madagascar, Malawi, Mauritania, Mozambique, Nepal, Niger, Pakistan, Rwanda, Senegal, Somalia, Sudan, Tanzania, Togo, Viet Nam, Zaire, Zambia

[c]category includes Angola, Bolivia, Botswana, Cameroon, Chile, Colombia, Congo, Egypt, Jamaica, Lebanon, Mauritius, Monglia, Morocco, Paraguay, Peru, Senegal, Syrian Arab Republic, Thailand, Tunisia, Turkey, Yemen Arab Republic, Yemen PDR, Zimbabwe

[d]category includes Algeria, Gabon, Greece, Hong Kong, Hungary, Iran, Iraq, Korea (Rep.), Malaysia, Oman, Panama, Poland, Portugal, Romania, Singapore, South Africa, Trinidad and Tobago, Uruguay, Yugoslavia

[e]category includes Libya, United Arab Emirates

[f]category includes Austria, Belgium, Denmark, Federal Republic of Germany, Finland, France, Ireland, Italy, Netherlands, Norway, Spain, Sweden, Switzerland

[g]category includes Albania, Bulgaria, German Democratic Republic

Table 2. Basic Indicators of Health in the United States

States	per capita income[a]	infant mortality[b] all races	whites	blacks	per capita[c] hospital care	health care	physicians[d] per 100,000 population	nurses[e]	dentists[f]
United States average	10,798	10.9	9.5	18.6	$577	$1,220	207	641	57
New England		9.4	8.8	18.4	669	1,356	267	972	69
Connecticut	14,090	10.1	8.9	19.9	578	1,348	276	853	76
Maine	9,042	8.7	8.8	n.a.	517	1,091	187	751	49
Massachusetts	12,510	9.0	8.5	17.3	810	1,508	302	1,109	75
New Hampshire	11,659	9.4	9.4	n.a.	458	986	181	865	56
Rhode Island	10,892	9.9	9.5	16.2	623	1,351	233	935	54
Vermont	9,619	8.6	8.6	n.a.	443	978	238	920	62
Middle Atlantic		11.0	9.5	18.1	641	1,310	261	749	67
New Jersey	13,129	11.0	9.2	18.9	498	1,115	234	712	68
New York	11,765	11.1	9.7	16.8	679	1,417	290	739	73
Pennsylvania	10,288	10.9	9.4	20.9	675	1,273	236	787	59
East North Central		11.2	9.5	20.9	615	1,249	193	688	58
Illinois	11,302	12.1	9.5	22.2	700	1,308	205	703	58
Indiana	9,978	11.1	10.3	18.9	512	1,101	147	623	47
Michigan	10,902	11.6	9.4	23.0	628	1,281	208	647	62
Ohio	10,302	10.6	9.5	18.1	599	1,247	199	730	54
Wisconsin	10,298	9.6	8.9	17.5	539	1,219	177	712	67
West North Central		9.7	9.1	17.3	592	1,241	183	737	58
Iowa	10,096	9.1	8.9	16.3	536	1,176	156	837	57
Kansas	10,684	9.9	9.4	16.0	593	1,271	173	681	50
Minnesota	11,186	9.2	9.1	16.6	540	1,229	205	803	69
Missouri	10,283	10.5	9.1	18.1	679	1,285	205	647	54
Nebraska	10,546	9.7	9.3	16.6	568	1,216	157	713	68
North Dakota	9,635	8.5	8.2	n.a.	624	1,325	158	824	52
South Dakota	8,553	10.2	8.7	n.a.	530	1,154	134	738	52
South Atlantic		12.3	9.7	19.3	539	1,115	197	586	48
Delaware	11,375	11.9	9.1	20.8	552	1,153	197	773	47
District of Columbia	13,530	20.4	9.9	23.1	2,021	2,838	553	1,455	92

South Atlantic	per capita income[a]	infant mortality[b] all races	whites	blacks	per capita[c] hospital care	health care	physicians[d] per 100,000 population	nurses[e]	dentists[f]
Florida	11,271	11.4	9.2	18.5	569	1,228	202	628	45
Georgia	10,191	13.0	9.8	19.1	492	1,048	162	486	43
Maryland	12,967	11.8	9.3	18.2	606	1,232	304	762	66
North Carolina	9,517	12.4	9.9	18.7	428	931	169	527	42
South Carolina	8,890	14.6	10.6	21.1	397	857	147	431	41
Virginia	11,894	11.8	9.6	19.6	506	1,054	195	521	53
West Virginia	8,141	10.9	10.6	18.2	564	1,057	163	554	44
East South Central		12.6	10.2	19.1	507	1,025	150	500	46
Alabama	8,681	12.9	10.1	18.2	541	1,033	142	512	39
Kentucky	8,614	11.4	10.8	19.0	433	957	151	472	51
Mississippi	7,483	14.4	10.0	19.5	431	897	118	426	34
Tennessee	9,290	12.0	9.8	19.8	578	1,144	177	551	53
West South Central		10.9	9.8	16.7	500	1,096	164	445	42
Arkansas	8,389	11.1	9.7	15.5	443	994	138	442	38
Louisiana	8,836	12.5	9.1	18.1	549	1,106	173	394	42
Oklahoma	9,754	10.9	10.9	16.1	498	1,086	161	418	43
Texas	10,373	10.4	9.7	15.9	495	1,110	168	465	42
Mountain		9.8	9.6	15.3	483	1,070	178	593	55
Arizona	10,561	9.6	9.1	16.5	498	1,112	202	614	45
Colorado	11,713	9.9	9.7	16.1	557	1,209	207	690	64
Idaho	8,567	10.3	10.4	n.a.	335	868	121	544	54
Montana	8,781	9.9	9.9	n.a.	445	1,036	140	616	63
Nevada	11,200	9.9	9.9	14.8	630	1,380	160	547	45
New Mexico	8,814	10.1	9.9	11.7	449	904	170	548	47
Utah	8,535	9.2	9.2	n.a.	399	896	172	459	65
Wyoming	9,782	11.0	11.1	n.a.	398	873	129	457	52
Pacific		9.7	9.4	16.3	583	1,380	225	596	64
Alaska	13,650	11.5	9.8	19.1	552	1,187	130	658	57
California	11,885	9.6	9.2	16.2	626	1,451	237	563	62
Hawaii	11,003	9.4	8.6	16.5	479	1,228	215	657	65
Oregon	9,925	9.8	9.8	15.3	468	1,165	197	701	73
Washington	10,866	10.1	10.0	17.4	434	1,165	202	703	70

[a]1985 figures from U.S. Department of Commerce, Bureau of the Census, *Statistical Abstract of the United States: 1988* (Washington, D.C.: GPO, 1988), p. 431.

[b]1983-85 figures from U.S. Department of Health and Human Services, Public Health Service, *Health—United States: 1987* (Washington, D.C.: GPO, 1987), pp. 46-47.

[c]1982 figures from *Health—United States: 1987*, pp. 150-51, 162-63.

[d]1985 figures from *Health—United States: 1987*, pp. 126-27.

[e]1985 figures from American Nurses' Association, *Facts about Nursing: 86–87* (Kansas City, Mo.: American Nurses' Association, 1987), p. 4.

[f]1984 figures from U.S. Department of Commerce, Bureau of the Census, *Statistical Abstract of the United States: 1987* (Washington, D.C.: GPO, 1987), p. 94.

Table 3. Basic Indicators of Health in Canada[a]

	per family income[b]	per capita hospital[c]	per capita insur.[d]	population per[e]		
				physician	nurse	dentist
Canada	30,440	401	1,210	538	104	2,133
Newfoundland		398	1,059	640	118	4,638
Prince Edward Island	24,659	332	1,081	794	109	3,075
Nova Scotia		429	1,260	532	104	2,707
New Brunswick		464	1,123	857	97	3,564
Quebec	28,124	388	1,161	511	115	2,502
Ontario	32,170	391	1,191	509	88	1,869
Manitoba		453	1,233	539	119	2,325
Saskatchewan	31,723	418	1,155	662	114	2,918
Alberta		434	1,376	641	111	2,164
British Columbia	32,835	402	1,299	514	104	1,602
Yukon		—	1,443	850	—	1,831
Northwest Territories		108	1,443	1,107	150	2,906

[a]data compiled from Minister of Supply and Services, *Canada Yearbook 1985* (Ottawa: Statistics Canada, 1985), pp. 51, 85-119. The national infant mortality rate for both sexes is 9.1 per 1,000 births; the national life expectency at birth for 1981 was 71.9 years for males and 79.0 years for females.

[b]income in Canadian dollars for the year 1981

[c]figures calculated by dividing the reported public expenditures by public general hospitals in each province in 1982 by the 1983 population per province

[d]figures calculated by dividing the total national health expenditures, both public and private, for each province for 1982 by the 1983 population per province

[e]1981 figures as reported, except the figure for nurses, which was calculated by dividing the provincial population by the number of licenses issued to professional nurses per province in 1981

Table 4. Allocations of Government Dollars for Health and Leading Causes of Morbidity and Mortality in Some Third World Countries[a]

Country	health expenditures			water[b]	Causes of morbidity and mortality
	nat'l budget	total current expend.	per capita		
Bangladesh	2.2%	5.3%	$1	53%	smallpox, cholera, tuberculosis, typhoid, diphtheria
Bolivia	8.6	2.0	$9	34	malaria, influenza, dysentery, tuberculosis, venereal disease
Brazil	8.5	7.8	$27	>77	influenza, dysentery, tuberculosis, measles, whooping cough
Columbia	6.9	4.0	$12	>56	malaria, goiter, anemia, scurvy, pellagra, typhoid, hookworm
Costa Rica	5.1	32.8	$27	77	gastroenteritis, tuberculosis
Cuba	?	?	?	?	heart diseases, cancer, cerebro-vascular diseases, respiratory diseases
Dominica	8.8	8.8	$22	?	tuberculosis, intestinal infections, anemias
Dominican Republic	9.0	10.7	$17	>40	gastroenteritis, cancer, tetanus, pneumonia, influenza, malaria
Ecuador	8.7	7.7	$20	>34	respiratory ailments, parasitic diseases, gastrointestinal diseases
El Salvador	8.7	7.1	$11	>55	gastroenteritis, influenza, malaria, measles, pneumonia, bronchitis
Ethiopia	4.0	?	$1	6	malaria, tuberculosis, leprosy, venereal diseases, smallpox, typhus
Guatemala	10.9	?	$15	40	gastroenteritis, measles, whooping cough, anemia, dysentery
Guinea	?	?	$3	10	malaria, venereal diseases, tuber-culosis, leprosy, schistosomiasis
Haiti	9.8	?	$2	14	malaria, tuberculosis, dermatosis, parasite worms, respiratory ail-ments
Honduras	14.7	?	$10	5	gastritis, enteritis, tuberculosis
India	1.7	2.2	$1	16	malaria, filaria, tuberculosis, leprosy, venereal diseases
Indonesia	2.5	2.5	$3	12	yaws, trachoma, plague, venereal diseases
Ivory Coast	3.9	3.9	$15	19	malaria, smallpox, yellow fever, measles
Liberia	7.6	?	$13	20	malaria, tuberculosis, leprosy, bilharziasis, trypanosomiasis

| Country | health expenditures | | | water[b] | Causes of morbidity and mortality |
	nat'l budget	total current expend.	per capita		
Mexico	2.4	1.3	$13	50	diarrhea, pneumonia, heart disease, malaria, poliomyelitis
Nicaragua	14.6	?	$34	38	gastritis, duodenitis, enteritis, colitus, cardiovascular and respiratory diseases
Nigeria	2.4	1.3	$2	?	yellow fever, smallpox, malaria, tuberculosis, bilharziasis, Guinea worm, trachoma
Papua New Guinea	8.7	9.2	$25	20	malaria, tuberculosis, leprosy, venereal diseases
Philippines	3.5	5.3	$4	43	pneumonia, tuberculosis, malaria
Sierra Leone	4.1	6.2	$4	12	parasitic and infectious diseases, schistosomiasis, gastroenteritis
Sri Lanka	3.3	3.3	$4	20	gastritis, pneumonia, cancer, heart disease, anemia
Uganda	6.1	?	$4	35	malaria, sleeping sickness, leprosy, kwashiorkor, hookworm, schistosomiasis

[a]data from George Thomas Kurian, *Encyclopedia of the Third World,* 3 vols., rev. ed. (New York: Facts on File, 1982).

[b]water: percentage of population with access to safe drinking water

Table 5. Leading Causes of Death in Canada (1982) and the United States (1981), Age-adjusted for All Ages

Cause of death	Canada[a]	United States[b]
cardiovascular disease	326.1	224.0
cancer	170.3	133.6
accidents	38.1	34.7
pneumonia	21.3	32.1
suicide	n.a.	11.5
chronic liver disease	n.a.	9.6
diabetes mellitus	12.3	9.6
homicide	n.a.	8.3

[a]data from Minister of Supply and Services, *Canada Yearbook 1985* (Ottawa: Statistics Canada, 1985), p. 99. This source listed only the five leading causes of mortality; values are rates per 100,000 population.

[b]data from U.S. Department of Commerce, Bureau of the Census, *Statistical Abstract of the United States: 1987* (Washington, D.C.: GPO, 1987), p. 77; values are rates per 100,000 population.

Appendix D: Codes of Ethics

The Hippocratic Oath*

I swear by Apollo Physician and Asclepius and Hygeia and Panacea and all the gods and goddesses, making them my witnesses, that I will fulfill according to my ability and judgment this oath and this covenant:

To hold him who has taught me this art as equal to my parents and to live my life in partnership with him, and if he is in need of money, to give him a share of mine, and to regard his offspring as equal to my brothers in male lineage and to teach them this art—if they desire to learn it—without fee and covenant; to give a share of precepts and oral instruction and all the other learning to my sons and to the sons of him who has instructed me and to pupils who have signed the covenant and have taken an oath according to the medical law, but to no one else.

I will apply dietetic measures for the benefit of the sick according to my ability and judgment; I will keep them from harm and injustice.

I will neither give a deadly drug to anybody if asked for it, nor will I make a suggestion to this effect. Similarly I will not give to a woman an abortive remedy. In purity and holiness I will guard my life and my art.

I will not use the knife, not even on sufferers from stone, but will withdraw in favor of such men as are engaged in this work.

Whatever houses I may visit, I will come for the benefit of the sick, remaining free of all intentional injustice, of all mischief and in particular of sexual relations with both female and male persons, be they free or slaves.

Whatever I may see or hear in the course of the treatment or even

*Taken from Ludwig Edelstein, *The Hippocratic Oath: Text, Translation, and Interpretation,* Supplements to *The Bulletin of the History of Medicine,* 1 (Baltimore: Johns Hopkins, 1943), p. 3.

outside of the treatment in regard to the life of men, which on no account one must spread abroad, I will keep to myself, holding such things shameful to be spoken about.

If I fulfill this oath and do not violate it, may it be granted to me to enjoy life and art, being honored with fame among all men for all time to come; if I transgress it and swear falsely, may the opposite of all this be my lot.

American Medical Association Principles of Medical Ethics (adopted in 1980)

Preamble:

The medical profession has long subscribed to a body of ethical statements developed primarily for the benefit of the patient. As a member of this profession, a physician must recognize responsibility not only to patients, but also to society, to other health professionals, and to self. The following Principles adopted by the American Medical Association are not laws, but standards of conduct which define the essentials of honorable behavior for the physician.

I. A physician shall be dedicated to providing competent medical service with compassion and respect for human dignity.

II. A physician shall deal honestly with patients and colleagues, and strive to expose those physicians deficient in character or competence, or who engage in fraud or deception.

III. A physician shall respect the law and also recognize a responsiblity to seek changes in those requirements which are contrary to the best interests of the patient.

IV. A physician shall respect the rights of patients, of colleagues, and of other health professionals, and shall safeguard patient confidences within the constraints of the law.

V. A physician shall continue to study, apply and advance scientific knowledge, make relevant information available to patients, colleagues, and the public, obtain consultation, and use the talents of other health professionals when indicated.

VI. A physician shall, in the provision of appropriate patient care, except in emergencies, be free to choose whom to serve, with whom to associate, and the environment in which to provide medical services.

VII. A physician shall recognize a responsibility to participate in activities contributing to an improved community.

American Nurses' Association Code for Nurses* (adopted in 1976)

1. The nurse provides services with respect for human dignity and the uniqueness of the client, unrestricted by considerations of social or economic status, personal attributes, or the nature of health problems.

2. The nurse safeguards the client's right to privacy by judiciously protecting information of a confidential nature.

3. The nurse acts to safeguard the client and the public when health care and safety are affected by the incompetent, unethical, or illegal practice of any person.

4. The nurse assumes responsibility and accountability for individual nursing judgments and actions.

5. The nurse maintains competence in nursing.

6. The nurse exercises informed judgment and uses individual competence and qualifications as criteria in seeking consultation, accepting responsibilities, and delegating nursing activities to others.

7. The nurse participates in activities that contribute to the ongoing development of the profession's body of knowledge.

8. The nurse participates in the profession's efforts to implement and improve standards of nursing.

9. The nurse participates in the profession's efforts to establish and maintain conditions of employment conducive to high quality nursing care.

10. The nurse participates in the profession's efforts to protect the public from misinformation and misrepresentation and to maintain the integrity of nursing.

11. The nurse collaborates with members of the health professions and other citizens in promoting community and national efforts to meet the health needs of the public.

---

* Taken from American Nurses' Association, *Code for Nurses with Interpretive Statements* (Kansas City: American Nurses' Association, 1976), p. 3.

References

Aaron, Henry J., and William B. Schwartz. *The Painful Prescription: Rationing Hospital Care.* Washington: Brookings Institution, 1984.

"Abortion Done on Comatose Woman Patient." *Grand Rapids Press,* 9 Oct. 1985, Sec. A, p. 6.

Abrams, Frederick R. "Caring for the Sick: An Emerging Industrial By-Product." *Journal of the American Medical Association* 255 (1986): 937-38.

Ad Hoc Committee of the Harvard Medical School. "A Definition of Irreversible Coma." *Journal of the American Medical Association,* 1968, pp. 337-40.

Alexander, Shana. "They Decide Who Lives, Who Dies." *Life,* 9 Nov. 1962, pp. 102+.

Allen, James R. "Health Care Workers and the Risk of HIV Transmission." *Hastings Center Report,* Special Supplement: *AIDS: The Responsibilities of Health Professionals* 18.2 (1988): 2-5.

Allen, Joseph L. *Love and Conflict: A Covenantal Model of Christian Ethics.* Nashville: Abingdon Press, 1984.

American Medical Association. *Physician Characteristics and Distribution in the United States.* Chicago: AMA, 1984.

———. "Report of the Council on Long-range Planning and Development." In *The Environment of Medicine,* p. 116. Chicago: AMA, 1985.

American Nurses' Association. *Code for Nurses with Interpretive Statements.* Kansas City: American Nurses' Association, 1976.

———. *Facts about Nursing: 86-87.* Kansas City, Mo.: American Nurses' Association, 1987.

Amundsen, Darrel W. "The Physician's Obligation to Prolong Life: A Medical Duty without Classical Roots." *Hastings Center Report* 8.4 (1978): 23-30.

Amundsen, Darrel W., and Gary B. Ferngren. "Medicine and Religion: Early Christianity through the Middle Ages." In *Health/Medicine and the Faith Traditions,* ed. Martin E. Marty and Kenneth L. Vaux, pp. 93-131. Philadelphia: Fortress Press, 1982.

Anderson, Peggy. *Nurse.* New York: St. Martin's Press, 1979.

Andrews, L. B. *New Conceptions.* New York: St. Martin's Press, 1984.

Andrusko, Dave. "The Pro-Life Momentum." *Cresset,* May 1986, pp. 5-10.

Angell, Marcia. "The Baby Doe Rules." *New England Journal of Medicine* 314 (1986): 642-44.

————. "Respecting the Autonomy of Competent Patients." *New England Journal of Medicine* 309 (1984): 1115-16.

Annas, George. "Adam Smith in the Emergency Room." *Hastings Center Report* 15.4 (1985): 16-18.

————. "AIDS, Judges, and the Right to Medical Care." *Hastings Center Report* 18.4 (1988): 20-22.

————. "Forced Cesareans: The Most Unkindest Cut of All." *Hastings Center Report* 12.3 (1982): 16-17.

————. "Legal Risks and Responsibilities of Physicians in the AIDS Epidemic." *Hastings Center Report*, Special Supplement: *AIDS: The Responsibilities of Health Professionals* 18.2 (1988): 26-32.

————. "Nonfeeding: Lawful Killing in California, Homicide in New Jersey." *Hastings Center Report* 13.6 (1983): 19-20.

Annis, Edward R. "Joseph Ward Hooper Lecture: 'It Was the Best of Times. It Was the Worst of Times.'" *North Carolina Medical Journal* 44 (1983): 701-5.

Appelbaum, Paul S., and Joel Klein. "Therefore Choose Death?" *Commentary*, Apr. 1986, pp. 23-29.

Aries, Philippe. *The Hour of Our Death.* New York: Random House, 1981.

Arras, John D. "The Fragile Web of Responsibility: AIDS and the Duty to Treat." *Hastings Center Report*, Special Supplement: *AIDS: The Responsibilities of Health Professionals* 18.2 (1988): 10-20.

"Baby David: Alive, Well and Waiting." *Science News* 105 (1974): 335.

Backer, Barbara A., et al. *Death and Dying: Individuals and Institutions.* New York: Wiley, 1982.

Bajema, Clifford E. *Abortion and the Meaning of Personhood.* Grand Rapids: Baker Book House, 1974.

Bandstra, Barry, and Allen Verhey. "Sex; Sexuality." In vol. 4 of *The International Standard Bible Encyclopedia.* Ed. Geoffrey W. Bromiley, pp. 429-39. Rev. ed. Grand Rapids: Eerdmans, 1988.

Banks, Peter J. "Medicine in the '80s—Can We Afford It?" *Canadian Medical Association Journal* 123 (1980): 1247-56.

Banks, Taunga Lovel. "AIDS and the Right to Health Care." *Issues in Law & Medicine* 4 (Fall 1988): 151-73.

Barbour, John. *Tragedy as a Critique of Virtue.* Chico, Calif.: Scholars Press, 1984.

Baron, Richard J. "An Introduction to Medical Phenomenology: I Can't Hear You While I'm Listening." *Annals of Internal Medicine* 103 (1985): 606-11.

Barry, Michele. "Ethical Considerations of Human Investigation in Developing Countries: The AIDS Dilemma." *New England Journal of Medicine* 319 (1988): 1083-86.

Barth, Karl. *Church Dogmatics.* III/4. Trans. A. T. Mackey et al. Edinburgh: T. & T. Clark, 1961.

Bayles, Michael D. *Professional Ethics.* Belmont, Calif.: Wadsworth, 1981.

Bayles, Michael D., and Arthur Caplan. "Medical Fallibility and Malpractice." *Journal of Medicine and Philosophy* 3 (1978): 169-86.

Beach, George K. "Covenantal Ethics." In *The Life of Choice*, ed. Clark Kucheman, pp. 107-25. Boston: Beacon Press, 1978.

Beauchamp, Dan E. "Community: The Neglected Tradition of Public Health." *Hastings Center Report* 15.6 (1985): 28-36.

———. "Morality and the Health of the Body Politic." *Hastings Center Report, Special Supplement: Aids: Public Health and Civil Liberties* 16.6 (1986): 30-36.

Beauchamp, Tom L., and James F. Childress. *Principles of Biomedical Ethics.* 2nd ed. New York: Oxford University Press, 1983.

Becker, Ernst. *The Structure of Evil.* New York: Braziller, 1968.

Begley, Sharon. "The Troubling Question of 'Fetal Rights.'" *Newsweek,* 8 Dec. 1986, p. 87.

Belloc, Nedra B. "Relation of Health Practices and Mortality." *Preventive Medicine* 2 (1973): 67.

Belloc, Nedra B., and Lester Breslow. "Relationship of Physical Health Status and Health Practices." *Preventive Medicine* 1 (1972): 409.

Benjamin, Martin. "Compromise and Integrity in Ethics and Politics." Manuscript, 1987.

Benn, L. I. "Abortion, Infanticide, and Respect for Persons." In *The Problem of Abortion,* ed. Joel Feinberg, pp. 135-44. 2nd ed. Belmont, Calif.: Wadsworth, 1984.

Bennett, Ivan L., Jr. "Technology as a Shaping Force." In *Doing Better and Feeling Worse: Health in the United States,* ed. John H. Knowles, pp. 125-33. New York: W. W. Norton, 1977.

Bentham, Jeremy. *An Introduction to the Principles of Morals and Legislation.* 1780; rpt. in *A Bentham Reader,* ed. Mary Peter Mack, pp. 78-144. New York: Western Publishing Co., 1969.

Berger, Patrick F., and Carol Altekruse Berger. "Death on Demand." *Commonweal* 102 (1975): 585-89.

Berlin, Elois Ann, and William C. Fowkes, Jr. "A Teaching Framework for Cross-cultural Health Care." *Western Journal of Medicine* 139.6 (1983): 934-38.

Berlyne, G. M. "Over 50 and Uremic = Death." *Nephron* 31 (1982): 189-90.

Binger, C. M., et al. "Childhood Leukemia: Emotional Impact on Patient and Family." In *Understanding Death and Dying: An Interdisciplinary Approach,* ed. Sandra Galdieri Wilcox and Marilyn Sutton, pp. 314-27. Port Washington, N.Y.: Alfred Publishing Co., 1977.

Blackburn, Will R., et al. "Comparative Studies of Infants with Mosaic and Complete Triploidy: An Analysis of 55 Cases." *Birth Defects: Original Article Series* 18.3B (1982): 251-74.

Blendon, R. J., and D. E. Rogers. "Cutting Medical Care Costs: Primum Non Nocere." *Journal of the American Medical Association* 250 (1983): 1880-85.

Blendon, Robert J., et al. "Uncompensated Care by Hospitals or Public Insurance for the Poor: Does It Make a Difference?" *New England Journal of Medicine* 314 (1986): 1160-63.

Boer, Harry. *An Ember Still Glowing: Humankind as the Image of God.* Grand Rapids: Eerdmans, forthcoming.

Bok, Sissela. "Ethical Problems of Abortion." *Hastings Center Studies* 2.1 (1974): 33-52.

————. "Personal Directions for the Care at the End of Life." *New England Journal of Medicine* 295 (1976): 367-69.

————. *Secrets: On the Ethics of Concealment and Revelation.* New York: Vintage, 1984.

Bondi, Richard, and Stanley Hauerwas. "Memory, Community, and the Reasons for Living: Reflections on Suicide and Euthanasia." In *Truthfulness and Tragedy,* ed. Stanley Hauerwas, pp. 101-15. South Bend: University of Notre Dame Press, 1977.

Boue, Andre, et al. "Cytogenetics of Pregnancy Wastage." In vol. 14 of *Advances in Human Genetics.* 15 vols. Ed. Harry Harris and Kurt Hirschhorn. New York: Plenum, 1985.

Boy or Girl: Should the Choice Be Ours? Dir. Patrick A. Woodley. 1st of 6 episodes in film series *Hard Choices.* PBS video, 1980.

Brandt, R. B. "The Morality of Abortion." *Monist* 56 (1972): 504-26.

Brody, Baruch. "Legal Models of the Patient-Physician Relation." In *The Clinical Encounter,* ed. Earl E. Shelp, pp. 117-31. Dordrecht, Netherlands: Reidel, 1983.

Brody, Howard. *Ethical Decisions in Medicine.* 2nd ed. Boston: Little, Brown, 1981.

Bromiley, G. W. "Anthropology." In *The International Standard Bible Encyclopedia,* ed. G. W. Bromiley. 4 vols. Rev. ed. Grand Rapids: Eerdmans, 1979-1988, 1: 131-36.

"Bubble Boy's Lost Battle, The." *Time,* 5 March 1984, p. 51.

Bube, Richard. "Abortion." *Journal of the American Scientific Affiliation* 33 (1981): 158-65.

Buchanan, Allen. "The Right to a Decent Minimum of Health Care." In *Securing Access to Health Care,* vol. 2: *Appendices, Sociocultural and Philosophical Studies,* pp. 201-38. President's Commission for the Study of Ethical Problems in Medicine and Biomedical and Behavioral Research. Washington: GPO, 1983.

Bursztain, Harold, et al. *Medical Choices, Medical Chances.* New York: Delacorte/Lawrence, 1981.

Burt, Robert A. *Taking Care of Strangers: The Rule of Law in Doctor-Patient Relations.* New York: Free Press, 1979.

Burtchaell, James Tunstead. *Rachel Weeping: And Other Essays on Abortion.* Kansas City: Andrews McMeel & Parker, 1982.

————. "A Response [to Beverly Harrison's 'How to Argue about Abortion']." In *Comprehensive Theological Perspectives on Abortion,* ed. Gary N. McLean, pp. 64-67. Minneapolis: Planned Parenthood of Minnesota, 1983. (First published in *Christianity and Crisis,* 26 Dec. 1977, pp. 313-16.)

Cahill, Lisa. *Between the Sexes.* Philadelphia: Fortress Press, 1985.

Calabresi, Guido, and Philip Bobbitt. *Tragic Choices.* New York: W. W. Norton, 1978.

Callahan, Daniel. "How Technology Is Reframing the Abortion Debate." *Hastings Center Report* 16.1 (1986): 33-42.

————. "On Feeding the Dying." *Hastings Center Report* 13.5 (1983): 22.

380   *References*

———. "The Sanctity of Life." In *Updating Life and Death*. Ed. Donald R. Cutler, pp. 181-250. Boston: Beacon Press, 1968.

———. "Science: Limits and Prohibitions." *Hastings Center Report* 3.5 (1973): 5-7.

Callahan, Sidney. "Abortion and the Sexual Agenda." *Commonweal*, 25 Apr. 1986, pp. 232-38.

Calvin, John. *Institutes of the Christian Religion*. 2 vols. Trans. Ford Lewis Battles, ed. John T. McNeill. Philadelphia: Westminster Press, 1960.

Campbell, Courtney S. "Plague, Piety, and Policy." *Second Opinion* 9 (1988): 71-89.

Caplan, Arthur, and Michael D. Bayles. "A Response to Professor Gorovitz." *Journal of Medicine and Philosophy* 3 (1978): 192-95.

Carrell, Steve. "Professions Now Face New Version of Gray Zone." *American Medical News*, 3 Oct. 1986, pp. 20-21.

Cassell, Eric J. *The Healer's Art*. New York: Penguin Books, 1976.

———. "What Is the Function of Medicine." In *Death and Decision*, ed. E. McMullin, pp. 35-44. Boulder, Colo.: Westview Press, 1978.

Centers for Disease Control. "Update: Acquired Immunodeficiency Syndrome—United States, 1981-1988." *Morbidity and Mortality Weekly Report*, 14 Apr. 1989, pp. 229-36.

Chambers, Marcia, et al. "Dead Baby's Mother Faces Criminal Charges on Acts in Pregnancy." *New York Times*, 9 Oct. 1986, Sec. A, p. 22.

Chandler, William U. "Banishing Tobacco." In *State of the World 1986: A Worldwatch Institute Report on Progress toward a Sustainable Society*, ed. Linda Starke, pp. 139-58. New York: W. W. Norton, 1986.

Charmas, Kathy. *The Social Reality of Death*. Reading, Mass.: Addison-Wesley, 1980.

Chervenak, Frank, et al. "Advances in the Diagnosis of Fetal Defects." *New England Journal of Medicine* 315.5 (1986): 305-7.

Chesterton, Gilbert K. *Orthodoxy*. Garden City, N.Y.: Image Books, 1959.

Childress, James F. "The Art of Technology Assessment." In *Priorities in Biomedical Ethics*, pp. 98-118. Philadelphia: Westminster Press, 1981.

———. "Love and Justice in Christian Biomedical Ethics." In *Theology and Bioethics*, ed. Earl E. Shelp, pp. 225-42. Dordrecht, Netherlands: Reidel, 1985.

———. "Priorities in the Allocation of Health Care Resources." In *Biomedical Ethics*, ed. Thomas A. Mappes and Jane S. Zembaty, pp. 561-68. New York: McGraw-Hill, 1981.

———. "Who Shall Live When Not All Can Live?" *Soundings* 53 (1970): 339-55.

Childs, J. M., Jr. "Genetic Screening and Counseling." In *Questions about the Beginnings of Life*, ed. Edward D. Schneider. Minneapolis: Augsburg, 1985.

Christakis, Nicholas A. "The Ethical Design of an AIDS Vaccine Trial in Africa." *Hastings Center Report* 18.3 (1988): 31-37.

Christian Reformed Church in North America. *Acts of Synod: 1972*. Grand Rapids: Board of Publications of the Christian Reformed Church, 1972.

Clark, Matt, and Mariana Gosnell. "The New Gene Doctors." *Newsweek*, 18 May 1981, pp. 120-24.

Clouser, K. Danner. "Veatch, May, and Models: A Critical Review and a New

View." In *The Clinical Encounter,* ed. Earl E. Shelp, pp. 89-103. Dordrecht, Netherlands: Reidel, 1983.

Cluff, L. F. "Chronic Disease: Function and Quality of Care." *Journal of Chronic Disease* 34 (1981): 299-301.

Cooper, John. "Dualism and the Biblical View of Human Beings." *Reformed Journal,* Sept. 1982, pp. 13-16; Oct. 1982, pp. 16-18.

Council on Medical Service. "Closing the Gaps in Health Insurance Coverage." *Journal of the American Medical Association* 255 (1986): 790-93.

"Council Report." *Journal of the American Medical Association,* 14 Feb. 1986.

Crane, Diane. *The Sanctity of Social Life.* New Brunswick, N.J.: Transaction Books, 1975.

Curran, James W., et al. "Epidemiology of HIV Infection and AIDS in the United States." *Science* 239 (1988): 610-16.

Daniels, Norman. "Health-Care Needs and Distributive Justice." *Philosophy and Public Affairs,* 2 Oct. 1981, pp. 146-79.

————. "Why Saying No to Patients in the United States Is So Hard." *New England Journal of Medicine* 314 (1986): 1380-83.

"David's Debut into the World." *Science News* 112 (1977): 314-15.

Davis, Karen. "Cost Containment and Health Care in the United States." In *Contemporary Issues in Health Care,* ed. Daniel J. Schnall and Carl L. Figliola, pp. 37-59. New York: Praeger, 1984.

Davis, Karen, et al. "Is Cost Containment Working?" *Health Affairs* 4.3 (1985): 81-94.

Day, Patricia, and Rudolf Klein. "Towards A New Health Care System." *British Medical Journal* 291 (1985): 1291-93.

Deardon, R. W. "Inequalities in Health: Can They Be Corrected?" *British Medical Journal* 288 (1984): 1625-27.

Denes, Magna. *In Necessity and Sorrow: Life and Death in an Abortion Hospital.* New York: Penguin Books, 1977.

Dennett, Daniel. "Conditions of Personhood." In *The Identities of Persons,* ed. Amelie Oksenberg Rorty, pp. 175-96. Berkeley: University of California Press, 1976.

de Pouvourville, Gerard, and Marc Renaud. "Hospital System Management in France and Canada: National Pluralism and Provincial Centralism." *Social Science and Medicine* 20.2 (1985): 153-66.

Devlin, Patrick. *The Enforcement of Morals.* Oxford: Oxford University Press, 1965.

DeVries, Raymond G. "Christian Responsibility in Professional Society." *Christian Scholar's Review* 13 (1984): 151-57.

Dickman, Robert L. "Comments on 'Toward a Reconstruction of Medical Morality.'" *Journal of Medicine and Philosophy* 5 (1980): 201-7.

Dillon, William P., et al. "Life Support and Maternal Brain Death During Pregnancy." *Journal of the American Medical Association* 248 (1982): 1089-91.

Dinman, Bertram D. "The Reality and Acceptance of Risk." *Journal of the American Medical Association* 244 (1980): 1226-28.

Donagan, Alan. *The Theory of Morality.* Chicago: University of Chicago Press, 1977.

Donovan, Patricia. "New Reproductive Technologies: Some Legal Dilemmas." *Family Planning Perspective* 18.2 (1986): 56-60.

Dresser, Rebecca S., and Eugene V. Boisaubin, Jr. "Ethics, Law, and Nutritional Support." *Archives of Internal Medicine* 45.1 (1985): 122-24.

Drinan, Robert F. "Should There Be a Legal Right to Die?" In *Ethical Issues in Death and Dying,* ed. Robert F. Weir, pp. 297-307. New York: Columbia University Press, 1977.

Drummond, M. F., and G. H. Mooney. "Essentials of Health Economics," Part II: "Financing Health Care." *British Medical Journal* 285 (1982): 1191-92.

————. "Essentials of Health Economics, Part VI: Challenges for the Future." *British Medical Journal* 285 (1982): 1727-28.

Dubos, Rene. *Man Adapting.* New Haven: Yale University Press, 1980.

Dworkin, Gerald. "Autonomy and Behavior Control." *Hastings Center Report* 6.1 (1976): 23-28.

Dyck, Arthur J. "An Alternative to the Ethic of Euthanasia." In *To Live and to Die,* ed. Robert Williams, pp. 98-112. New York: Springer-Verlag, 1973.

Eckholm, Erik P. *The Picture of Health.* New York: W. W. Norton, 1977.

Edelstein, Ludwig. *The Hippocratic Oath: Text, Translation, and Interpretation.* Supplements to *The Bulletin of the History of Medicine,* 1, p. 3. Baltimore: Johns Hopkins, 1943.

Edwards, R. G. "Mammalian Eggs in the Laboratory." *Scientific American* 214 (1966): 73-81.

Edwards, R. G., and D. J. Sharpe. "Social Values and Research in Human Embryology." *Nature* 231 (1971): 87-91.

Elshtain, Jean Bethke. "Reflections on Abortion, Values, and the Family." In *Abortion: Understanding Differences,* ed. Sidney Callahan and Daniel Callahan, pp. 47-72. New York: Plenum, 1984.

"Emerging from the Bubble." *Time,* 20 Feb. 1984, p. 72.

Emson, H. E. "Rationing Health Care: Where Does the Buck Stop?" *Canadian Medical Journal* 128 (1983): 435-38.

Engel, George. "Clinical Application of the Biopsychosocial Model." In *Medicine as a Human Experience,* ed. David Reiser and David Rosen, pp. 43-60. Baltimore: University Park Press, 1984.

Engelhardt, H. Tristram, Jr. *The Foundations of Bioethics.* New York: Oxford University Press, 1986.

Essex, Max, and Phyllis J. Kanki. "The Origins of the AIDS Virus." *Scientific American* 259.4 (1988): 64-71.

Ethics Advisory Board. "Report and Conclusions: HEW Support of Research Involving Human in Vitro Fertilization and Embryo Transfer." *Federal Register,* 18 June 1979, pp. 35-57.

Euthanasia Educational Council. "A Living Will." New York: Euthanasia Educational Council, 1974.

Evans, C. Stephen. "Healing Old Wounds and Recovering Old Insights." *Christian Faith and Practice in the Modern World,* ed. Mark A. Noll and David F. Wells. Grand Rapids: Eerdmans, 1988.

————. "Human Persons as Substantial Achievers." Third International Symposium of the Association for Calvinist Philosophy. Zeist, Netherlands, 12 Aug. 1986.

———. "Separable Souls: A Defense of Minimal Dualism." *Southern Journal of Philosophy* 19 (1981): 313-31.

Faix, Roger G., et al. "Triploidy: Case Report of a Live-Born Male and an Ethical Dilemma." *Pediatrics* 74 (1984): 296-99.

Falloon, Judith, et al. "Human Immunodeficiency Virus Infection in Children." *Journal of Pediatrics* 114 (Jan. 1989): 1- 30.

Farley, Margaret. "Sexual Ethics." In *Encyclopedia of Bioethics.* ed. Warren Reich, pp. 1575-87. New York: Free Press, 1978.

Feinberg, Joel. "Abortion." In *Matters of Life and Death,* ed. Tom Regan, pp. 256-92. 2nd ed. New York: Random House, 1986.

———. "Sentiment and Sentimentality in Practical Ethics." *Prereadings and Addresses of the American Philosophical Association* 56 (1982): 19-46.

Ferrieri, Patricia. "AIDS, Children, and Primary Care Physicians." *Journal of Diseases in Children,* March 1988, p. 272.

Fielding, Jonathan E. "Smoking: Health Effects and Control." *New England Journal of Medicine* 312 (1985): 491+, 555-61.

Fielding, Jonathan E., and Kenneth J. Phenow. "Health Effects of Involuntary Smoking." *New England Journal of Medicine* 319 (1988): 1452-60.

"58% Oppose Reversing Abortion Decision." *Star Tribune* (Minneapolis), 22 Jan. 1989, Sec. D, p. 18.

Filkins, Karen. "Fetoscopy." *Clinical Obstetrics and Gynecology* 26 (1983): 339-46.

Final Report: For the Children of Tomorrow. Southern Regional Task Force on Infant Mortality. Columbia, S.C.: The Governor's Office, Nov. 1985.

Fineberg, Harvey V. "The Social Dimensions of AIDS." *Scientific American* 259.4 (1988): 128-34.

A Fiscal Imperative: Prenatal and Infant Care. Southern Regional Task Force on Infant Mortality. Columbia, S.C.: The Governor's Office, Feb. 1985.

Fisher, Margaret C. "Transfusion-associated Acquired Immunodeficiency Syndrome—What Is the Risk?" *Pediatrics* 79.1 (1987): 157-60.

Fletcher, John. "The Brink: The Parent-Child Bond in the Genetic Revolution." *Theological Studies* 33 (1972): 457-85.

Fletcher, Joseph. "Ethical Aspects of Genetic Controls." *New England Journal of Medicine* 285 (1971): 776-83.

Flores, Albert, and Deborah G. Johnson. "Collective Responsibility and Professional Roles." *Ethics* 93 (1983): 537-45.

Fox, Maurice, and Helene Levens Lipton. "The Decision to Perform Cardio-pulmonary Resuscitation." *New England Journal of Medicine* 309 (1983): 607-8.

Francke, Linda Bird. *The Ambivalence of Abortion.* New York: Random House, 1978.

Frankfurt, Harry G. "Freedom of the Will and the Concept of a Person." *Journal of Philosophy* 68 (1971): 5-20.

Freedman, Benjamin. "Health Professions, Codes, and the Right to Refuse to Treat HIV-infectious Patients." *Hastings Center Report,* Special Supplement: *AIDS: The Responsibilities of Health Professionals* 18.2 (1988): 20-25.

Freeman, David. "Some Christian Thoughts on Death and Dying." *Reformed Journal*, May-June 1976, pp. 22-24.

Freeman, Howard, et al. "Americans Report on Their Access to Care." *Health Affairs* 6.1 (1987): 6-18.

Freidson, Eliot. "The Theory of Professions: State of the Art." In *The Sociology of the Professions*, ed. Robert Dingwall and Philip Lewis, pp. 19-37. New York: St. Martin's Press, 1983.

Freund, Paul. "Introduction." *Daedalus* 98 (1969): viii-xiv.

Fried, Charles. "Equality and Rights in Medical Care." *Hastings Center Report* 6.1 (1976): 29-34.

Friedmann, Theodore. *Gene Therapy—Fact and Fiction*. Cold Spring Harbor, N.Y.: Cold Spring Harbor Laboratory, 1983.

Friedrich, Otto. "One Miracle, Many Doubts." *Time*, 10 Dec. 1984, pp. 70-77.

Fuchs, Fritz. "Genetic Amniocentesis." *Scientific American* 242.6 (1980): 47-53.

Fuchs, R., and S. Scheidt. "Improved Criteria for Admission to Cardiac Care Units." *Journal of the American Medical Association* 247 (1982): 2037-41.

Fuchs, Victor R. *Who Shall Live?* New York: Basic Books, 1974.

Fuchs, Victor R., and Leslie Perreault. "Expenditures for Reproduction-related Health Care." *Journal of the American Medical Association* 255 (1986): 76-81.

Fulton, Robert, and Julie Fulton. "A Psychosocial Aspect of Terminal Care: Anticipatory Grief." In *Death and Identity*, ed. Robert Fulton. Rev. ed. Bowie, Md.: Charles Press, 1976.

Furnish, Victor Paul. *The Moral Teachings of Paul*. Rev. ed. Nashville: Abingdon Press, 1985.

Gadow, Sally. "Body and Self: A Dialectic." In *The Humanity of the Ill: Phenomenological Perspectives*, ed. Victor Kestenbaum, pp. 86-100. Knoxville: University of Tennessee Press, 1982.

Gallo, Robert C., and Luc Montagnier. "AIDS in 1988." *Scientific American* 259.4 (1988): 41-48.

Gaylin, Willard. "Harvesting the Dead." *Harper's Magazine*, Sept. 1974, pp. 23-30.

———. "In Defense of the Dignity of Being Human." *Hastings Center Report* 14.4 (1984): 18-22.

Gervais, Karen. *Redefining Death*. New Haven: Yale University Press, 1986.

Gewirth, Alan. *Reason and Morality*. Chicago: University of Chicago Press, 1978.

Glaser, Barney, and Anselm Strauss. *Awareness of Dying*. Chicago: Aldine, 1965.

Goodin, Robert E. *Protecting the Vulnerable: A Reanalysis of Our Social Responsibilities*. Chicago: University of Chicago Press, 1985.

Gorovitz, Samuel. "Medical Fallibility: A Rejoinder." *Journal of Medicine and Philosophy* 3 (1978): 187-91.

Gorovitz, Samuel, and Alasdair MacIntyre. "Toward a Theory of Medical Fallibility." *Journal of Medicine and Philosophy* 1 (1976): 51-71.

Grady, Denise. "The Cruel Price of Cutting Medical Expenses." *Discover*, May 1986, pp. 25-43.

Green, Michael B., and Daniel Wikler. "Brain Death and Personal Identity." *Philosophy and Public Affairs* 9 (1980): 105-33.

Green, Ronald M. "Conferred Rights and the Fetus." *Journal of Religious Ethics* 2.1 (1974): 65-75.

Greenberg, Hayim. "The Right to Kill?" In *Jewish Reflections on Death*, ed. Jack Riemer, pp. 107-16. New York: Schocken Books, 1974.

Grobstein, Clifford. "The Early Development of Human Embryos." *Journal of Medicine and Philosophy* 10 (1985): 213-36.

———. "External Human Fertilization." *Scientific American* 240.6 (1979): 57-67.

Gustafson, James M. *The Contributions of Theology to Medical Ethics.* Milwaukee: Marquette University Press, 1975.

———. *Ethics and Theology,* vol. 2 of *Ethics from a Theocentric Perspective.* Chicago: University of Chicago Press, 1984.

———. "Mongolism, Parental Desires, and the Right to Life." In *Bioethics*, ed. Thomas Shannon, pp. 95-121. New York: Paulist Press, 1976.

———. "Theology Confronts Technology and the Life Sciences." *Commonweal,* 16 June 1978, pp. 386-92.

Haggerty, Robert J. "The Limits of Medical Care." *New England Journal of Medicine* 313 (1985): 383-84.

Hamilton, Allan J. "Who Shall Live and Who Shall Die." *Newsweek,* 26 Mar. 1984, p. 15.

Hare, R. M. *Moral Thinking.* Oxford: Clarendon, 1981.

Harris, Curtis E. "AIDS and the Future." *Issues in Law & Medicine* 4.2 (1988): 141-49.

Harrison, Beverly Wildung. *Our Right to Choose: Toward a New Ethic of Abortion.* Boston: Beacon Press, 1983.

Harrison, Geoffrey. "Relativism and Tolerance." *Ethics* 86 (1976): 122-35.

Haseltine, William A., and Flossie Wong-Staal. "The Molecular Biology of the AIDS Virus." *Scientific American* 259.4 (1988): 52-62.

Hasker, William. *Metaphysics: Constructing a World View.* Downers Grove, Ill.: InterVarsity Press, 1983.

Hauerwas, Stanley. "Can Ethics Be Theological?" *Hastings Center Report* 8.5 (1978): 47-49.

———. "Care." In *Encyclopedia of Bioethics.* 4 vols. Ed. Warren T. Reich, 1:145-50. New York: Free Press, 1978.

———. *A Community of Character: Toward a Constructive Christian Social Ethic.* South Bend: Notre Dame University Press, 1981.

———. "Medicine as a Tragic Profession." In *Truthfulness and Tragedy,* pp. 184-202. South Bend: Notre Dame University Press, 1977.

———. "Salvation and Health: Why Medicine Needs the Church." In *Theology and Bioethics,* ed. Earl E. Shelp, pp. 205-24. Dordrecht, Netherlands: Reidel, 1985.

———. *Suffering Presence.* South Bend: Notre Dame University Press, 1986.

———. *Vision and Virtue.* South Bend: Fides/Claretian, 1974.

Hauerwas, Stanley, and Allen Verhey. "From Conduct to Character—A Guide to Sexual Adventure." *Reformed Journal,* Nov. 1986, pp. 12-16.

Hellegers, Andre E. "Fetal Development." *Theological Studies* 31.1 (1970): 3-9.

Hewitt, Thomas. *The Epistle to the Hebrews.* Grand Rapids: Eerdmans, 1960.

Heyward, William L., and James W. Curran. "The Epidemiology of AIDS in the U.S." *Scientific American* 259.4 (1988): 72-81.

Hilbert, Richard. "Abortion and Rights." *Minneapolis Star and Tribune,* 27 Sept. 1986, Sec. A, p. 18.

Hilfiker, David. *Healing the Wounds.* New York: Pantheon, 1985.

Himmelstein, David U., and Steffie Woolhandler. "Cost without Benefit—Administrative Waste in U.S. Health Care." *New England Journal of Medicine* 314 (1986): 441-45.

Hippocrates. "The Art." In *Hippocrates.* 4 vols. Trans. W. H. S. Jones, 1:317. Cambridge, Mass.: Harvard University Press, 1923.

"HIV Risk Too Rare to Affect Breast Feeding." *Pediatric News* 22.11 (1988): 16a.

Hobbes, Thomas. *Leviathan.* 1651; rpt. Oxford: Clarendon, 1909.

Hoekema, Anthony A. *Created in God's Image.* Grand Rapids: Eerdmans, 1986.

Hoeksema, Thomas B. "Christian Responses to the Handicapped." *Banner,* 24 Dec. 1976, pp. 4-6.

Hoitenga, Dewey J., Jr. "Christianity and the Professions." *Christian Scholar's Review* 10 (1981): 296-309.

Humphrey, Derek. *Let Me Die Before I Wake: Hemlock's Book of Self-Deliverance for the Dying.* New York: Grove Press, 1984.

Huxley, Aldous. *Brave New World.* New York: Bantam Books, 1946.

Illich, Ivan. *Medical Nemesis.* New York: Bantam Books, 1976.

Inglehart, John K. "Health Policy Report: Canada's Health Care System." *New England Journal of Medicine* 315 (1986): 202-8, 778-84, 1623-28.

———. "Medical Care of the Poor—A Growing Problem." *New England Journal of Medicine* 313 (1985): 59-63.

Jackson, Laird. "First-Trimester Diagnosis of Fetal Genetic Disorders." *Hospital Practice* 20.3 (1985): 39-48.

James, Frank E. "Medical Expenses Resist Controls and Keep Going One Way: Higher." *Wall Street Journal,* 29 Feb. 1987, p. 41.

Jenson, Robert W. "Man as Patient." In *Man, Medicine, and Theology.* New York: Board of Social Ministry, Lutheran Church in America, 1967.

Jewett, Robert. *Letter to Pilgrims.* New York: Pilgrim Press, 1981.

Jewkes, John, and Sylvia Jewkes. *The Genesis of the British National Health Service.* Oxford: Blackwell, 1962.

Jonas, Hans. "Philosophical Reflections on Experimenting with Human Subjects." *Daedalus* 98 (1969): 219-47.

Jonas, Steven. *Health Care Delivery in the United States.* 3rd ed. New York: Springer, 1986.

Jones, D. Gareth. "Abortion: An Exercise in Biomedical Ethics." *Journal of the American Scientific Affiliation* 34.2 (1982): 6-17.

———. *Brave New People.* Grand Rapids: Eerdmans, 1985.

"Judge Dismisses Pregnancy Abuse Case." *Minneapolis Star and Tribune,* 27 Feb. 1987, Sec. A, p. 3.

Kane, Robert, et al. "A Randomised Controlled Trial of Hospice Care." *Lancet* 1.8382 (1984): 890-94.

Kane, Robert L., and Rosalie A. Kane. *A Will and a Way: What the United States*

Can Learn from Canada about Caring for the Elderly. New York: Columbia University Press, 1985.

Kant, Immanuel. *Groundwork of the Metaphysics of Morals.* Trans. H. V. Paton. New York: Harper, 1965.

Kass, Leon R. "Death as an Event: A Commentary on Robert Morison." *Science,* 20 Aug. 1971, pp. 698-702.

———. "New Beginnings in Life." In *The New Genetics and the Future of Man,* ed. Michael P. Hamilton, pp. 15-63. Grand Rapids: Eerdmans, 1972.

———. "The New Biology: What Price Relieving Man's Estate?" *Science,* 19 Nov. 1971, pp. 779-88.

———. "Regarding the End of Medicine and the Pursuit of Health." *Public Interest* 40 (1975): 11-42.

Katz, Jay. *The Silent World of Doctor and Patient.* New York: Free Press, 1984.

Kelly, Gerald. "The Duty to Preserve Life." *Theological Studies* 12 (1951): 550.

———. *Medico-Moral Problems.* St. Louis: Catholic Hospital Association, 1958.

Kleinig, John. "Good Samaritanism." *Philosophy and Public Affairs* 5 (1976): 382-407.

Kleinman, Arthur, et al. "Culture, Illness, and Care: Clinical Lessons from Anthropologic and Cross-cultural Research." *Annals of Internal Medicine* 88 (1978): 251-58.

Knowles, John H. "The Responsibility of the Individual." In *Doing Better and Feeling Worse: Health in the United States,* ed. John H. Knowles, pp. 57-80. New York: W. W. Norton, 1977.

Kopelman, Loretta. "On Disease: Theories of Disease and the Description of Disease." In *Evaluation and Explanation in the Biomedical Sciences,* ed. H. T. Engelhardt, Jr., and S. F. Spicker, pp. 143-50. Dordrecht, Netherlands: Reidel, 1975.

Krafrissen, Michael E., et al. "Abortion: Incidence, Mortality, and Morbidity." In *Perspectives on Abortion,* ed. Paul Sachdev, pp. 130-47. Metuchen, N.J.: Scarecrow Press, 1985.

Kübler-Ross, Elisabeth. *On Death and Dying.* New York: Macmillan, 1969.

Kurian, George Thomas. *Encyclopedia of the Third World.* 3 vols. Rev. ed. New York: Facts on File, 1982.

Kuyvenhoven, Andrew. "The Protection of the Unborn." *Banner,* 5 Sept. 1983, pp. 7-8.

Lamanna, Mary Ann. "Social Science and Ethical Issues: The Policy Implications of Poll Data on Abortion." In *Abortion: Understanding Differences,* ed. Sidney Callahan and Daniel Callahan, pp. 1-23. New York: Plenum, 1984.

Lamb, David. *Death, Brain Death, and Ethics.* Albany: State University of New York Press, 1985.

Lammers, Stephen E., and Allen Verhey. *On Moral Medicine: Theological Perspectives on Medical Ethics.* Grand Rapids: Eerdmans, 1987.

Langerak, Edward. "Abortion: Listening to the Middle." *Hastings Center Report* 9.5 (1979): 24-28.

———. "Teaching How to Disagree." In *Values in Teaching and Professional Ethics,* ed. Carlton T. Mitchell. Macon: Mercer University Press, forthcoming.

————. "Tolerance, Cooperation, and Respect for Wrong Views." American Philosophical Association Convention, New York, 29 Dec. 1984.

Lappe, Marc. "Blaming the Victim." In *Hard Choices.* Seattle: Regents of University of Washington, 1980.

Lawrence, Raymond J. "David the 'Bubble Boy' and the Boundaries of Being Human." *Journal of the American Medical Association* 253 (1985): 74-76.

Leaf, Alexander. "The Doctor's Dilemma — And Society's Too." *New England Journal of Medicine* 310 (1984): 718-21.

Lebacqz, Karen. *Genetics, Ethics, and Parenthood.* New York: Pilgrim Press, 1983.

Lemp, George. "Model Suggests 100% of HIV Infected May Progress to AIDS." *Medical World News,* 8 Feb. 1988, p. 56.

Levine, Carol. "More Money for AIDS, Less for Rural Health." *Hastings Center Report,* Special Supplement: *AIDS: The Emerging Ethical Dilemmas* 15.4 (1985): 26.

Levinsky, Norman G. "The Doctor's Master." *New England Journal of Medicine* 311 (1984): 1573-75.

Lewis, Charles E., et al. *A Right to Health: The Problem of Access to Primary Medical Care.* New York: John Wiley, 1976.

Lewis, C. S. *The Abolition of Man.* New York: Collier, 1962.

Lindsay, Almont. *Socialized Medicine in England and Wales.* Chapel Hill, N.C.: University of North Carolina Press, 1962.

Linton, Adam L. "Who's Afraid of an HMO?" *Ontario Medical Review* 54.3 (1987): 194-201.

Linton, Adam L., and David Naylor. "Problems of Health Care in Canada." *Medical Journal of Australia* 142 (1985): 556-58.

Lohr, Kathleen N., and M. Susan Marquis. *Medicare and Medicaid: Past, Present, and Future.* Santa Monica: Rand Corp., 1984.

Lomasky, Loren E. "Being a Person—Does It Matter?" In *The Problem of Abortion,* ed. Joel Feinberg, pp. 161-72. 2nd ed. Belmont, Calif.: Wadsworth, 1984.

Loop, F. O., et al. "A Strategy for Cost Containment in Coronary Surgery." *Journal of the American Medical Association* 250 (1983): 63.

Los, Roger. *Between Heaven and Earth.* New York: Holt, Rinehart, 1969.

Luker, Kristin. *Abortion and the Politics of Motherhood.* Berkeley: University of California Press, 1984.

————. *Taking Chances: Abortion and the Decision Not to Contracept.* Berkeley: University of California Press, 1978.

Lundberg, George D. "Rationing Human Life." *Journal of the American Medical Association* 249 (1983): 2223-24.

Lurie, Nicole, et al. "Termination of Medi-Cal Benefits: A Follow-up Study One Year Later." *New England Journal of Medicine* 314 (1986): 1266-68.

Lynn, Joanne, and James F. Childress. "Must Patients Always Be Given Food and Water?" *Hastings Center Report* 13.5 (1983): 17-21.

McCormick, Richard A., S.J. *Health and Medicine in the Roman Catholic Tradition: Tradition in Transition.* New York: Crossroad, 1984.

————. *How Brave a New World?: Dilemmas in Bioethics.* Garden City, N.Y.: Doubleday, 1981.

————. "The New Medicine and Morality." *Theology Digest* 21 (1973): 308-21.

McCormick, Richard A., S.J., and Paul Ramsey, eds. *Doing Evil to Achieve Good.* Chicago: Loyola University Press, 1978.

MacIntyre, Alasdair. *After Virtue.* 2nd ed. Notre Dame: University of Notre Dame Press, 1984.

————. "How Virtues Become Vices: Values, Medicine, and Social Context." In *Evaluation and Explanation in the Biomedical Sciences,* ed. H. Tristram Engelhardt, Jr., and Stuart Spicker. Dordrecht, Netherlands: Reidel, 1975.

————. "Seven Traits for the Future." *Hastings Center Report* 9.1 (1979): 5-7.

————. "Theology, Ethics, and the Ethics of Medicine and Health Care." *Journal of Medicine and Philosophy* 4 (1979): 435-43.

Mackenzie, Thomas B., and Theodore C. Nagel. "Commentary on When a Pregnant Woman Endangers Her Fetus." *Hastings Center Report* 16.1 (1986): 24-25.

McKusick, Victor A. *Mendelian Inheritance in Man: Catalogues of Autosomal Dominant, Autosomal Recessive, and X-Linked Phenotypes.* 6th ed. Baltimore: Johns Hopkins University Press, 1983.

Macrae, Norman. "Health Care International." *The Economist,* 23 Apr. 1984, pp. 17-34.

Maguire, Daniel. *Death by Choice.* New York: Schocken Books, 1973.

Mann, Jonathan M., et al. "The International Epidemiology of AIDS." *Scientific American* 259.4 (1988): 82-89.

Mannes, Marya. *Last Rights.* New York: William Morrow, 1974.

Mappes, Thomas A., and Jane S. Zembaty, eds. *Biomedical Ethics.* New York: McGraw-Hill, 1981.

Martin, J., D. Dolkart, and D. Freko. "Reasons for the Downturn in Under-65 Admissions." Policy Brief No. 52. Chicago: American Hospital Association, 1984.

Martin, Michael. "On a New Theory of Medical Fallibility: A Rejoinder." *Journal of Medicine and Philosophy* 2 (1977): 84-88.

Marty, Martin E. *Health and Medicine in the Lutheran Tradition: Being Well.* New York: Crossroad, 1983.

Marty, Martin E., and Kenneth L. Vaux, eds. *Health/Medicine and the Faith Traditions.* Philadelphia: Fortress Press, 1982.

Marzuk, Peter M. "The Right Kind of Paternalism." *New England Journal of Medicine* 312 (1985): 1474-76.

Masters, Roger D. "Is Contract an Adequate Basis for Medical Ethics?" *Hastings Center Report* 5.6 (1975): 24-38.

Matthews, Thomas J., and Dani P. Bolognesi. "AIDS Vaccines." *Scientific American* 259.4 (1988): 120-27.

Mattingly, Susan S. "Viewing Abortion from the Perspective of Transplantation: The Ethics of the Gift of Life." *Soundings* 67 (1984): 399-410.

May, William F. "Attitudes toward the Newly Dead." In *Death Inside Out,* ed. Peter Steinfels and Robert M. Veatch, pp. 139-49. New York: Harper, 1975.

————. "Code and Covenant or Philanthrophy and Contract?" *Hastings Center Report* 5.6 (1975): 29-38.

——. "Parenting, Bonding, and Valuing the Retarded." In *Ethics and Mental Retardation*, ed. Loretta Kopelman and John C. Moskop, pp. 141-60. Dordrecht, Netherlands: Reidel, 1984.

——. *The Physician's Covenant*. Philadelphia: Westminster Press, 1983.

——. "The Right to Know and the Right to Create." In *Science and the Public Interest*, ed. Robert P. Bareikis, pp. 192-205. Bloomington, Ind.: University Foundation, 1978.

——. "The Virtues in a Professional Setting." The Third Annual Memorial Lecture presented to the Society for Values in Higher Education at Vassar College, Poughkeepsie, New York, 6 Aug. 1984. Rpt. in *Soundings* 67 (1984): 245-66.

"MD, Nurse Teamwork Saves Lives: Study." *American Medical News*, 18 Apr. 1986, p. 24.

Meehan, Mary. "More Trouble Than They're Worth?" In *Abortion: Understanding Differences*, ed. Sidney Callahan and Daniel Callahan, pp. 145-70. New York: Plenum, 1984.

Meilaender, Gilbert. "Euthanasia and Christian Vision." *Thought* 57 (1983): 465-75.

Meisel, Alan, and H. Loren Roth. "Must a Man Be His Cousin's Keeper?" *Hastings Center Report* 8.5 (1978): 5-6.

Mellema, Gregory. *Individuals, Groups, and Shared Moral Responsibility*. Bern, Switzerland: Verlag Peter Lang, 1988.

Merritt, Deborah Jones. "The Constitutional Balance between Health and Liberty." *Hastings Center Report,* Special Supplement: *Aids: Public Health and Civil Liberties* 16.6 (1986): 2-10.

Mesthene, Emmanuel G. "Technology and Values." In *Who Shall Live?* ed. Kenneth Vaux, pp. 25-48. Philadelphia: Fortress Press, 1970.

Metcalfe, D. H. H. "Health Services in the United Kingdom: Trends in Provisions and Utilization 1971-80." *Family Practice* 1.3 (1984): 140-46.

Midgley, Mary. *Beast and Man*. Ithaca: Cornell University Press, 1978.

Mill, John Stuart. *Utilitarianism*. 1861; rpt. Indianapolis: Bobbs-Merrill, 1957.

Miller, Bruce. "Autonomy and the Refusal of Lifesaving Treatment." *Hastings Center Report* 11.4 (1981): 22-28.

Miller, Frances H., and Graham A. H. Miller. "The Painful Prescription: A Procrustean Perspective?" *New England Journal of Medicine* 314 (1986): 1383-85.

Minister of Supply and Services. *Canada Yearbook 1985*. Ottawa: Statistics Canada, 1985.

Minogio, Brendon P. "Error, Malpractice, and the Problem of Universals." *Journal of Medicine and Philosophy* 7 (1982): 239-50.

Momeyer, Richard. "Medical Decisions concerning Noncompetent Patients." *Theoretical Medicine* 3 (1983): 275-90.

"Monoclonal Antibodies Correct Severe Immune Deficiency." *Science News* 122 (1982): 244.

Mooney, G. H., and M. F. Drummond. "Essentials of Health Economics," Part IV — "Organizing Health Care Resources." *British Medical Journal* 285 (1982): 1485-86.

Moreno, Jonathan D., and Ronald Bayer. "The Limits of the Ledger in Public Health Promotion." *Hastings Center Report* 15.6 (1985): 37-42.

Morison, Robert S. "Death: Process or Event?" *Science*, 20 Aug. 1971, pp. 694-98.

"Mother Charged after Baby Born Brain-dead with Drugs in System." *Minneapolis Star and Tribune*, 2 Oct. 1986, Sec. A, p. 20.

Mouw, Richard V. "Biblical Revelation and Medical Decisions." *Journal of Medicine and Philosophy* 4 (1979): 367-83.

————. *When the Kings Come Marching In.* Grand Rapids: Eerdmans, 1983.

Muller, H. J. *Studies in Genetics: The Selected Papers of H. J. Muller.* Bloomington, Ind.: Indiana University Press, 1962.

Mundinger, Mary O'Neil. "Health Service Funding Cuts and the Declining Health of the Poor." *New England Journal of Medicine* 313 (1985): 44-47.

Munson, Ronald. "Why Medicine Cannot Be a Science." *Journal of Medicine and Philosophy* 6 (1981): 183-208.

Muyskens, James L. *Moral Problems in Nursing: A Philosophical Investigation.* Totowa, N.J.: Rowman & Littlefield, 1982.

Nathanson, Bernard N. *Aborting America.* New York: Doubleday, 1979.

National Center for Health Statistics. "Advanced Report of Final Mortality Statistics: 1984." *Monthly Statistics Report.* Hyattsville, Md.: Public Health Service, 1986.

"National Hospice Study." *Journal of Chronic Diseases* 39 (1986): 1-62.

Navarro, Vincent. "The Public/Private Mix in the Funding and Delivery of Health Services: An International Survey." *American Journal of Public Health* 75 (1985): 1318-20.

Nelson, J. Robert. *Human Life.* Philadelphia: Fortress Press, 1984.

Newland, Kathleen. *Worldwatch Paper #47: Infant Mortality and the Health of Societies.* Washington: Worldwatch Institute, United Nations Fund for Population Activities, 1981.

Newman, Jay. *Foundations of Religious Tolerance.* Toronto: University of Toronto Press, 1982.

Noonan, John T., Jr. "An Almost Absolute Value in History." In *The Morality of Abortion,* ed. John T. Noonan, Jr., pp. 1-59. Cambridge, Mass.: Harvard University Press, 1970.

Noyes, Russell, and John Clancy. "The Dying Role: Its Relevance to Improved Patient Care." *Death and Dying: Theory, Research, Practice,* ed. Larry Bugen, pp. 301-8. Dubuque: William C. Brown, 1979.

Nozick, Robert. *Anarchy, State, and Utopia.* New York: Basic Books, 1974.

Oberg, Charles N. "Health Care and the Corridor Poor." *Pediatrics* 76 (1985): 461-63.

————. "Pediatrics and Poverty." *Pediatrics* 79 (1987): 567-69.

O'Connor, June. "The Debate Continues: Recent Works on Abortion." *Religious Studies Review* 11 (1985): 105-14.

O'Donovan, Oliver. "Again: Who Is a Person?" In *Abortion and the Sanctity of Human Life,* ed. J. H. Channer, pp. 125-37. Exeter, Eng.: Paternoster, n.d.

————. *Begotten or Made?* Oxford: Clarendon, 1984.

Office of Technology Assessment. *Life-Sustaining Technologies and the Elderly.* Washington: GPO, 1987.

Oken, Donald. "What to Tell Cancer Patients: A Study of Medical Attitudes." In *Ethical Issues in Death and Dying,* ed. Robert F. Weir, pp. 9-25. New York: Columbia University Press, 1977.

"Oldest SCID Survivor Dies." *Science News* 125 (1984): 133.

Oleske, James M., Edward M. Conner, and Mary M. Boland. "A Perspective on Pediatric AIDS." *Pediatric Annals* 17.5 (1988): 319-21.

Owen, David. "Medicine, Morality, and the Market." *Canadian Medical Association Journal* 130 (1984): 1341-45.

Palmiter, Richard, et al. "Dramatic Growth of Mice That Develop from Eggs Microinjected with Metallothionein-Growth Hormone Fusion Genes." *Nature* 300 (1982): 611-15.

———. "Metallothionein-Human GH Fusion Genes Stimulate Growth of Mice." *Science,* 18 Nov. 1983, pp. 809-14.

Paris, John J., and Frank E. Reardon. "Court Responses to Withholding or Withdrawing Artificial Nutrition and Fluids." *Journal of the American Medical Association* 253 (1985): 2243-45.

Parsons, Talcott. "Illness and the Role of the Physician: A Sociological Perspective." In *Personality in Nature, Society, and Culture,* ed. Clyde Kluckhohn and Henry Murray, pp. 609-17. Rev. ed. New York: Knopf, 1956.

Paul VI. "The Pope Speaks." *Humanae Vitae* 14 (1969): 330-46. Rpt. in Stephen E. Lammers and Allen Verhey. *On Moral Medicine.* Grand Rapids: Eerdmans, 1987.

Pellegrino, Edmund D. "Being Ill and Being Healed." In *The Humanity of the Ill,* ed. Victor Kestenbaum, pp. 157-66. Knoxville: University of Tennessee Press, 1982.

———. *Humanism and the Physician.* Knoxville: University of Tennessee Press, 1979.

———. "Medical Morality and Medical Economics." *Hastings Center Report* 81.4 (1978): 8-12.

Pellegrino, Edmund D., and David Thomasma. *A Philosophical Basis of Medical Practice: Toward a Philosophy and Ethic of the Healing Professions.* New York: Oxford University Press, 1981.

Petres, Robert E., and Fay O. Redwine. "Ultrasound in the Intrauterine Diagnosis and Treatment of Fetal Abnormalities." *Clinical Obstetrics and Gynecology* 25.4 (1982): 753-71.

Pius XII. "Apostolate of the Midwife: An Address by His Holiness to the Italian Catholic Union of Midwives." *29 Oct. 1951. Rpt. in Catholic Mind* 50 (1952): 61.

———. "To Catholic Doctors: An Address by His Holiness to the Fourth International Convention of Catholic Doctors," Castelgandolfo, Italy, 29 Sept. 1949. Rpt. in *Catholic Mind* 48 (1950): 250-53.

Plantinga, Cornelius, Jr. "Images of God." In *Christian Faith and Practice in the Modern World,* ed. Mark A. Noll and David F. Wells, pp. 51-67. Grand Rapids: Eerdmans, 1988.

Plantinga, Cornelius, Jr. "The Justification of Rock Hudson: AIDS Has a Dual Message for Christians." *Christianity Today,* 18 Oct. 1985, pp. 16-17.

President's Commission for the Study of Ethical Problems in Medicine and Biomedical and Behavioral Research. *Deciding to Forego Life-Sustaining Treatment.* Washington: GPO, 1983.

————. *Making Health Care Decisions.* 3 vols. Washington: GPO, 1982.

————. *Screening and Counseling for Genetic Conditions.* Washington: GPO, 1983.

————. *Securing Access to Health Care: A Report on the Ethical Implications of Differences in Availability of Health Services.* 3 vols. Washington: GPO, 1983.

Press, Aric, and Frank Maier. "A Surrogate Mother's Story." *Newsweek,* 14 Feb. 1983, p. 76.

Preston, Thomas A. "Who Benefits from the Artificial Heart?" *Hastings Center Report* 15.1 (1985): 5-7.

Quinn, Warren. "Abortion: Identity and Loss." *Philosophy and Public Affairs* 13.1 (1984): 24-54.

Rachels, James. "Active and Passive Euthanasia." *New England Medical Journal* 292 (1975): 4-5.

Ramsey, Paul. *Ethics at the Edges of Life.* New Haven: Yale University Press, 1978.

————. *Fabricated Man.* New Haven: Yale University Press, 1970.

————. "The Indignity of 'Death with Dignity.'" In *Death Inside Out,* ed. Peter Steinfels and Robert M. Veatch, pp. 81-96. New York: Harper, 1975.

————. "The Morality of Abortion." In *Life or Death: Ethics and Options,* ed. Daniel H. Labby. Seattle: University of Washington Press, 1968.

————. "The Nature of Medical Ethics." In *The Teaching of Medical Ethics,* ed. Robert M. Veatch, Willard Gaylin, and Councilman Morgan, pp. 14-28. Hastings-on-Hudson, New York: Hastings Center, 1973.

————. *The Patient as Person.* New Haven: Yale University Press, 1970.

Raphael, D. D. *The Paradox of Tragedy.* London: Allen & Unwin, 1960.

Ravenholt, R. T. "Addiction Mortality in the United States, 1980: Tobacco, Alcohol, and Other Substances." *Population and Development Review* 10.4 (1984): 697-724.

————. "The Children's Fate." *Natural History,* Apr. 1986, pp. 41-68.

Rawls, John. *A Theory of Justice.* Harvard University Press, 1971.

Redfield, Robert R., and Donald S. Burke. "HIV Infections: The Clinical Picture," *Scientific American* 259.4 (1988): 90-98.

Reformed Churches in the Netherlands. "Euthanasia and the Pastorate." Trans. Sierd Woudstra. N.p.: n.p., 1985.

Reich, Warren Thomas. "Care of the Handicapped." In *The Westminster Dictionary of Christian Ethics,* ed. James F. Childress and John Macquarrie, pp. 258-60. Philadelphia: Westminster Press, 1986.

Reinhardt, Uwe E. Keynote address, 34th Annual Meeting of the American College of Obstetricians and Gynecologists, New Orleans, 5 May 1986.

Reinherz, E., et al. "Reconstitution after Transplantation with T-Lymphocyte-Depleted HLA Haplotype-Mismatched Bone Marrow for Severe Combined Immunodeficiency." *Proceedings of the Natural Academy of Sciences of the United States of America* 79 (1982): 6047-51.

Relman, Arnold S. "The Future of Medical Practice." The Merriman Lecture, presented at the University of North Carolina School of Medicine, Chapel Hill, 19 Oct. 1982.

————. "The New Medical-Industrial Complex." *New England Journal of Medicine* 303 (1980): 963-70.

————. "Texas Eliminates Dumping—A Start Toward Equity in Hospital Care." *New England Journal of Medicine* 314 (1986): 578-79.

————. "The United States and Canada: Different Approaches to Health Care." *New England Journal of Medicine* 315 (1986): 1608-10.

Rescher, Nicholas. "Philosophical Disagreement." *Review of Metaphysics* 32 (1978): 217-51.

Richard, Leon. "Medicare Is Financially Sick." *Canadian Medical Association Journal* 126 (1982): 838-42.

Rogers, Martha F. "Pediatric HIV Infections: Epidemiology, Etiopatho-genesis, and Transmission." *Pediatric Annals* 17.5 (1988): 324-30.

Rosemann, Kenneth. "God, AIDS, and Community Responsibility." *Second Opinion,* March 1988, pp. 128-41.

Rosner, Fred. "Hemophilia in the Talmud and Rabbinic Writings." *Annals of Internal Medicine* 70 (1969): 833-37.

Ross, David. *The Right and the Good.* Oxford: Clarendon, 1930.

Rothman, Barbara Katz. "Commentary on When a Pregnant Woman Endangers Her Fetus." *Hastings Center Report* 16.1 (1986): 25.

Rozovsky, Lorne Elkin. *The Canadian Patient's Book of Rights.* Toronto: Doubleday-Canada, 1980.

Rust, George. "What Can I Do? 50 Ways to Love Your Neighbor." *Christian Medical Society Journal* 17 (1986): 23-25.

Rust, Marik. "Quinlan Lawyer Files Artificial Feeding Suit." *American Medical News,* 18 Oct. 1985, pp. 1+.

Sade, Robert M. "Medical Care as a Right: A Refutation." *New England Journal of Medicine* 285 (1971): 1288-92.

Santurri, Edmund. "Prenatal Diagnosis: Some Moral Considerations." In *Questions about the Beginning of Life,* ed. Edward Schneider, pp. 120-50. Minneapolis: Augsburg, 1985.

Sargent, Douglas A. "Treating the Condemned to Death." *Hastings Center Report* 16.6 (1986): 5-6.

Saunders, Cicely. Taped interview: *Dr. Cicely Saunders: A Medical Pioneer.* Bowie, Md.: Charles Press, 1975.

Schieber, George J., and Jean-Pierre Poullier. "International Health Care Spending." *Health Affairs* 5.3 (1986): 111-22.

Schiff, Robert L., et al. "Transfers to a Public Hospital: A Prospective Study of 467 Patients." *New England Journal of Medicine* 314 (1986): 552-56.

Schneider, Edward D., ed. *Questions about the Beginning of Life.* Minneapolis: Augsburg, 1985.

Schroeder, Steven A. "Doctors and the Medical Cost Crisis: Culprits, Victims, or Solution?" *Pharos* 48.2 (1985): 12-18.

Schwartz, William B., and Henry J. Aaron. "Rationing Hospital Care: Lessons from Britain." *New England Journal of Medicine* 310 (1984): 52-56.

Scott, Nathan A., Jr. *The Tragic Vision and the Christian Faith.* New York: Association Press, 1957.

Selwyn, Peter A. "AIDS: What Is Now Known," Part II. *Epidemiology Hospital Practice,* 15 June 1986, pp. 127-64.

Selzer, Richard. *Mortal Lessons.* New York: Simon & Schuster, 1978.

Seybold, Klaus, and Ulrich B. Mueller. *Sickness and Healing,* trans. Douglass W. Stott. Nashville: Abingdon Press, 1981.

Shah, Chandrakant P., and Carrol Spindell Farkas. "The Health of Indians in Canadian Cities: A Challenge to the Health Care System." *Canadian Medical Association Journal* 133 (1985): 859-63.

Shelp, Earl E., and Ronald H. Sunderland. *AIDS and the Church.* Philadelphia: Westminster Press, 1987.

Shenson, Douglas. "When Fear Conquers." *New York Times Magazine,* 2 Feb. 1988, pp. 34-36, 38, 48.

Shock, Nathan W. "The Physiology of Aging." *Scientific American,* Jan. 1962, pp. 100-110.

Showstack, J. A., et al. "The Role of Changing Clinical Practices in the Rising Costs of Hospital Care." *New England Journal of Medicine* 313 (1985): 1201-7.

Shrader, Douglas. "On Dying More than One Death." *Hastings Center Report* 16.1 (1986): 12-16.

Shriver, Donald W., Jr. "The Interrelationships of Religion and Medicine." In *Medicine and Religion: Strategies of Care,* ed. Donald W. Shriver, Jr. Pittsburgh: University of Pittsburgh Press, 1980.

Sider, Ronald J. "AIDS: An Evangelical Perspective." *Christian Century,* 6-13 Jan. 1988, pp. 11-14.

Siegler, Mark. "A Physician's Perspective on a Right to Health Care." *Journal of the American Medical Association* 244 (1980): 1591-96.

Silverman, William A. "Mismatched Attitudes toward Neonatal Death." *Hastings Center Report* 11.6 (1981): 12-16.

Simmons, Paul D. *Birth and Death: Bioethical Decision Making.* Philadelphia: Westminster Press, 1983.

Simmons, Roberta J., and Susan Klein Marine. "The Regulation of High Cost Technology Medicine: The Case of Dialysis and Transplantation in the United Kingdom." *Journal of Health and Social Behavior* 25 (1984): 320-34.

Smedes, Lewis. "The Law and Karen Quinlan." *Reformed Journal,* Feb. 1975, pp. 4-5.

———. *Mere Morality.* Grand Rapids: Eerdmans, 1983.

———. *Sex for Christians.* Grand Rapids: Eerdmans, 1975.

Smith, Anthony. *The Mind.* New York: Viking Press, 1984.

Smith, David H. "The Abortion of Defective Fetuses: Some Moral Considerations." In *No Rush to Judgment*, ed. David H. Smith and Linda M. Bernstein, pp. 126-51. Bloomington: Indiana University Foundation, 1978.

———. "Suffering, Medicine, and Christian Theology." In *On Moral Medicine*, ed. Stephen Lammers and Allen Verhey, pp. 255-61. Grand Rapids: Eerdmans, 1986.

———. "A Theological Context for the Relationship between Patient and Physician." In *The Clinical Encounter*, ed. Earl E. Shelp, pp. 289-301. Dordrecht, Netherlands: Reidel, 1983.

Snow, John. *Mortal Fear: Meditation on Death and AIDS*. Cambridge, Mass.: Cowley, 1987.

Southall, Hilary A. "The Canadian Medical Association Membership Survey: Opinions on Issues Facing the Medical Profession." *Canadian Medical Association Journal* 133 (1985): 1029-39.

"Special Report: America's Abortion Dilemma." *Newsweek*, 14 Jan. 1985, pp. 20-29.

Spicer, Michael W. "British and American Health Care Systems: A Comparative Economic Perspective." *British Medical Journal* 282 (1981): 1334-36.

Sprague, Elmer. *Metaphysical Thinking*. New York: Oxford University Press, 1978.

Starr, Paul. *The Social Transformation of American Medicine*. New York: Basic Books, 1982.

Stinson, Robert, and Peggy Stinson. *The Long Dying of Baby Andrew*. Boston: Little, Brown, 1983.

Stith, Richard. "Toward Freedom from Value." *Bioethics Digest* 3.1 (1978): 1-10; 3.2 (1978): 1-10.

Stob, Henry. *Ethical Reflections*. Grand Rapids: Eerdmans, 1978.

Stoeckle, J., et al. "The Quantity and Significance of Psychological Distress in Medical Patients." *Journal of Chronic Disease* 17 (1964): 959-70.

Sturm, Douglas. "Contextuality and Covenant: The Pertinence of Social Theory and Theology to Bioethics." In *Theology and Bioethics*, ed. Earl E. Shelp, pp. 135-61. Dordrecht, Netherlands: Reidel, 1985.

Sullivan, Thomas. "Active and Passive Euthanasia: An Impertinent Distinction?" *Human Life Review* 3.3 (1977): 40-46.

Sun, Marjorie. "Will Growth Hormone Swell Milk Surplus?" *Science*, 11 July 1986, pp. 150-51.

Sunderland, Ronald H., and Earl E. Shelp. *AIDS: A Manual for Pastoral Care*. Philadelphia: Westminster Press, 1987.

Task Force on Pediatric AIDS. "Pediatric Guidelines for Infection Control of Human Immunodeficiency Virus (Acquired Immunodeficiency Virus) in Hospitals, Medical Offices, Schools, and Other Settings." *Pediatrics* 82.5 (1988): 801-7.

Taylor, Stuart. "Justices Hear Debate Over Pregnancy Leave." *New York Times*, 9 Oct. 1986, Sec. A, p. 30.

Temkin, Ousei. "Health and Disease." In vol. 2 of *Dictionary of the History of Ideas*, ed. Philip Wiener. New York: Scribner's, 1973.

Thielicke, Helmut. *The Ethics of Sex*, trans. John W. Doberstein. New York: Harper, 1964.

Thomas, Lewis. "Notes of a Biology Watcher: The Technology of Medicine." *New England Journal of Medicine* 285 (1971): 1366-68.

———. "On the Science and Technology of Medicine." In *Doing Better and Feeling Worse: Health in the United States,* ed. John H. Knowles, pp. 35-46. New York: W. W. Norton, 1977.

———. *The Youngest Science.* New York: Viking Press, 1983.

Thompson, Judith Jarvis. "A Defense of Abortion." In *The Problem of Abortion,* ed. Joel Feinberg, pp. 173-87. 2nd ed. Belmont, Calif.: Wadsworth, 1984.

"Times Mirror: AIDS and the Real Electorate." *Newsweek,* 1 Feb. 1988, p. 7.

Tooley, Michael. *Abortion and Infanticide.* Oxford: Clarendon, 1983.

"'Totally Awesome': The Valley Bible." *The Wittenberg Door,* Apr.-May 1982, p. 22.

Traub, James. "Goodbye, Dr. Spock." *Harper's,* Mar. 1986, pp. 57-64.

Tripp, Paivi. "A Comparative Analysis of the Health Care Cost of Three Selected Countries: The United States, the United Kingdom, and Australia." *Social Science and Medicine* 15 (1984): 19-30.

Uken, Robert. "My Teachers—The Retarded." *Banner,* 1 Sept. 1978, pp. 7-8.

U.S. Department of Commerce. Bureau of the Census. *Statistical Abstract of the United States: 1985.* Washington: GPO, 1985.

———. Bureau of the Census. *Statistical Abstract of the United States: 1987.* Washington: GPO, 1987.

———. Bureau of the Census. *Statistical Abstract of the United States: 1988.* Washington: GPO, 1988.

U.S. Department of Health and Human Services. Public Health Service. *Health—United States: 1984.* Washington: GPO, 1984.

———. Public Health Service. *Health—United States: 1987.* Washington: GPO, 1987.

———. Public Health Service. *Nurse Supply, Distribution, and Requirements.* 3rd Report to Congress. Washington: GPO, 1977.

———. Public Health Service. *The Surgeon General's Report on Acquired Immune Deficiency Syndrome.* Washington: GPO, 1986.

U.S. Department of Health, Education, and Welfare. Public Health Service. *Healthy People: The Surgeon General's Report on Health Promotion and Disease Prevention.* Washington: GPO, 1979.

U.S. Food and Drug Administration. "Human Growth Hormone Distribution Discontinued." *FDA Drug Bulletin* 15.2 (1985): 17-18.

VanDeVeer, Donald. "Whither Baby Doe?" In *Matters of Life and Death,* ed. Tom Regan, pp. 213-55. 2nd ed. New York: Random House, 1986.

Vanier, Jean. "How the Weak Heal Us, " *Sojourners,* 17 Jan. 1982, pp. 16-19.

Van Leeuwen, Mary Stewart. *The Person in Psychology.* Grand Rapids: Eerdmans, 1985.

Van Peursen, C. A. *Body, Soul, Spirit: A Survey of the Body-Mind Problem.* London: Oxford University Press, 1966.

Van Regenmorter, John, and Sylvia Van Regenmorter. "Infertility: Everyone's Problem." *Banner,* 12 May 1985, pp. 14-15.

Vaux, Kenneth L. *Health and Medicine in the Reformed Tradition: Promise, Providence, and Care.* New York: Crossroad, 1984.

Vayda, Eugene, and Rowsa Deber. "The Canadian Health Care System: An Overview." *Social Science and Medicine* 15 (1984): 19-30.

Veatch, Robert M. "Against Virtue: A Deontological Critique of Virtue Theory in Medical Ethics." In *Virtue and Medicine,* ed. Earl E. Shelp, pp. 329-45. Dordrecht, Netherlands: Reidel, 1985.

————. "The Case for Contract in Medical Ethics." In *The Clinical Encounter,* ed. Earl E. Shelp, pp. 105-12. Dordrecht, Netherlands: Reidel, 1983.

————. "Choosing Not to Prolong Dying." *Medical Dimensions* 40 (1972): 8-10.

————. *Death, Dying, and the Biological Revolution: Our Last Quest for Responsibility.* New Haven: Yale University Press, 1976.

————. "Models for Ethical Medicine in a Revolutionary Age." *Hastings Center Report* 2.3 (1972): 5-7.

————. "The Physician as Stranger: The Ethics of the Anonymous Patient-Physician Relationship." In *The Clinical Encounter,* ed. Earl E. Shelp, pp. 187-207. Dordrecht, Netherlands: Reidel, 1983.

————. *A Theory of Medical Ethics.* New York: Basic Books, 1981.

Verhey, Allen. "Calvin's Treatise 'Against the Libertines,'"*Calvin Theological Journal* 15 (Nov. 1980): 190-219.

————. "Christian Community and Identity: What Difference Do They Make to Patients and Physicians Finally?" *Linacre Quarterly* 52 (May 1985): 149-69.

————. "Evil." In *The International Standard Bible Encyclopedia,* ed. G. W. Bromiley. 4 vols. Rev. ed. Grand Rapids: Eerdmans, 1979-1988, 2: 206-10.

————. "In Defense of Theocracy." *Reformed Review* 34 (1984): 98-104.

————. *The Great Reversal.* Grand Rapids: Eerdmans, 1984.

————. *Living the Heidelberg: The Heidelberg Catechism and the Moral Life.* Grand Rapids: CRC Publications, 1986.

————. "The Morality of Genetic Engineering." *Christian Scholar's Review* 14 (1985): 124-39.

————. "Organs for Transplant: Technology and Tragedy." *Banner,* 31 Dec. 1984, pp. 8-10.

————. "Sanctity and Scarcity: The Makings of Tragedy." *Reformed Journal,* Feb. 1975, pp. 10-14.

————. "The Strange World of Sickness in Scripture," *Perspectives,* May 1986, pp. 4-8.

————. "The Test-Tube Baby Boom: Technology and Parenting." *Banner,* 14 Nov. 1983, pp. 8-10.

Verhey, Allen, and Hessel Bouma III. "Genetic Control: On Celebration and Caution." *Banner,* 24 Mar. 1986, pp. 12-14.

Wade, Francis C. "Potentiality in the Abortion Discussion." *Review of Metaphysics* 29 (1975): 239-55.

Wadhera, S. N., and C. R. Nair. "Trends in Legal Abortions and Abortion Rates in Canada, 1970-1980." In *Perspectives on Abortion,* ed. Paul Sachdev. Metuchen, N.J.: Scarecrow Press, 1985.

Wallis, Claudia, et al. "The Stormy Legacy of Baby Doe." *Time,* 26 Sept. 1983, p. 58.

Walters, Leroy. "Religion and the Renaissance of Medical Ethics in the United

States." In *Theology and Bioethics: Exploring the Foundations and the Frontiers,* ed. Earl E. Shelp, pp. 3-16. Dordrecht, Netherlands: Reidel, 1985.

Ward, John W., et al. "Transmission of Human Immunodeficiency Virus (HIV) by Blood Transfusions Screened as Negative for HIV Antibody." *New England Journal of Medicine* 318 (1988): 473-78.

Warnock Report: *Report of the Committee of Inquiry into Human Fertilization and Embryology.* London: HMSO, 1984.

Warren, Mary Anne. "On the Moral and Legal Status of Abortion." *Monist* 57 (1973): 43-61.

Weber, Leonard. "Ethics and Euthanasia: Another View." *American Journal of Nursing* 73 (1973): 1228-31.

Weber, Jonathan N., and Robin A. Weiss. "HIV Infection: The Cellular Picture." *Scientific American* 259.4 (1988): 100-9.

Weir, Robert. "Genetic Counseling and Truthtelling." In *No Rush to Judgment,* ed. David H. Smith and Linda M. Bernstein, pp. 87-125. Bloomington: Indiana University Foundation, 1978.

Weiss, Ken. "Corporate Medicine—What's the Bottom Line for Physicians and Patients." *The New Physician* 9 (1982): 19-25.

Weller, Geoffrey R., and Pranlal Manga. "The Push for Reprivatization of Health Care Services in Canada, Britain, and the United States." *Health Politics, Policy and Law* 8 (1983): 495-518.

Wennberg, Robert. "Euthanasia: A Sympathetic Appraisal." *Christian Scholar's Review* 6 (1977): 281-302.

————. *Life in the Balance: Exploring the Abortion Controversy.* Grand Rapids: Eerdmans, 1985.

"When Doctors Refuse to Treat AIDS." *New York Times,* 3 Aug. 1987, Sec. A, p. 16.

Whol, Stanley. *The Medical Industrial Complex.* New York: Harmony, 1984.

Wilensky, Gail. "Viable Strategies for Dealing with the Uninsured." *Health Affairs* 6.2 (1987): 34-35.

Wilensky, G. R., and M. L. Berk. "Poor, Sick, and Uninsured." *Health Affairs* 2 (1983): 91-95.

Wilensky, Harold L. "The Professionalization of Everyone?" *American Journal of Sociology,* Sept. 1964, pp. 137-58.

Williams, Alan. "Economics of Coronary Artery Bypass Grafting." *British Medical Journal* 291 (1985): 326-29.

Williamson, Bob. "Thalassemia: From Theory to Practice." *Nature* 292 (1981): 405.

Wilson, Florence A., and Duncan Neuhauser. *Health Services in the United States.* Cambridge, Mass.: Ballinger, 1981.

Winslow, Gerald R. "From Loyalty to Advocacy: A New Metaphor for Nursing." *Hastings Center Report* 14.3 (1984): 32-39.

Wolterstorff, Nicholas. *Reason within the Bounds of Religion.* 2nd ed. Grand Rapids: Eerdmans, 1984.

World Bank. *World Development Report: 1988.* New York: Oxford University Press, 1988.

Wyngaarden, James B. "Human Heredity." In *Cecil Textbook of Medicine,* ed.

James B. Wyngaarden and Lloyd H. Smith, pp. 117-22. 17th ed. Philadelphia: Saunders, 1985.

Yarchoan, Robert, Hiroaki Mitsuya, and Samuel Broder. "AIDS Therapies." *Scientific American* 259.4 (1988): 110-19.

Yule, Brian, and Garth Mooney. "Perspectives on Health Economics. 1. An Introduction to Economics in Health Care." *Family Practice* 1.3 (1984): 136-39.

Zaner, Richard M. "Embodiment." In *The Westminister Dictionary of Christian Ethics*, ed. James R. Childress and John Macquarrie, pp. 187-90. Philadelphia: Westminster Press, 1986.

Zerwekh, Joyce V. "The Dehydration Question." *Nursing 83* (1983): 47-51.

Zuck, Thomas F. "Transfusion-transmitted AIDS Reassessed." *New England Journal of Medicine* 318 (1988): 511-12.

Zuger, Abigail, and Steven Miles. "Physicians, AIDS, and Occupational Risk: Historical Traditions and Ethical Obligations." *Journal of the American Medical Association* 258.4 (1987): 1924-28.